OCCUPATIONAL
HEALTH AND SAFETY

FOR THE 21ST CENTURY

ROBERT H. FRIIS, PhD

Professor, Emeritus and Chair, Emeritus
Health Science Department
California State University
Long Beach, California

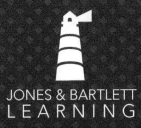

JONES & BARTLETT
LEARNING

World Headquarters
Jones & Bartlett Learning
5 Wall Street
Burlington, MA 01803
978-443-5000
info@jblearning.com
www.jblearning.com

Jones & Bartlett Learning books and products are available through most bookstores and online booksellers. To contact Jones & Bartlett Learning directly, call 800-832-0034, fax 978-443-8000, or visit our website, www.jblearning.com.

Substantial discounts on bulk quantities of Jones & Bartlett Learning publications are available to corporations, professional associations, and other qualified organizations. For details and specific discount information, contact the special sales department at Jones & Bartlett Learning via the above contact information or send an email to specialsales@jblearning.com.

Production Credits

VP, Executive Publisher: David Cella
Publisher: Michael Brown
Editorial Assistant: Nicholas Alakel
Associate Production Editor: Rebekah Linga
Rights and Media Manager: Joanna Lundeen
Media Development Assistant: Shannon Sheehan
Senior Marketing Manager: Sophie Fleck Teague
Manufacturing and Inventory Control Supervisor:
    Amy Bacus

Composition: Cenveo Publisher Services
Cover Design: Kristin E. Parker
Rights and Media Coordinator: Mary Flatley
Cover Image: Construction Workers: © sculpies/
    ShutterStock, Inc.; Warning Stripes: © Eky
    Studio/ShutterStock, Inc.; Abstract Metal:
    © DinoZ/Shutterstock, Inc.
Printing and Binding: Edwards Brothers Malloy
Cover Printing: Edwards Brothers Malloy

9852-2

Library of Congress Cataloging-in-Publication Data
Friis, Robert H., author.
  Occupational health and safety for the 21st century / Robert H. Friis.
    p. ; cm.
  Includes bibliographical references and index.
  ISBN 978-1-284-04603-8 (paper.)
  I. Title.
  [DNLM: 1. Occupational Health. 2. Accidents, Occupational—prevention & control.
3. Occupational Diseases—prevention & control. WA 400]
  RC964
  613.6'2—dc23
                                2014038077
6048

Printed in the United States of America
19 18 17 16 15   10 9 8 7 6 5 4 3 2 1

To C.A.F.

Contents

Preface

For the majority of the world's inhabitants, work is the major focus of our existence. Since the beginnings of organized society, continuing with the Industrial Revolution, and now in the present era—and always in a changing landscape of employment, occupational exposures, and working conditions—employment has been highly salient for people's health. My goal in this text is to increase readers' awareness of the crucial role played by occupational factors in the health of workers and the many connections between occupational and environmental exposures. To this end, key topics and issues related to occupational health and safety are introduced here.

As a result of my practical experience as a health department epidemiologist, research on chronic diseases, and participation in seminars and lectures, I have become cognizant of the impact of work-related exposures on employees' health. These experiences called attention to an acute need for an accessible text that would cover the major topics in the field.

Occupational Health and Safety for the 21st Century is intended for graduate and undergraduate students enrolled in occupational health and safety courses in a variety of settings. This text should also be of interest to public health, epidemiology, and health science students who want to delve more deeply into occupational health issues. Frequently, courses that explore this topic are offered by schools of public health and college health science programs. The text can also be adapted for use in online courses and intensive courses offered in a nontraditional format. Taking a nontechnical approach, it is accessible to and should intrigue students with little or no previous introductory background in the occupational health field or related disciplines. At the same time, the text should appeal to more advanced students as well.

To better elucidate the subject matter, this text includes many examples and illustrations of occupational health issues. Text boxes provide detailed information on selected topics. Other learning aids include a list of learning objectives at the beginning of each chapter and study questions and exercises at its conclusion.

—*Robert H. Friis*

Acknowledgments

First, I express my gratitude to my teachers and colleagues at the settings where I have worked during the past four decades. Among these individuals are the late Dr. Sidney Cobb and the late Dr. John R. P. French, Jr., who were my postdoctoral supervisors at the University of Michigan's Institute for Social Research. The late Dr. Mervyn Susser was responsible for offering me my first professional employment in public health (epidemiology) at the School of Public Health, Columbia University.

I also thank many generations of students in my various classes, most recently at California State University, Long Beach (CSULB). Over the years, students' probing questions have helped me sharpen my focus and think about public health. CSULB Health Science Department faculty member Claire Garrido-Ortega helped conduct background literature research for this text.

My wife, Carol Friis, was involved extensively with this project: She proofread the manuscript, provided detailed editorial comments, verified the accuracy of the references, and helped with many other aspects of the project. Without her support and assistance, completion of this text would not have been possible.

Finally, I would like to thank the dedicated and anonymous reviewers whose insightful comments greatly enhanced the quality of this text. Mike Brown, publisher for Jones & Bartlett Learning, provided continuing encouragement and motivation for completion of the project; Jones & Bartlett Learning staff offered much helpful technical publishing expertise.

—*Robert H. Friis*

Introduction

This text provides a broad and concise overview of the topics that make up the field of occupational health and safety. These areas include important occupational policies, legislative acts, and laws for protection of workers. A crucial issue for occupational health research is defining exposures to potentially dangerous agents found in the work environment and delineating the effects of such exposures. Epidemiology and toxicology are examples of two fields that make contributions to exposure assessments and illuminate the adverse health effects associated with work-related exposures. Broad categories of agents of occupational disease include physical hazards, biological and microbial agents, and hazardous chemicals. Among the adverse health outcomes that have been linked with the work environment are cancer, respiratory illness, and reproductive abnormalities. Unintentional injuries are one of the leading causes of work-related morbidity and mortality, but the psychological and social environment can also affect the health of workers by influencing levels of stress and morale. Methods have been developed to reduce exposures to hazards and increase occupational safety through redesign of the work environment, introduction of engineering controls, and limiting exposures to physical, microbial, and chemical agents.

Introduction to Occupational Health and Safety

Occupational health is concerned with protecting workers from diseases and injuries associated with hazardous work-related exposures. More broadly, the field is perceived to include improvement of the work environment and promotion of employees' health in general. The Introduction to Occupational Health and Safety chapter traces the history of adverse working conditions and highlights the achievements of leaders who were instrumental in addressing occupational health. In addition, it presents findings regarding human impacts and economic costs of significant occupational diseases and injuries. The intimate connection between the fields of occupational health and safety and public health is reinforced. National objectives for occupational health developed by *Healthy People 2020* are provided.

Occupational Health Policy and the Regulatory Climate

Occupational health policies are statements of plans for actions recommended to protect the health and safety of workers. Many contemporary health policies and legislative acts for protection of workers' health originated during the Industrial Revolution, when the deleterious effects of hazardous exposures and dangerous occupational environments became starkly apparent. Examples of key occupational laws in the United States include the Occupational Safety and Health Act of 1970 and the Federal Mine Safety and Health Act of 1977. Policies and legislative acts rely on government agencies such as the Occupational Safety and Health Administration (OSHA) to ensure their enforcement. These activities are supported by international and private organizations that promote occupational health and safety. Given the importance of policy issues for the field, many of the source documents are provided in their original wording in the Occupational Health Policy and the Regulatory Climate chapter.

Epidemiologic and Toxicologic Aspects of Occupational Health and Safety

The Epidemiologic and Toxicologic Aspects of Occupational Health and Safety chapter describes applications of methods derived from epidemiology and toxicology to occupational health and safety. Occupational epidemiology provides a body of methods for assessing hazards and risks from occupational exposures, identifying associations between exposures and adverse health outcomes from work-related factors, developing standards for permissible levels of exposures, and suggesting methods for protecting workers from occupational hazards. In comparison with other fields concerned with job-related health issues, occupational epidemiology is unique with respect to maintaining a focus on an entire population of workers. Toxicology provides methods for assessing and characterizing the effects of exposures to hazards such as toxic chemicals. Occupational epidemiology and toxicology are complementary disciplines, with toxicology providing methods for examining the toxic effects of agents and exposures that may impact the work environment.

Hazards from Chemicals and Toxic Metals

Chemicals are essential to the functioning of society and modern industrial operations. Furthermore, the number of chemicals in use continues to increase each year. Hazardous chemicals encountered in the work environment include toxic metals and gases, pesticides, and solvents. From an international perspective, thousands of injuries associated with unsafe chemical use occur each year. Some chemicals have cancer-causing properties; others have been linked to a variety of unwanted human health effects such as adverse birth outcomes.

Physical Hazards in the Workplace

Physical hazards encountered at work include radiation (both ionizing and non-ionizing), noise and vibration, extreme temperatures, and atmospheric variations (high and low atmospheric pressures). Examples of ionizing radiation are radiation from X-ray and imaging devices and radiation from cancer treatment. Examples of non-ionizing radiation are radiation from microwave ovens and intense light beams from lasers. Physical hazards are a feature of many work settings—for example, in the construction, healthcare, food processing, and transportation fields. Affected employees include physicians and nurses who may be exposed to ionizing radiation from imaging procedures and cancer treatments. Nurses who monitor hyperbaric chambers may need to accompany patients inside these devices and consequently be placed under high atmospheric pressures. Construction workers are exposed to noise and vibration from power tools and often are required to work outdoors in frigid temperatures during the winter months and, conversely, in torrid conditions during the summer. The Physical Hazards in the Workplace chapter presents information on the nature of these hazards and their potential health effects.

Biological and Microbial Hazards in the Workplace

Biological and microbial hazards include infectious disease agents such as bacteria, viruses, and fungi. Healthcare personnel, veterinarians, laboratory technicians, and sanitation workers are among the groups of workers who may come into contact with infectious disease agents during the course of their work-related activities. For example, healthcare personnel can become infected as a result of direct contact with patients and through indirect contact with infectious agents from blood and bodily fluids.

Examples of Major Occupational Diseases

Examples of adverse health outcomes associated with the occupational environment include dermatologic conditions (skin diseases/occupational dermatoses), cancer (e.g., breast cancer, liver cancer, and skin cancer), respiratory diseases (e.g., lung cancer and asbestosis), neurologic conditions, and reproductive abnormalities. Associations between these conditions and specific occupational exposures are discussed in the Examples of Major Occupational Diseases chapter.

Work-Related Injuries and Fatalities

Work-related unintentional injuries kill more than 4500 individuals each year in the United States. The most frequent cause of such deaths is transportation fatalities on the job. Also a crucial factor in the occupational environment is the risk of nonfatal injuries—a major source of worker morbidity and lost work time. Nonfatal injuries include falls and musculoskeletal injuries. Workplace violence is another cause of both fatal and nonfatal injuries.

Psychosocial Aspects of Work: Job Stress and Associated Conditions

Approximately two-thirds of all U.S. workers indicate that they experience stress in the workplace. Stress is associated with a changing work environment—for example, workers' inability to obtain and maintain employment, reduction of salary and benefits, increased emphasis on productivity, and globalization of the workforce. The way in which work is organized can lead to isolation and demoralization of workers. Other psychosocial influences on workers include lifestyle factors such as the level of physical activity at work (e.g., being sedentary due to the requirement for long hours of sitting), dietary changes, and abuse of alcohol and other substances.

Occupational Safety and the Prevention of Occupational Disease

As noted elsewhere in this text, occupational injuries and illnesses are a global phenomenon, being especially common in the developing world. A substantial proportion of these tragic events are preventable. The Occupational Safety and the Prevention of Occupational Disease chapter describes methods for increasing the safety of the work environment. For example, surveillance of occupational injuries and illnesses can aid in the development of descriptive epidemiologic studies that identify settings with high frequencies of adverse health outcomes. Related to occupational safety is risk assessment, which aids in targeting high-risk work environments. Another section in this chapter presents information on occupational health career specializations that contribute to the improvement of worker health and safety.

About the Author

Robert H. Friis, PhD, is Professor Emeritus of Health Science and Chair Emeritus of the Department of Health Science at California State University, Long Beach (CSULB), and former Director of the CSULB-VA Long Beach Healthcare System Joint Studies Institute. He is also a former Clinical Professor of Community and Environmental Medicine at the University of California at Irvine. Previously, he was an Associate Clinical Professor in the Department of Medicine, Department of Neurology, and School of Social Ecology, University of California at Irvine. Dr. Friis was also on the faculty at the Columbia University School of Public Health, Albert Einstein College of Medicine, and Brooklyn College. He was employed as an epidemiologist in a local health department, where he obtained applied public health experience. Dr. Friis is past president and a member of the Governing Council of the Southern California Public Health Association. Currently, he serves on the advisory boards of several health-related organizations, including the California Health Interview Survey. He is an epidemiologist by training and profession.

Dr. Friis has conducted research and published and presented papers related to tobacco use, mental health, nursing home infections, chronic disease, disability, minority health, and psychosocial epidemiology. He has been principal investigator or co-investigator on grants and contracts from the University of California's Tobacco-Related Disease Research Program, the National Institutes of Health, the joint CSULB and University of Southern California METRANS program, and other agencies. He has been a visiting professor at the Center for Nutrition and Toxicology, Karolinska Institute, Stockholm, Sweden; the Max Planck Institute, Munich, Germany; and twice at the Technical University of Dresden, Germany. Dr. Friis is a fellow of the Royal Society for Public Health and a member of the International Editorial Board of the journal *Public Health.* He is also a member of the Society for Epidemiologic Research and the American Public Health Association. Early in his career, he was awarded a postdoctoral fellowship for study at the Institute for Social Research, University of Michigan, and later the Achievement Award for Scholarly and Creative Activity from California State University, Long Beach.

Dr. Friis is the author of several books and textbooks, including *Epidemiology 101* (Jones and Bartlett), *Essentials of Environmental Health, Second Edition* (Jones and Bartlett), *Epidemiology for Public Health Practice, Fifth Edition* (senior author; Jones & Bartlett Learning), *Introductory Biostatistics for the Health Sciences* (co-author; Wiley), *Praeger Handbook of Environmental Health* (editor; Praeger), and *Community and Public Health* (senior author; Bridgepoint Education).

List of Abbreviations

Abbreviation	Definition
ABIH	American Board of Industrial Hygiene
AIDS	acquired immunodeficiency syndrome
ATSDR	Agency for Toxic Substances and Disease Registry
BBF	blood and body fluids
BEI	biological exposure indices
BLBA	Black Lung Benefits Act
BLL	blood lead level
BLS	Bureau of Labor Statistics
BO	bronchiolitis obliterans
BSL	biosafety level
CBSM	cognitive behavioral stress management
CDC	Centers for Disease Control and Prevention
CERCLA	Comprehensive Environmental Response, Compensation, and Liability Act, 1980
CFOI	Census of Fatal Occupational Injuries
CHD	coronary heart disease
CHP	chemical hygiene plan
Ci	Curie
CNS	central nervous system
CO	carbon monoxide
COHb	carboxyhemoglobin
COPD	chronic obstructive pulmonary disease

Cr VI	hexavalent chromium
CTD	cumulative trauma disorder
CTS	carpal tunnel syndrome
CWP	coal workers' pneumoconiosis
dB	decibel
DCS	decompression sickness
DDT	dichlorodiphenyltrichloroethane
DHHS	Department of Health and Human Services
DNA	deoxyribonucleic acid
DON	dysbaric osteonecrosis
EAP	Employee Assistance Program
EEOC	U.S. Equal Employment Opportunity Commission
ELF	extremely low frequency radiation
EMF	electromagnetic field
EMT	emergency medical technician
EPA	U.S. Environmental Protection Agency
ERI	effort-reward imbalance model
EU	European Union
EU-OSHA	European Agency for Safety and Health at Work
FDA	Food and Drug Administration
FECA	Federal Employees' Compensation Act
FLSA	Fair Labor Standards Act of 1938
FTE	full-time equivalent
GHS	Globally Harmonized System of Classification and Labelling of Chemicals
H_2S	hydrogen sulfide
HAV	hepatitis A virus
HAVs	hand-arm vibration syndrome
HBV	hepatitis B virus
HCV	hepatitis C virus
HIV	human immunodeficiency virus
HPS	hantavirus pulmonary syndrome
HP	hypersensitivity pneumonitis
HTV	hand-transmitted vibration
Hz	hertz

IDHL	immediately dangerous to life or health
ILO	International Labor Organization
IARC	International Agency for Research on Cancer
IR	infrared
JD-C	job demand-control model
LBP	low back pain
LD_{50}	lethal dose 50
MESA	Mine Enforcement and Safety Administration
MEK	Methyl ethyl ketone
MFF	metal fume fever
MRI	magnetic resonance imaging
MRSA	methicillin-resistant *Staphylococcus aureus*
MSD	musculoskeletal disorder
MSDS	material safety data sheet
MSFWs	migrant and seasonal farm workers
MSHA	Mine Safety and Health Administration
MW	microwave
NAFTA	North American Free Trade Agreement
NaSH	National surveillance system for health care workers
NCHS	National Center for Health Statistics
NCI	National Cancer Institute
NIEHS	National Institute of Environmental Health Sciences
NIH	National Institutes of Health
NIHL	noise-induced hearing loss
NIOSH	National Institute for Occupational Safety and Health
NMSC	non-melanoma skin cancer
NOA	new-onset asthma
NOAA	National Oceanographic and Atmospheric Administration
NOMS	National Occupational Mortality Surveillance
OEL	occupational exposure limit
OHN	occupational health nurse
OR	odds ratio
OSH	Occupational Safety and Health
OSHA	Occupational Safety and Health Administration

OSH Act	Occupational Safety and Health Act of 1970
OWCP	Office of Workers' Compensation Program
PAHs	polycyclic aromatic hydrocarbons
PCBs	polychlorinated biphenyls
PCDDs	polychlorinated dibenzodioxins
PELs	permissible exposure limits
PCDFs	polychlorinated dibenzofurans
P-E	person-environment
PEP	post-exposure prophylaxis
POPs	persistent organic pollutants
PPE	personal protective equipment
PTS	permanent threshold shift
PTSD	post-traumatic stress disorder
PVC	polyvinyl chloride
RCF	refactory ceramic fibers
REC	respirable elemental carbon
REL	recommended exposure limit
RF	radio frequency
RMD	repetitive motion disorder
RR	relative risk
SCE	sister chromatid exchange
SDSs	safety data sheets
SHE	sentinel health event
SI	System International
SLM	sound level meter
SMR	standardized mortality ratio
SOII	Survey of Occupational Injuries and Illnesses
SSA	Social Security Administration
SSI	Supplemental Security Income
TCDD	2,3,7,8-tetrachlorodibenzo-p-dioxin
TLV	threshold limit value
TSCA	Toxic Substances Control Act, 1976
TTS	temporary threshold shift
TWA	8-hour time weighted average
USDOL	U.S. Department of Labor

UV	ultraviolet
VOCs	volatile organic compounds
WBV	whole body vibration
WHO	World Health Organization
WLL	work-related asthma
WNV	West Nile virus
WRMSD	work-related musculoskeletal disorders
YPLL	years of potential life lost

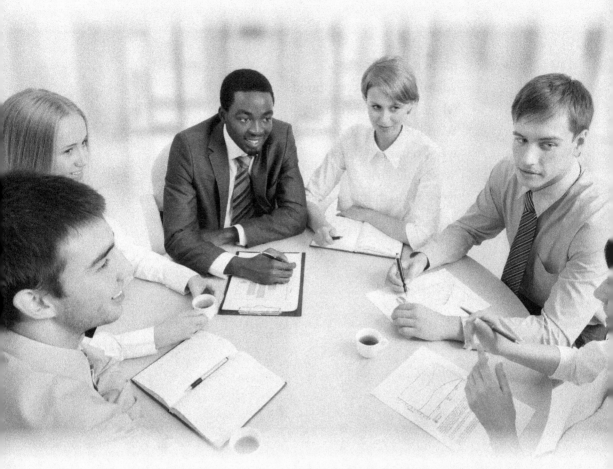

FIGURE 1.1 People at work

© Konstantin Chagin/Shutterstock

Each day millions of workers in America enter a battlefield, but they fight no foreign enemy and conquer no lands. No borders are in dispute. The war they are fighting is against the poisonous chemicals they work with and the working conditions that place serious mental and physical stress upon them. The battlefield is the American workplace, and the casualties of this war are higher than those of any other in the nation's history.

—Jeanne M. Stellman and Susan M. Daum, in the 1973 edition of their book, *Work Is Dangerous to Your Health*[1(p. 3)]

Reprinted from Stellman JM, Daum SM. Work Is Dangerous to Your Health. New York, NY: Vintage Books, a division of Random House; 1973.

CHAPTER 1

Introduction to Occupational Health and Safety

Learning Objectives

By the end of this chapter you will be able to:

- Define the term *occupational health.*
- State five historical developments in occupational health.
- Explain the social and economic significance of workers' illnesses and injuries for society.
- Describe at least three current issues in the field of occupational health and safety.
- Explain how the core functions of public health (assessment, policy development, and assurance) may be applied to occupational health.

Chapter Outline

- Introduction
- Occupational Health
- Landmarks in the History of Occupational Health
- Significance of the Occupational Environment for Health
- Twenty-First Century Occupational Trends and Challenges
- The Public Health Model for Occupational Health and Safety
- *Healthy People 2020* Objectives for Occupational Health and Safety
- Summary
- Study Questions and Exercises

Introduction

Occupational health is concerned with protecting the health of workers from diseases and injuries associated with hazardous work-related exposures; in addition, the field pursues the improvement of the work environment and the promotion of workers' health in general. As applied to individuals, occupational health is "the ability of a worker to function at an optimum level of well-being at a worksite as reflected in terms of productivity, work attendance, disability compensation claims, and employment longevity."[2]

Occupational health and safety are significant to society in view of the large percentage of the population that is currently employed and the numerous waking hours that the typical employed person spends on the job. Given the scale of the workforce, then, occupational health constitutes a major public health issue. Also, occupational health issues can extend beyond the time of active employment. In particular, retired persons may be afflicted by the sequelae of work-related conditions acquired when they were actively employed.

Since the formation of complex human societies supported by farming and nonagricultural activities, the relationship between work and the health of workers has been a concern for many people:

> Throughout recorded history, there have been references to work under a variety of conditions. The Old Testament includes rules about safe practices with regards to agriculture and how to treat workers. The Greeks and Romans used slaves, generally those captured in battle, to do both domestic work and to work in especially hazardous conditions, such as mining. The writings of the ancients even discussed some early preventive measures such as using pig bladders to breathe into to avoid dusty atmospheres.[3]

Occupational health emerged as an important issue for humanity beginning with ancient societies; it expanded as a concern in the Renaissance, during the Industrial Revolution, and into the 21st century. Unfortunately, society's attitudes toward occupational safety and health have evolved very slowly over time, with the economic viability of industry sometimes at odds with workers' health.[4]

During the 21st century, global trends such as rapid changes in the nature of work and technological advances are expected to have continuing impacts on occupational health. Adverse health outcomes and worker fatalities are significant issues for employees in both developed countries and the developing world. One of the most important policy statements for expressing occupational health goals for U.S. workers is *Healthy People 2020*.

Occupational Health

The field of occupational health is concerned with "identification and control of the risks arising from physical, chemical, and other workplace hazards in order to establish and maintain a safe and healthy working environment. These hazards may include chemical agents and solvents, heavy metals such as lead and mercury, physical agents such as loud noise or vibration, and physical hazards such as electricity or dangerous machinery."[5] In addition to identifying and controlling job-related risks, occupational health specializes in "the recognition, diagnosis, treatment, and prevention of illnesses, injuries resulting from hazardous exposures in the work-place."[6 (p. 3)] The field maintains an interdisciplinary approach, which includes the application of medicine, epidemiology, toxicology, engineering, and management to occupational health issues within an organizational context. [7] In addition, the field is closely aligned with the traditional concerns of preventive medicine and public health. Linked with occupational health is occupational medicine, "[t]he branch of medicine that deals with the prevention and treatment of diseases and injuries occurring at work or in specific occupations."[8] Other examples of related disciplines include occupational health nursing and industrial hygiene.

According to the Twelfth Session of the Joint International Labour Organization (ILO)/World Health Organization (WHO) Committee on Occupational Health (from 1995), occupational health has "three key objectives:

1. The maintenance and promotion of workers' health and working capacity;
2. The improvement of working environment and work, to become conducive to safety and health; and
3. The development of work organization and working cultures in a direction which supports health and safety at work, and in doing so also, promotes a positive social climate and smooth operation, and may enhance the productivity of the undertaking."[9(p. 2)]

Occupational Safety

The term *safety* refers to "the state of being safe; freedom from the occurrence or risk of injury, danger, or loss."[10] Occupational safety pertains to "the health and well-being of people employed in a work environment."[11] A safe work environment is free from hazardous conditions that might be linked with injuries and illnesses that originate from the workplace. One method to promote occupational safety is by formulating and enforcing regulations such as those developed by the U.S. federal government—for example, the Occupational Health and Safety Act of 1970. Promotion of occupational safety is a systematic process that involves ongoing monitoring of occupational hazards (surveillance), hazard identification, communication of information about risks, and collaboration between employers and workers.

Occupational Exposures and Hazards

Some types of occupational health specialists attempt to find linkages between specific exposures and adverse health outcomes in the workplace. Occupational exposures "include physical conditions (for example, structural insecurity or deficient lighting), physical stress (for example, lifting heavy weights or repetitive strain injuries), physical agents (for example, noise, vibration, or radiation), chemicals (for example, dusts or solvents), biological agents (for example, bacteria or viruses) and psychosocial stressors."[12(p. 7)]

An exposure "that may adversely affect health" is called a *hazard*.[13] Hazard identification is "the process of determining whether exposure to an agent can cause an increase in the incidence of a health condition (cancer, birth defect, etc.)"[14(p. 19)] According to the National Institute of Environmental Health Sciences, nearly all work settings have associated hazards, even though in some cases they can be minimal.[15] **EXHIBIT I.I** provides an example of job-related hazards.

Work-Related Diseases

The term work-related diseases (or injuries or illnesses) refers to adverse health events that arise from the work environment. The Occupational Safety and Health Administration classifies an injury or illness as work-related "if an event or exposure in the work environment either caused or contributed to the resulting condition or significantly aggravated a preexisting condition."[16] Examples of the main work-related diseases include "occupational lung diseases, dermatological conditions, cardiovascular diseases, musculoskeletal injuries, disorders of reproduction and development, noise induced hearing loss, occupational cancer, neurological disorders, and psychological disorders."[12(p. 7)] The National Library of Medicine points out that in addition to the foregoing adverse health outcomes, other conditions associated with occupations can include lacerations, fractures, amputations, sprains, and vision problems as severe as loss of sight. Also, a wide range of work-related hazardous exposures can occur—for example, to germs, unsafe substances, and radiation.[17]

Landmarks in the History of Occupational Health

Occupational hazards have been noted since the classical period of human history and, in fact, were a subject of early Greek and Roman writers. However, during the Dark Ages, humankind's attention to health issues temporarily became quiescent. A resurgence of interest in the topic occurred later, during the early and late Renaissance periods, when Agricola wrote about the dangers that affected workers in trades such as metal working. Paracelsus elaborated some of the crucial principles of toxicology, a field that now makes vital contributions to occupational health. Ramazzini, who is often called the father of occupational medicine, expounded upon the diseases of workers. Toward the end of the 17th century, Pott described the occurrence of scrotal cancer among chimney sweeps. Awareness of the growing tide of occupational illnesses grew during the 19th-century Industrial Revolution. Since the early 1900s, several major industrial calamities have elicited public alarm and riveted the attention of policy makers on occupational hazards. The 20th century was a time of great expansion of medical knowledge: "More medical advances have been made during the 20th century than in all the other centuries combined."[18] (p. 171) TABLE 1.1 provides an abridged list of noteworthy figures in the history of occupational health.

Occupational Health During the Classical Period (500 BCE–500 CE)

The classical period, which spanned approximately 500 BCE to 500 CE, marked the time when the ancient Greeks and Romans made important contributions to the history of occupational health. In addition to theorizing about the causes of disease, a major contribution of the ancients was the recognition of the hazards of chemicals used in the production of metals.

TABLE 1.1   Abridged List of Noteworthy Figures in the History of Occupational Health

Name	Dates (Birth–Death)	Contribution
Hippocrates	460–370 BCE	Discussed hazards of metal working and lead
Pliny the Elder	23–79 CE	Described hazards of dust
Galen	129–200 CE (estimated)	Described hazards to miners
Paracelsus	1493–1541	Wrote book on occupational diseases
Agricola	1494–1555	Described hazards of mining and producing gold and silver
Bernardino Ramazzini	1633–1714	"Father of occupational medicine"
Sir Percival Pott	1714–1788	Identified scrotal cancer among chimney sweeps
Dr. Alice Hamilton	1869–1970	Publicized dangerous occupational conditions (e.g., phossy jaw)
Charles Turner Thackrah	1795–1833	Among the first to recommend the principle of substitution for hazardous agents

Hippocrates (460–370 BCE)

Hippocrates wrote about the role of environmental and climatic factors in human health. These factors were thought to include weather, seasons, prevailing winds, the quality of air and water, and geographic location. Hippocrates's theories regarding the influence of environment were expressed in his work titled *On Airs, Waters, and Places*, published around 400 BCE. He is also said to have recognized the toxic properties of lead. At present, in agreement with the prescient thinking of Hippocrates, occupational health specialists have determined that many environmental exposures are salient for workers' health.

Pliny the Elder (23–79 CE)

During the first century, Pliny noted the toxic properties of sulfur and zinc. In addition, he invented a mask constructed from the bladder of an animal for protection against dusts and metal fumes.

Galen (129–200 CE)

Galen, a renowned Greek physician, outlined the pathological aspects of lead toxicity and suggested that mists from acids could endanger the health of copper miners. His work advanced the field of occupational medicine and contributed ideas that influenced the field for 1500 years.

Occupational Health Developments from 1500 to the Mid-1800s

From about 1500 to the mid-1800s, recognition grew regarding the contribution of occupationally related exposures to adverse health conditions. During this era, many investigators examined the impacts of unsafe and hazardous working environments on the health of workers, especially the effects of exposures to toxic metals and hazards that occurred among miners. Among the historically important figures in occupational health were Paracelsus (1493–1541), Agricola (1494–1555), Bernardino Ramazzini (1633–1714), Percival Pott (1714–1788), Charles Turner Thackrah (1795–1833), and Alice Hamilton (1869–1970). Although his contributions were not limited specifically to occupational health, John Graunt (one of the early compilers of vital statistics data) published *Natural and Political Observations Made upon the Bills of Mortality* in 1662. Sometimes Graunt is referred to as "the Columbus of statistics" because his book made a fundamental contribution by attempting to demonstrate the quantitative characteristics of birth and death data.

Paracelsus (1493–1541)

Paracelsus (**FIGURE 1.2**) is regarded as the founder of toxicology, a discipline that examines the toxic effects of chemicals found in environmental venues such as the workplace. A contemporary of da Vinci, Martin Luther, and Copernicus,[19] Paracelsus was active during the early 16th century. Among his contributions was the concept of a dose-response relationship, meaning that the effects of a poison are related to the amount of the dose that has been administered. Another conceptual breakthrough was Paracelsus's notion of target organ specificity of chemicals.

Agricola (1494–1555)

Georgius (Georg) Agricola (**FIGURE 1.3**) lived in Germany. In 1556, *De Re Metallica*, his book that described the environmental and occupational hazards of mining, was published posthumously (**FIGURE 1.4**).

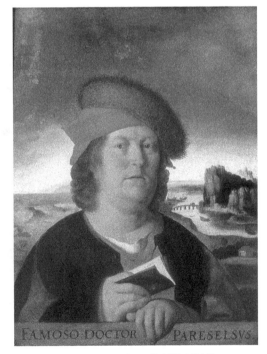

FIGURE 1.2   Paracelsus (1493-1541)
© Photos.com/Thinkstock

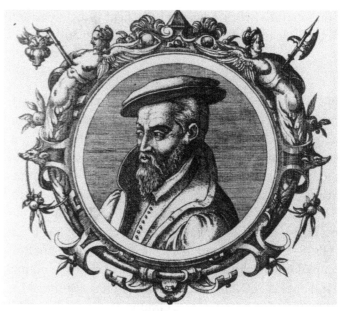

FIGURE 1.3   Georg Agricola (1494–1555)

Courtesy of National Library of Medicine.

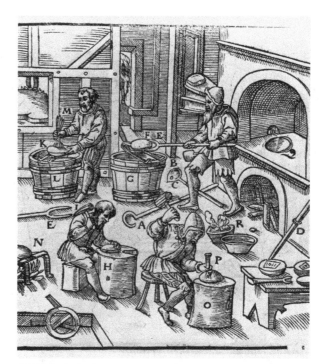

FIGURE 1.4   Interior view of a workshop showing four men at various stages of the metallurgical process during the mid-fourteenth century.

Courtesy of National Library of Medicine.

Ramazzini (1633–1714)

Bernardino Ramazzini (FIGURE 1.5) has been called the father of the field of occupational medicine.[20] "The name of Ramazzini marks the beginning of society's concern with the well-being and physical and emotional health of its workers from the shops of the crafts to the offices of the executives." [21(p. 167)] In his seminal works, Ramazzini created elaborate descriptions of the manifestations of occupational diseases among many different types of workers.[22] His descriptions covered a plethora of occupations, ranging from miners to cleaners of privies to fabric workers. Ramazzini is also considered to be a pioneer in the field of ergonomics, as he pointed out the hazards associated with postures assumed in various occupations. Ramazzini authored *De Morbis Artificum Diatriba (Diseases of Workers)*, published in 1700 (FIGURE 1.6), which highlighted the risks posed by hazardous chemicals, dusts, and metals used in the workplace.

Percival Pott (1714–1788)

Sir Percival Pott (FIGURE 1.7), a London surgeon, made the astute observation in 1775 that chimney sweeps had a high incidence of scrotal cancer. He argued that chimney sweeps were prone to this malady as a consequence of their contact with soot. "Sagely, he connected this observation to their occupational history. 'Climbing boys,' Pott knew, were recruited at ages as young as five to eight. . . . From this fact, he further deduced that the continuous exposure to soot implied a long latency period. (*3-4 Benzpyrene*, the responsible chemical agent in soot, was identified a century and a half later, in 1934.)" [23(pp. 28–29)] After reaching his conclusions about the relationship between scrotal cancer and chimney sweeping, Pott established an occupational hygiene control measure—the recommendation that chimney sweeps bathe once a week. EXHIBIT 1.2 describes chimney sweepers' cancer (scrotal cancer).

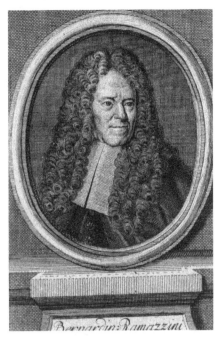

FIGURE 1.5   Bernardino Ramazzini, father of occupational medicine, 1633–1714

Courtesy of National Library of Medicine.

D E

MORBIS ARTIFICUM

D I A T R I B A

BERNARDINI RAMAZZINI

IN PATAVINO ARCHI-LYCEO

Practicæ Medicinæ Ordinariæ
Publici Profefforis,

ET NATURÆ CURIOSORUM COLLEGÆ.

Illuftrifs., & Excellentifs. DD. Ejufdem

ARCHI-LYCEI

MODERATORIBUS.

D.

MUTINÆ M.DCC.

Typis Antonii Capponi, Impreſſoris Epiſcopalis.
Supriorum Confenfu.

FIGURE 1.6   *De Morbis Artificum Diatriba* by Ramazzini

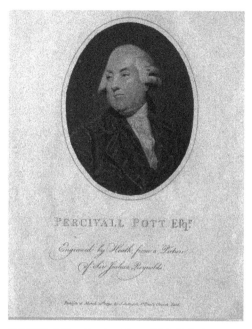

FIGURE 1.7   Percival Pott, FRS (1714–1788)

Courtesy of Wellcome Library, London.

Charles Turner Thackrah (1795–1833)

Thackrah was an early-19th-century innovator in occupational health. His book *The Effects of the Principal Arts, Trades and Professions . . . on Health and Longevity* (abridged title) raised the public's awareness of the difficult conditions under which factory workers labored. Examples of the adversities experienced by these workers included the deleterious effects of child labor, exposures to hazardous dusts in mines and metal working factories, the connection between occupational exposures to dusts and tuberculosis, and the consequences of workers' contact with lead. Thackrah also noted the general social and economic distresses that confronted many

---

EXHIBIT 1.2   Sir Percival Pott (1714–1788) Chimney Sweepers' Cancer

In a book entitled *Chirurgical Observations Relative to the Cataract, the Polypus of the Nose, the Cancer of the Scrotum, the Different Kinds of Ruptures, and the Mortification of the Toes and Feet*, Pott developed a chapter called "A Short Treatise of the Chimney Sweeper's Cancer." This brief work of only 725 words is noteworthy because "it provided the first clear description of an environmental cause of cancer, suggested a way to prevent the disease, and led indirectly to the synthesis of the first known pure carcinogen and the isolation of the first carcinogenic chemical to be obtained from a natural product. No wonder therefore that Pott's observation has come to be regarded as the foundation stone on w[h]ich the knowledge of cancer prevention has been built!"[24 (p. 521)] In Pott's own words:

[E]very body . . . is acquainted with the disorders to which painters, plummers, glaziers, and the workers in white lead are liable; but there is a disease as peculiar to a certain set of people which has not, at least to my knowledge, been publickly noteced; I mean the chimney-sweepers' cancer. . . . The fate of these people seems singularly hard; in their early infancy, they are most frequently treated with great brutality, and almost starved with cold and hunger; they are thrust up narrow, and sometimes hot chimnies, where they are bruised, burned, and almost suffocated; and when they get to puberty, become peculiary [sic] liable to a noisome, painful and fatal disease. Of this last circumstance there is not the least doubt though perhaps it may not have been sufficiently attended to, to make it generally known. Other people have cancers of the same part; and so have others besides lead-workers, the Poictou colic, and the consequent paralysis; but it is nevertheless a disease to which they are particularly liable; and so are chimney-sweepers to the cancer of the scrotum and testicles. The disease, in these people . . . seems to derive its origin from a lodgment of soot in the rugae of the scrotum.[24(pp. 521–522)]

factory workers. In addition, he was among the first occupational health experts to advocate for the substitution of more hazardous materials with less dangerous ones. Substitution is regarded as the first principle of industrial hygiene, meaning that substitution is one of the most important procedures for protecting workers from hazardous materials and remains relevant today.

At the young age of 31, Thackrah established the Leeds University School of Medicine, which provided an alternative to London's medical schools. These institutions dominated English medical education at that time.[22]

Unusual Occupational Diseases of the Past

Some of the occupational illnesses and injuries that were common in the past occurred in jobs that have, for the most part, fallen by the wayside in the modern world. To illustrate, work-associated lung conditions such as coal workers' pneumoconiosis and byssinosis in the textile industry occur much less frequently now than they did in the past; in their place, asthma, dermatoses, and injuries have risen to the forefront as important occupational conditions.[25] Names of occupational disorders from the past include "coal miners' nystagmus, scrotal cancer in chimney sweeps, phossy jaw, hatters' shakes, painters' colic, potters' rot, chauffers' [sic] knee, glanders, [and] caisson disease."[26] Coal miners' nystagmus is an example of an occupational disease that became unusual after the mid-20th century. This condition "was one of the first occupational illnesses ever recognized as being due to a hazardous working environment. It aroused great concern and much controversy in Great Britain in the first half of the 20th century but was not seen in the United States."[27] Another occupational condition, mule spinner's disease, referred to scrotal cancer from exposure to mineral oils among textile workers who operated textile spinning machines called "mules."[28] TABLE 1.2 lists examples of other unusual occupational conditions from past eras.

Industrial Revolution and Early 20th Century

During the Industrial Revolution in England, when the population moved to cities in search of employment and large numbers of persons toiled for long hours in crowded factories, health issues connected with the work environment became apparent. Later, in the early 20th century, awareness grew regarding occupational illnesses associated with workers' exposure to hazardous chemicals (e.g., white phosphorus, mercury, and lead) and work environments.

Working conditions during the Industrial Revolution were deplorable for many types of employees, as the following graphic description illustrates.

TABLE 1.2   Names of Classic Occupational Diseases Found in the Historical Literature

Name of Disease	Definition/Etiology
Miners' asthma	The common name for pneumoconiosis among miners who were exposed to dusts such as coal dust.
Coal miners' nystagmus	A visual disturbance that occurred among underground miners who worked under low light levels for a period of years.
Potters' rot, miners' phthisis	Silicosis, respiratory disease from inhalation of silica dust.
Brass-founders' ague	A type of metal fume fever caused by inhalation of fumes from welding brass. This self-limiting condition is associated with fever and other symptoms that resolve after 24 hours.
Filecutters' paralysis	Paralysis of the hands caused by lead exposure.
Painters' colic	Abdominal pain associated with anemia caused by exposure to white lead in paint.
Bakers' itch	A skin reaction (eczema) caused by contact with the components of baked goods (e.g., sugar).
Mule spinners' cancer, also known as mule spinners' disease	The mule was a textile spinning machine; the disease referred to scrotal cancer that occurred among male cotton textile workers who were exposed to mineral oils over long time periods as they used the mule.
Hatters' shakes; mad hatter's disease	Mercury poisoning among millinery workers.
Caisson disease (decompression sickness)	A disease caused by decompression when workers emerged from caissons, which were used to construct the anchoring piers for the Brooklyn Bridge in New York City and for similar projects. The laborers were exposed to air under very high pressures for extended time periods.
Phossy jaw	Phosphorus necrosis of the jaw.
Chauffeurs' knee	Damage to the right knee caused by operating the engine crank of a motor vehicle.
Glanders	A zoonotic disease (disease transmitted from animals) that occurred among horsemen in Europe. Glanders caused lung diseases, skin problems, bone damage, and harm to other bodily organs. The chronic form was usually fatal.

Data from Cherniack, MG, Diseases of unusual occupations: an historical perspective, *Occup Med.*, 1992;7(3):369–384.

During the industrial revolution, the population of England more than doubled. Men, women and children unable to find work on farms moved to towns and cities to seek work in factories, mills, mines and shops. Working conditions and crowded unsanitary housing took a terrible toll on workers who toiled long hours, being poorly fed, poorly housed, and poorly paid. (Women and boys working the cotton mills in dreadful conditions were paid two shillings to two shillings and sixpence, a pittance, per week.) Working conditions were dangerous, accidents were rife, and workers were afflicted by industrial disease. Long shifts of 12 hours or more led to chronic fatigue that caused terrible accidents, especially for tired children working around machines with no guard rails.[29]

Alice Hamilton (1869–1970)

Dr. Alice Hamilton (**FIGURE 1.8**) created awareness of phosphorus necrosis of the jaw (phossy jaw) through her writings on this disabling condition. During the early 20th century, many countries passed laws that prohibited the use of white phosphorus in matches. Another one of Hamilton's crusades was to call attention to industrial plumbism (lead poisoning), which affected employees in pottery factories and battery factories as well as plumbers and painters.[30] By creating awareness of occupational hazards such as these, Hamilton became a renowned contributor to occupational health and is regarded as the mother of occupational medicine.

Phossy Jaw/Phosphorus Necrosis

Phosphorus necrosis of the jaw (phossy jaw) was a condition that became prevalent starting about 1858, but subsequently became very uncommon by 1906.[31] Although phosphorus necrosis once reached epidemic proportions, it is now almost extinct.[32] This condition, which affected the victims' jawbones, was accompanied by severe pain and abscesses that drained fetid-smelling pus. Over time, as the disease process unfolded, the victim gradually became disfigured; surgery—the only means available to save the life of the patient—entailed removal of the jaw bone and further disfigurement.

Phossy jaw was caused by exposure to white phosphorus among workers who used

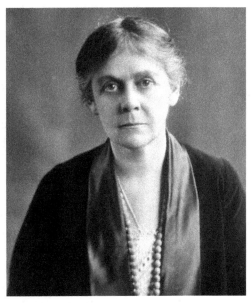

FIGURE 1.8   Alice Hamilton
© Science Source

it in the manufacture of matches. Affected workers were those who dipped matchsticks into white phosphorus paste. Many of the workers were children who labored in vapor-filled, poorly ventilated rooms. The condition, which developed slowly over a period of years, produced debilitation, neurologic disturbances, and lung hemorrhages. Remarkably, phossy jaw was a completely avoidable condition, because red phosphorus worked as well in matches as white phosphorus but was much safer.

Caisson Disease

Caisson disease is a form of decompression sickness that occurs among workers who have been laboring in underground pressurized chambers used in construction projects.[33] It is described further in the chapter *Physical Hazards in the Workplace.*

Historically Significant Incidents in Occupational Health and Safety, 1800s and Later

An example of a historically significant event for occupational health and safety was the Great Railroad Strike of 1877, which represented labor's response to the hazardous and unjust working conditions in the U.S. railroad industry at that time. Occupational hazards continued to plague workers into the early 20th century. A report in *Morbidity and Mortality Weekly Report* observed: "At the beginning of this century [the 20th century], workers in the United States faced remarkably high health and safety risks on the job."[34(p. 461)] Many workers remained on the job for 16-hour periods during 6- and 7-day work weeks.[35] Two major incidents—the Triangle Shirtwaist Company fire and the Gauley Bridge disaster—illustrated the deplorable conditions that workers were often forced to endure. These poor environmental conditions included contact with hazardous machinery, crowding, lack of ventilation, poor lighting, and infrequent protection against hazards. Such dangerous working conditions inspired reforms that resulted eventually in the improvement of workers' environments.

The Great Railroad Strike of 1877

The United States' railways expanded rapidly following the Civil War and continuing into the early 20th century. During this era, vast contingents of workers constructed thousands of miles of new track. At the onset of World War I, the railroads provided work for one out of every 25 employees in this country.[36]

Railway work—building new lines and operating the trains—was extremely dangerous. Construction tasks required that employees endure exceedingly harsh and demanding conditions. In the 1860s, immigrant Chinese laborers from Canton Province provided much of the railway construction workforce for the Central Pacific Railroad in California. They demonstrated an excellent work ethic and completed some of the more difficult construction tasks with admirable diligence.[37]

During the 19th and early 20th centuries in the United States, examples of injustice abounded in railway work. One of the landmarks in workers' disgruntlement regarding these conditions was the Great Railroad Strike of 1877, the first major national railway strike, which set the stage for subsequent labor unrest toward the end of the 19th century.[36] Following the Financial Panic of 1873, several railroads in 1877 initiated substantial wage cuts, reduced work hours, and increased workloads. Workers responded with the Great Railroad Strike, a national general strike that spread to major cities including Baltimore, Chicago, Kansas City, Philadelphia, Pittsburgh, St. Louis, and San Francisco. Some workers abandoned their jobs or blocked freight trains. In Baltimore, the Maryland National Guard killed 10 rioters who were among an angry mob of 14,000 demonstrators. Violence erupted also in Pittsburgh in response to the Philadelphia National Guard's firing into crowds of protestors and killing at least 20 persons. After enraged demonstrators set railroad facilities alight, the conflagration spread to other sections of Pittsburgh (FIGURE 1.9).

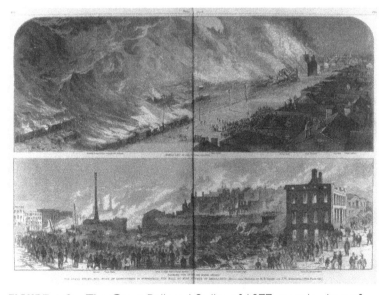

FIGURE 1.9   The Great Railroad Strike of 1877, steeple view of conflagration in Pittsburgh

Courtesy of Library of Congress.

Triangle Shirtwaist Company Fire

March 25, 1911, marks the date of New York City's worst factory fire, which occurred at a 10-story structure formerly named the Asch building (**FIGURE 1.10**). The disaster—one of the worst industrial accidents in U.S. history—claimed the lives of 146 women within the brief time span of 15 minutes. Several hundred women labored on the top three floors used by the Triangle Shirtwaist Factory. Doors were locked to prevent the women from leaving their sewing machines; fire escapes were nonfunctional. As a result, when a fire erupted about 4:30 in the afternoon, many of the women (especially on the ninth floor) perished from the fire when they were unable to escape or were killed when they jumped from windows or attempted to slide down elevator cables.[38,39]

Gauley Bridge Disaster

Beginning about 1931, workers began the Hawk's Nest Tunnel project near the small town of Gauley Bridge, West Virginia. During tunneling operations, workers were exposed to high levels of silica dust from which they did not have adequate protection. Estimates indicate that as many

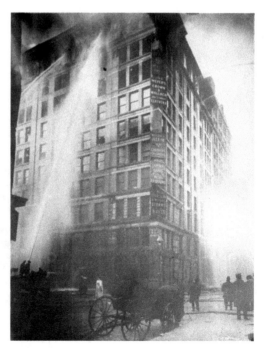

FIGURE 1.10   Triangle Shirtwaist Fire, March 25, 1911

Courtesy of the U.S. Department of Labor.

as 1500 workers contracted the lung disease known as silicosis and that 1000 ultimately died from this cause.[40]

Significance of the Occupational Environment for Health

Occupational health hazards and job-associated injuries affect workers in all countries around the world. Unhealthful working conditions are found in many developing countries and impact developed European countries as well as the United States. Currently, fatal and nonfatal occupational illnesses and injuries exact a significant social and economic toll in the United States.[41]

International Significance of Occupational Health and Safety

The international significance of occupational health and safety is reflected in the working conditions for many adults and children who labor in less developed countries. Occupational illnesses and injuries contribute substantially to global morbidity and mortality. Migration of persons in search of employment has become a global phenomenon. Often, immigrant workers experience increased risks of injuries and disease from their employment in host countries.[42]

Employment Conditions in Developing Countries

Employment conditions in some of the world's developing regions tend to be much more dangerous than in the United States, European countries, and other economically mature nations. According to the International Labour Organization, "Occupational deaths and injuries and work-related diseases take a particularly heavy toll in developing countries, where large numbers of workers are concentrated in primary and extractive activities. . . . [Examples are agriculture, construction, mining, breaking apart old ships.] It often happens that these countries are also those without adequate technical and economic capacities to maintain effective national OSH [occupational safety and health] systems, particularly regulatory and enforcement mechanisms."[43]

Media reports have documented dangerous working conditions in the developing world, particularly disasters in factories. For example, two incidents riveted global attention in 2013: A conflagration in a factory accompanied by the collapse of a building killed more than 1000 workers in Bangladesh, and an explosion and fire prompted a worker stampede in a Chinese poultry factory, resulting in the deaths of 119 trapped employees. EXHIBIT 1.3 describes these horrific incidents.

Global Burden of Occupationally Related Morbidity and Mortality

The number of work-related deaths that occurs worldwide is estimated at approximately 2 million annually, with disease likely to be the cause

---

EXHIBIT 1.3   Case Studies in Factories in Developing Countries

Case Study 1: Factory Collapse in Bangladesh, April 2013

When an eight-story factory building collapsed near Dhaka, more than 1000 people were killed and 2500 injured. The factory building was home to five garment factories that employed several thousand workers. One day before the collapse, cracks appeared in the walls of the building, which was evacuated briefly. Later, the employees returned to work inside the building. The factories located in the building supplied garments to some of the world's major retailers. After this incident, the Accord on Fire and Building Safety in Bangladesh was created. This accord, which is designed to improve safety of working conditions, had been signed by several global apparel companies—with Wal-Mart and Gap being notable exceptions—as of May 17, 2013.

Data from CBS News, Death toll tops 1000 in Banagladesh factory collapse, May 10 2013; BBC News, Bangladesh factory collapse toll passes 1000, May 10, 2013; James Brudney and Catherine Fisk, Opting out of worker protection, *Los Angeles Times*, May 17, 2013: p. A17.

Case Study 2: Fire and Stampede in Chinese Poultry Factory, June 2013

An explosion and fire in a poultry factory in northeastern China killed 119 workers and injured 54. The explosion, which was triggered by ammonia used as a refrigerant, caused a stampede. People were unable to escape through building entrances and the fire door, which had been blocked. According to a *Los Angeles Times* report, "Chinese workers often endure conditions more akin to those at military barracks than factories, with restrictions on their freedom of movement.... Workers, who made about $325 a month, were 'strictly controlled.'"

Data from Barbara Demick, Poultry workers tell of stampede, Los Angeles Times, June 4, 2013: p. A3.

---

of most of these deaths.[44] As a result of the imprecision of available data sources regarding occupational mortality, this figure is likely to be a major underestimate of the actual number of deaths.

Regarding occupational morbidity, five major occupationally associated risk factors are "workplace carcinogens, airborne particulates, hazards for injuries, ergonomic stressors for back pain, and noise."[45] These five risk factors contribute to a large percentage of the overall global burden of disease from back pain, hearing loss, chronic obstructive pulmonary disease, asthma, lung cancer, injuries, and leukemia. Sharps injuries among healthcare workers are a significant contributor to hepatitis and other blood-borne diseases. In summary, exposures to occupational hazards are important determinants of morbidity worldwide. According to Nelson et al., this burden "could be substantially reduced through replication of proven risk prevention strategies."[46]

The Burden of Occupational Illness and Injuries in the United States

Occupational illnesses and injuries are an important contributor to morbidity and mortality in the United States. Not only do they inflict suffering upon affected individuals, but also they disrupt the lives of the workers' family members. Loss of a wage earner from occupationally associated illnesses and injuries can result in economic impoverishment of workers and their families. In turn, such illnesses and injuries can produce devastating losses for society and for businesses.

In 2007, there were approximately 5600 work-related injury deaths and 8.6 million nonfatal injuries in the United States.[47] The number of fatal and nonfatal illnesses were approximately 53,000 and 427,000, respectively. In that same year, the total costs for occupational illnesses and injuries were estimated to be $250 billion—almost as great as the associated costs of cancer.

According to the Bureau of Labor Statistics (BLS), the number of cases of occupational illnesses and injuries reported by private industry employers has been declining since 2003.[48] For 2012 (the most recently available information from the BLS), private industry employers reported about 3.0 million workplace injuries and illnesses. Most of these cases (94.8%) involved injuries. Service-providing industries were responsible for approximately three-fourths of all injuries and employed about 80% of the private industry workforce; the remainder of injuries occurred in goods-producing industries.

Approximately 5.2% of workplace injury and illness cases in the United States involve workplace illnesses. These illnesses have the following distribution:

- Goods-producing industries: 34.3% of cases (29.5% of all illness cases in the manufacturing industry sector)
- Service-providing industries: 65.5% of cases (23.4% of all illness cases in the healthcare and social assistance sectors)

The direct costs of all occupational injuries and illnesses amounted to $45.8 billion and the indirect costs were as much as $229 billion.

Occupational Mortality and Fatal Occupational Injuries

Occupational deaths are regarded as an "epidemic" and "a pressing public issue in the United States and throughout the world."[49] (p. 541) Mortality from occupational causes is the eighth leading cause of death in this country.[50] As a representative case, consider the 2013 deaths of 19 Arizona firefighters. A violent wind gust caused a wildfire to change direction and overtake the crew.

The fire fighters, known as Hotshots, were attacking the conflagration in the town of Yarnell, Arizona.[51] Another example of work-related mortality is the death of six people and injury of two others from an explosion of a grain elevator in Atchison, Kansas, on October 30, 2011.[52]

Data on fatal occupational injuries are collected via the BLS's Census of Fatal Occupational Injuries (CFOI). The number of deaths from all work-related injuries and illnesses is difficult to determine precisely because of underreporting, underdiagnosis, and deficiencies of reporting mechanisms. One estimate of mortality from all work-related injuries and illnesses in the United States during the early 1990s was that 65,000 deaths occurred from such causes.[49(p. 541)] Other estimates have placed the total at 55,200 deaths, with a range of 32,200 to 78,200.[41] The BLS indicates that a total of 4690 workers died from occupational injuries in 2010.[53] **FIGURE I.II** shows the number of fatal work injuries in the United States from 1992 through 2010.

Iceberg Concept of Occupational Illness and Injuries

The iceberg concept gives credence to the unrecognized nature of most occupational illnesses and injuries. The burden of conditions recognized as being "work-related" represents the tip of the iceberg (**FIGURE I.I2**).[6] The following passage from Franklin Wallick's classic book, *The American Worker: An Endangered Species,* reinforces this notion of the iceberg.

We are dealing here with the tip of a treacherous ecological iceberg. Few exact studies have been made to measure the full dimensions

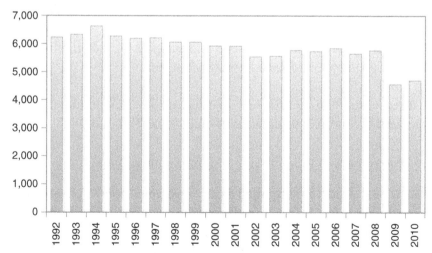

FIGURE I.II   Number of fatal work injuries in the United States, 1992–2010

Courtesy of U.S. Bureau of Labor Statistics.

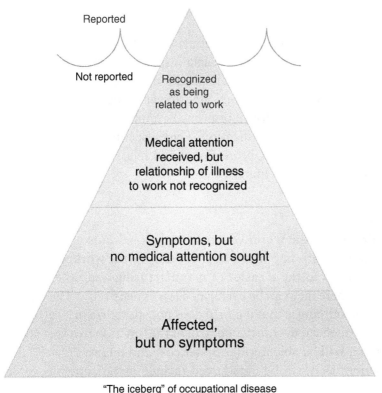

"The iceberg" of occupational disease

FIGURE 1.12   The "iceberg" of occupational disease

Reproduced from Levy BS, Wegman DH, Baron SL, Sokas RK, eds. Occupational and environmental health: twenty-first century challenges and opportunities. In: Levy BS, Wegman DH, Baron SL, Sokas RK Occupational and Environmental Health. 6th ed. New York, NY: Oxford University Press; 2011, p. 12.

of occupational illness, occupational pollution, [and] occupational exposures. It is, unhappily, mostly guess work. We do know, for instance, how certain occupations lead to a high rate of specific kinds of cancer. But there are only scant and fragmentary epidemiological studies of the health effects of chemical or noise pollution on whole groups of workers. Most of the data consists [*sic*] of broad hints of a far flung, unfathomed problem yet to be accurately measured.[54(p. 4)]

Wallick F., The American Worker: An Endangered Species, Ballantine Books; 1972.

Twenty-First Century Occupational Trends and Challenges

Presently, nearly half of the U.S. population engages in some level of employment. Challenges confronting workers during the current century include globalization of employment, adoption of new technologies, and development of green jobs. One of the consequences of changes in employment trends in the workplace has been increased salary disparities between service occupations and highly compensated professional occupations.

Trends in Numbers of Employed Americans

A large proportion of the U.S. population is employed either full or part time. Consequently, work is a crucial aspect of most people's lives in the United States and has important implications for the health of workers. As of July 2013, 145.1 million persons aged 16 years and older were employed.[55] FIGURE 1.13 presents information on the number of persons in the labor force according to job classification. The most common occupation categories in 2013 were service, professional and related occupations, and management, business, and financial.

Globalization and Global Outsourcing

Globalization of the world economy and global outsourcing are contemporary trends with important implications for the workplace. Global outsourcing refers to the transfer of manufacturing and other operations to countries where they can be performed less expensively. "The basic business idea of outsourcing is that if a firm does not specialize in a certain function it will be beneficial to transfer control of the function to a specialist organization that will be able to offer better cost and quality."[56 (p. 154)] Examples of functions that can be outsourced include manufacturing, information technology services, and customer support. Companies headquartered in the United States and other economically advanced countries such as those in Europe are able to gain economic advantages by relocating some of their activities to less developed regions, where wages and other costs are lower.

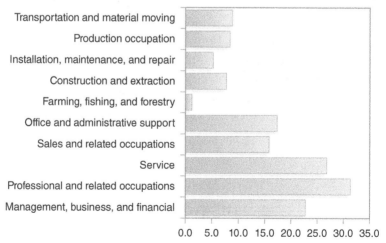

FIGURE 1.13   Number of persons (millions) in the labor force, U.S., July 2013

Data from U. S. Department of Labor. Bureau of Labor Statistics, The employment situation--July 2013. USDL-13-1527.

According to the European Agency for Safety and Health at Work (EU-OSHA), "This outsourcing trend [and] growing importance of supply chains has implications for the working conditions and health and safety of workers of supplier and contracting companies."[57] In developing countries, standards for occupational health and safety may be less rigorous than their counterparts in the developed world. In addition, child laborers may be involved with the manufacture of textiles and other goods and are required to labor under circumstances that would not be permitted in developed countries.

A potential impact of outsourcing in the United States is the weakening of labor unions and the rise of a generation of employees who have insecure employment situations (i.e., freelance workers, part-timers, and independent contractors). In the United States, greater integration of the domestic economy with the global economy has been accompanied by declining trends in rates of unionization.[58] This trend could weaken protections for U.S. workers.

Related to globalization of economic activities is the integration of regional economies. An example of economic integration is the North American Free Trade Agreement (NAFTA), which became effective on January 1, 1994, and created a free trade area among the United States, Canada, and Mexico (FIGURE 1.14).[59] Although NAFTA has had many

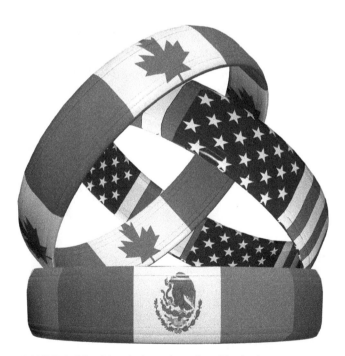

FIGURE 1.14   North American Free Trade Agreement (NAFTA)

© Sangoiri/Shutterstock

positive effects, such as lowering the costs of imports, the Economic Policy Institute argues that imports of automobiles and electronics from Mexico have caused the loss of hundreds of thousands of manufacturing jobs in the United States.[60]

New Technologies: Nanotechnologies and Nanoparticles

New technologies such as nanotechnologies hold much potential for supporting groundbreaking progress in diverse fields—for example, medicine, energy production, and products for the consumer. In fact, nanotechnologies "may revolutionize life in the future."[61(p. vii)] The word nanotechnology denotes "the manipulation of matter on a near-atomic scale [1 to 100 nanometers in length] to produce new structures, materials and devices."[62] These near-atomic scale materials are called nanomaterials. Because of their tiny size, nanomaterials have unique effects in terms of their physical, chemical, and biological behaviors.

Those persons who are most likely to be first exposed to nanomaterials are research workers. It is possible that nanomaterials may affect human health adversely, as some preliminary evidence has suggested.[61] According to Engeman et al., "the potential adverse human health effects of manufactured nanomaterial exposure are not yet fully understood and exposures in humans are mostly uncharacterized."[63 (p. 487)] The National Institute of Occupational Safety and Health (NIOSH) has developed a list of 10 critical topic areas for research on nanotechnology (FIGURE 1.15). Among these critical research topics are toxicity of nanomaterials, risk assessments with respect to their use, and epidemiologic studies and surveillance of workplace exposures to nanomaterials.[64] In addition, several ethical issues will need to be resolved with respect to workers involved with nanoparticles. These ethical issues deal with "identification and communication of hazards and risks by scientists, authorities, and employers; acceptance of risk by workers; implementation of controls; choice of participation in medical screening; and adequate investment in toxicologic and exposure control research."[65(p. 5)]

Growing Employment in Green Jobs

A growing employment field known as "green jobs" promises opportunities in the sustainable, low-carbon sector. The category of green jobs encompasses "work in agricultural, manufacturing, research and development (R & D), administrative, and service activities that contribute substantially to preserving and restoring environmental quality. Specifically, but not exclusively, this includes jobs that help to protect ecosystems and

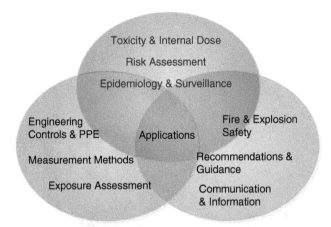

FIGURE 1.15 Ten critical topic areas in nanotechnology

Reproduced from Centers for Disease Control and Prevention, National Institute for Occupational Safety and Health, Nanotechnology: 10 critical topic areas, http://www.cdc.gov/niosh/topics/nanotech/critical.html. Accessed May 12, 2013.

biodiversity; de-carbonize the economy; and minimize or altogether avoid generation of all forms of waste and pollution."[66(p. 3)] **FIGURE 1.16** provides three examples of green jobs.

Although green jobs can contribute greatly to society, it will be necessary to assure the health and safety of the many workers who are likely to be employed in this new industry.[67] One category of green jobs focuses on the development of renewable energy sources and devices for increased energy efficiency. From the global perspective, the renewable energy sector has shown remarkable job growth, increasing by 21% each year and employing nearly 5 million persons early in the current decade.[68] However, green jobs are not without occupational health risks. For example, their installation of solar panels might expose workers to increased risks from electrical shocks and falls from working at heights. Occupational safety and health programs will need to identify hazards associated with green jobs and develop methods for controlling them.

Recycling operations help to preserve scarce resources and, therefore, can be considered part of the green economy. E-waste (electrical and electronic waste) is one of the fastest-growing categories of waste. This waste stream contains precious metals and other valuable materials; it is also contaminated with heavy metals and toxic chemicals. A large percentage of e-waste finds its way to developing nations, where recycling operations create employment for hundreds of thousands of impoverished people.[69] These individuals will need occupational safety and health protections from hazards in e-waste.

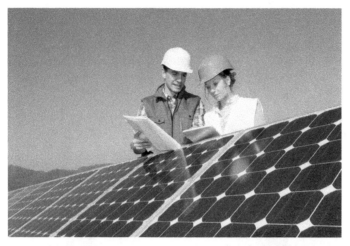

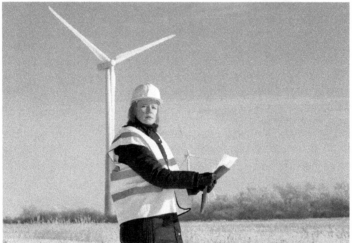

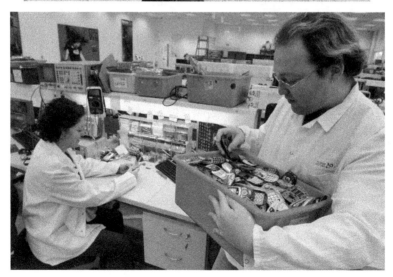

FIGURE 1.16   Examples of green jobs

© Goodluz/Shutterstock; © Andrei Merkulov/123RF; © ChameleonsEye/Shutterstock

Child Labor in Developing Countries

Child labor was common in England during the 19th-century Victorian era when the Industrial Revolution was in full swing. At that time, orphans constituted a major proportion of workers in the textile industry.[70] Currently, child labor is a problem of particular concern for developing countries. In these countries, poor children are often forced to leave school to work and support their families. These child laborers may be exposed to hazardous materials and deleterious chemicals, and are at great risk of injuries. Also, they may be subjected to sexual, physical, and verbal abuse.[71] Children are more vulnerable to injury and the effects of toxic chemicals because of their behaviors and developmental stages. The fact that child laborers typically come from backgrounds of extreme poverty, where they experience poor housing and environmental conditions as well as insufficient caloric intake, increases the likelihood that their development will be impacted by poor working conditions.[72]

Women Workers

Globally, participation of women in the workforce has increased steadily, especially in rapidly industrializing Asian countries.[73] Occupations typically associated with women are in the fields of electronics, textiles, and manufacturing of light-industrial goods for export. The working conditions for women in crowded factories may expose them to injuries such as amputations and burns. Fires in factories that are packed with trapped female employees who do not have access to building exits have caused massive deaths from conflagrations. Women who work in factories and in healthcare facilities may be exposed to toxic chemicals and radiation. The impact of such exposures upon reproductive function is a vital area of concern for occupational health research and will be explored later in this text. Given the expectation that women will manage their households in addition to working outside of the home, many female workers also experience high stress levels that stem from their multiple role responsibilities. Much of the work carried out by women is not documented formally and is unpaid.[73]

Immigrant Workers

In the future, racial and ethnic minorities (in aggregate) are projected to become a numerical majority in the United States.[74] As immigration is one of the forces driving population growth, immigrant workers are an important component of the U.S. labor force. Some groups of immigrant workers may be at increased risk for hazardous occupational exposures and working conditions; many of these exposures are thought to go unreported. For example, Southeast Asians employed in fields such as the electronics manufacturing industry are believed to have frequent and unreported exposures to hazardous dusts and solvents.[75] In the United States, many immigrants work less than full time[74] and may be employed as migrant and seasonal farm workers (MSFWs) who face frequent occupational hazards. These workers are confronted by cultural, legal, financial, and other barriers to obtaining health services.[76]

Occupational health hazards confronting MSFWs are noteworthy, as described by Hansen and Donohoe:

> MSFW's face numerous occupational hazards. Farm laborer is seasonal and intensive. Migrant workers labor in all seasons and weather conditions, including extreme heat, cold, rain, and bright sun. Work often requires stoop labor, working with soil and/or heavy machinery, climbing, and carrying burdensome loads, all of which lead to chronic musculoskeletal symptoms. Direct contact with plants can cause allergic rashes or, in the case of tobacco farmers, "green tobacco sickness" (i.e., transdermal nicotine poisoning).[77(p. 155)]

An Aging Workforce

The number of older workers (persons 55 years of age and older) in the U.S. labor force is increasing—a trend that is occurring in conjunction with the overall aging of the U.S. population. These older workers bring to the workplace a wealth of experience that is of great potential benefit to employers. Although occupational injuries and illnesses among older workers tend to be less frequent than among younger workers, older workers' injuries often are more serious.[78] Given increased number of older workers, comprehensive health promotion and health protection programs need to be developed for them to maximize the contribution of this cohort.[79]

The Public Health Model for Occupational Health and Safety

The field of public health is complex and has been defined in several ways. For example, Winslow, who founded the Yale University Department of Public Health, defined public health as follows:

> [T]he science and the art of preventing disease, prolonging life, and promoting physical health and efficiency through organized community efforts for the sanitation of the environment, the control of community infections, the education of the individual in principles of personal hygiene, the organization of medical and nursing service for the early diagnosis and preventive treatment of disease, and the development of the social machinery which will ensure to

every individual in the community a standard of living adequate for the maintenance of health.[80(p. 30)]

The field of public health has the following distinguishing characteristics:

- A focus on the health of entire populations rather than on the health of a single individual
- Emphasis on the prevention of disease
- Commitment to social justice as a core value

Occupational Health and Public Health

Occupational health experts recognize that occupational health is a part of public health.[81] The relevance of occupational health for public health stems from the fact that conditions in the work environment affect so many people in the United States (i.e., a large proportion of the population). In turn, the occupational environment is an important venue for health promotion.[82] Prevention of occupational illnesses and injuries can result from improving the work environment and educating employees and managers about work-related hazards.

Exposures that occur in the work environment can affect the larger community when toxic substances from factories are emitted into the community. In addition, many health disparities stem from workers' exposures in the occupational environment. According to Murray, "Workers of color generally are underrepresented in professional categories and overrepresented in blue-collar and service jobs, especially in certain occupations."[83] People who work in blue-collar occupations—such as garbage collectors, nursing aides, and farm workers—are disproportionately affected by the effects of exposures to hazardous biological agents, chemicals, and pesticides.

Health disparities between African American and white men in terms of occupational risks for some form of cancers (for example, non-Hodgkin's lymphoma) have been reported.[84] Possibly these disparities result from differential exposure levels to occupational carcinogens among different racial groups. Increasing awareness of the effects of work on health has encouraged the recognition of environmental determinants of heath disparities. The fields of occupational safety and health hold promise as "a way to reach a large portion of the population experiencing these disparities."[85(p. 526)]

In many respects, the workforce is a captive audience required to be in a place of employment for at least 40 hours each week. The workplace is an ideal setting in which to introduce health promotion activities. One of the benefits of wellness programs for businesses is increases in worker productivity—for example, by slowing or preventing chronic illnesses that might develop during the working years.[86] The process of improving workers' health can be facilitated through partnerships between employers and public health departments.

The Core Functions of Public Health Applied to Occupational Health

The Institute of Medicine has identified three core functions of public health: assessment, policy development, and assurance (**FIGURE 1.17**).[87,88] These functions are applicable to public health agencies at all levels of government, and they can be applied specifically to occupational health and safety. The assessment function pertains to the collection and analysis of health-related data. In occupational health, this function could involve the identification of populations and settings at high risk of adverse health conditions. The policy function is related to the development of health policies that limit occupational risks and promote workers' health. Finally, the assurance function means that needed occupational health regulations and health services for workers are being provided. Examples of these core functions of public health are emphasized throughout this text as they pertain to occupational health.

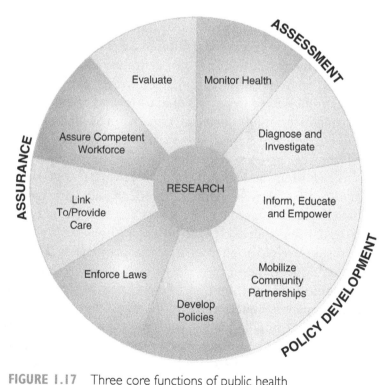

FIGURE 1.17   Three core functions of public health

Reproduced from Centers for Disease Control and Prevention, Environmental Health Services, Core functions of public health and how they relate to the 10 essential services, http://www.cdc.gov/nceh/ehs/ephli/core_ess.htm. Accessed August 17, 2013.

Healthy People 2020 Objectives for Occupational Health and Safety

The initiative known as Healthy People sets forth a comprehensive health promotion and disease prevention program for the United States. The publication *Healthy People 2020* identified a group of occupational safety and health objectives, shown in **EXHIBIT 1.4**.

EXHIBIT 1.4   *Healthy People 2020* Objectives for Occupational Safety and Health

- OSH-1 Reduce deaths from work-related injuries
  - OSH-1.1 Reduce deaths from work-related injuries in all industries
  - OSH-1.2 Reduce deaths from work-related injuries in mining
  - OSH-1.3 Reduce deaths from work-related injuries in construction
  - OSH-1.4 Reduce deaths from work-related injuries in transportation and warehousing
  - OSH-1.5 Reduce deaths from work-related injuries in agriculture, forestry, fishing, and hunting
- OSH-2 Reduce nonfatal work-related injuries
  - OSH-2.1 Reduce work-related injuries in private-sector industries resulting in medical treatment, lost time from work, or restricted work activity, as reported by employers
  - OSH-2.2 Reduce work-related injuries treated in emergency departments (EDs)
  - OSH-2.3 Reduce work-related injuries among adolescent workers aged 15 to 19 years
- OSH-3 Reduce the rate of injury and illness cases involving days away from work due to overexertion or repetitive motion
- OSH-4 Reduce pneumoconiosis deaths
- OSH-5 Reduce deaths from work-related homicides
- OSH-6 Reduce work-related assaults
- OSH-7 Reduce the proportion of persons who have elevated blood lead concentrations from work exposures
- OSH-8 Reduce occupational skin diseases or disorders among full-time workers
- OSH-9 (Developmental) Increase the proportion of employees who have access to workplace programs that prevent or reduce employee stress
- OSH-10 Reduce new cases of work-related, noise-induced hearing loss

OSH = Occupational safety and health (OSH).

Source: HealthyPeople.gov. Occupational safety and health: objectives. http://www.healthy-people.gov/2020/topicsobjectives2020/objectiveslist.aspx?topicId=30. Accessed May 13, 2013.

SUMMARY

Occupational health is concerned with protecting the health of workers from diseases and injuries associated with hazardous work-related exposures; in addition, the field pursues the improvement of the work environment and the promotion of workers' health in general. Work-related diseases are adverse health events that arise from the work environment. Occupational health hazards have been observed since the classical period of human history. Among the important names in occupational health history are Hippocrates, Georg Agricola, Bernardino Ramazzini, Paracelsus, Percival Pott, and Alice Hamilton. During the Industrial Revolution and the early 20th century, awareness of the causes and effects of hazardous working conditions increased.

Illnesses and injuries associated with work are leading sources of morbidity and mortality worldwide. Media reports have documented dangerous working conditions in the developing world, but occupational illnesses and injuries are significant concerns for the developed world as well. More than 50,000 deaths from work-related illness and 5000 deaths from injuries occur in the United States annually. Illnesses and injuries cost the U.S. economy approximately $250 billion per year. Among the forces that will continue to affect occupational health in the 21st century are changing trends in employment, adoption of new technologies, and alterations in the composition of the workforce.

With its potential to impact large numbers of people and aid in the prevention of disease, occupational health is closely allied with public health. In accordance with the goal to improve the health of employees, *Healthy People 2020* presents national objectives for occupational health.

STUDY QUESTIONS AND EXERCISES

1. Define the following terms:
    A. Occupational health
    B. Occupational safety
    C. Occupational exposures
    D. Work-related diseases
    E. Caisson disease
2. From a global perspective, what are some examples of risk factors for occupational morbidity and mortality?
3. What is the significance of adverse health outcomes associated with work for the United States? Describe the social, economic, and personal dimensions of work-related illnesses and injuries.
4. Hippocrates, Ramazzini, and Hamilton were important historical figures for occupational health. Briefly describe their most important contributions to the field.
5. Describe five unusual occupational diseases of the past, giving their definitions and information about their etiology.
6. Describe the Triangle Shirtwaist Factory fire and the Gauley Bridge disaster. What was the importance of these events for occupational health?
7. Give examples of three current trends that are relevant to the contemporary work environment. You could use examples from the text or find some other examples on the Web.

8. Describe three *Healthy People 2020* goals for occupational health, giving an example of each goal.
9. State five adverse health outcomes that have been linked to the work environment. What are some examples of agent factors that have been linked to these outcomes?
10. Compare and contrast traditional public health concerns with those of occupational health. Provide some examples of the similarities and differences between the fields of public health and occupational health. The Institute of Medicine has delineated three functions of the field of public health. How might these be implemented in the field of occupational health?

REFERENCES

1. Stellman JM, Daum SM. *Work is dangerous to your health*. New York, NY: Vintage Books; 1973.
2. *The Free Online Dictionary*. Definition of occupational health. n.d. http://medical-dictionary.thefreedictionary.com/Occupational health+and+safety. Accessed June 20, 2014.
3. Frank AL. Occupational safety and health: The history of work. In: *Gale encyclopedia of public health*. http://www.answers.com/topic/advisory-committee-on-construction-safety-and-health-accsh. Accessed September 27, 2012.
4. Radford EP. Evolution of attitudes toward occupational health in the U.S.A. *J UOEH*. 1986;8(1):1–9.
5. National Institute of Environmental Health Sciences. Occupational health. n.d. http://www.niehs.nih.gov/health/topics/population/occupational/. Accessed May 31, 2013.
6. Levy BS, Wegman DH, Baron SL, Sokas RK. Occupational and environmental health: twenty-first century challenges and opportunities. In: Levy BS, Wegman DH, Baron SL, Sokas RK, eds. *Occupational and environmental health*. 6th ed. New York, NY: Oxford University Press; 2011:3-22.
7. Macik-Frey M, Quick JC, Nelson DL. Advances in occupational health: from a stressful beginning to a positive future? *J Manage*. 2007;3(6):809–840.
8. *The Free Dictionary*. Occupational medicine. http://www.thefreedictionary.com/Occupational+safety+and+health. Accessed August 17, 2013.
9. Joint ILO/WHO Committee on Occupational Health, WHO Regional Office for Europe. *Good practice in occupational health services*. Copenhagen, Denmark: World Health Organization; 2002.
10. Dictionary.com. Safety. n.d. http://dictionary.reference.com/browse/safety. Accessed October 21, 2013.
11. BusinessDictionary.com. Occupational safety. n.d. http://www.businessdictionary.com/definition/occupational-safety.html. Accessed December 19, 2013.
12. Garcia AM, Checkoway H. A glossary for research in occupational health. *J Epidemiol Community Health*. 2003;57:7–10.
13. Porta M, ed. *A dictionary of epidemiology*. 5th ed. New York, NY: Oxford University Press; 2008.
14. National Research Council. *Risk assessment in the federal government: managing the process*. Washington, DC: National Academy Press; 1983.
15. National Institutes of Health. National Institute of Environmental Health Sciences. *Environmental diseases from A to Z*. 2nd Ed. NIH Publication No. 96-4145, June 2007.

16. U.S. Department of Labor, Bureau of Labor Statistics (BLS). Occupational safety and health definitions. n.d. http://www.bls.gov/iif/oshdef.htm. Accessed September 8, 2013.

17. National Institutes of Health, National Library of Medicine. Occupational health. *MedlinePlus*. n.d. http://www.nlm.nih.gov/medlineplus/occupationalhealth.html. Accessed August 13, 2013.

18. Cruse JM. History of medicine: the metamorphosis of scientific medicine in the ever-present past. *Am J Med Sci*. 1999;318(3):171–180.

19. Borzelleca JF. Paracelsus: herald of modern toxicology. *Toxicol Sci*. 2000;53:2–4.

20. Franco G. Ramazzini and workers' health. *Lancet*.1999;354:858–861.

21. Felton JS. The heritage of Bernardino Ramazzini. *Occup Med*. 1997;47(3):167–179.

22. Gochfeld M. Chronologic history of occupational medicine. *J Occup Environ Med*. 2005;47:96–114.

23. Susser M, Stein Z. *Eras in epidemiology: the evolution of ideas*. New York, NY: Oxford University Press; 2009.

24. Doll R. Pott and the path to prevention. *Arch Geschwulstforsch*. 1975;45:521–531.

25. Parker G. Hazard! Health in the workplace over 200 years. *Occup Med*. 2005;55:337–339.

26. Cherniack MG. Diseases of unusual occupations: an historical perspective. *Occup Med*. 1992;7(3):369–384.

27. Fishman RS. Dark as a dungeon: the rise and fall of coal miners' nystagmus. *Arch Ophthalmol*. 2006;124:1637–1644.

28. Castiglione FM, Selikowitz SM, Dimond RL. Mule spinner's disease. *Arch Dermatol*. 1985;121:370–372.

29. Kartenmeister.com. The social fabric. n.d. http://www.kartenmeister.com/preview/html/the_social_fabric.html. Accessed September 5, 2013.

30. Hamilton A. Lead poisoning in the United States. *Am J Public Health*. 2009;99(53): S547–S549. [Reprinted from Hamilton A. Lead poisoning in the United States. *Am J Public Health*. 1914;4(6):477–480.]

31. Marx RE. Uncovering the cause of "fossy jaw" circa 1858 to 1906: oral and maxillofacial surgery closed case files—case closed. *J Oral Maxillofac Surg*. 2008;6:2356–2363.

32. Felton JS. Classical syndromes in occupational medicine: phosphorus necrosis—a classical occupational disease. *Am J Ind Med*. 1982;3(1):77–120.

33. Butler WP. Caisson disease during the construction of the Eads and Brooklyn Bridges: a review. *Undersea Hyperb Med*. 2000;31(4):445–459.

34. Centers for Disease Control and Prevention. Improvements in workplace safety—United States, 1900–1999. *MMWR*. 1999;48(22):461–469.

35. Rosner D, Markowitz G. Labor Day and the war on workers. *Am J Public Health*. 1999;89:1310–1321.

36. *Digital History*. The Great Railroad Strike. n.d. http://www.digitalhistory.uh.edu/disp_textbook.cfm?smtID=2&psid=3189. Accessed June 4, 2014.

37. PBS.org. *WGBH American Experience*. Workers of the Central Pacific Railroad. Transcontinental Railroad. n.d. http://www.pbs.org/wgbh/americanexperience/features/general-article/tcrr-cprr/. Accessed June 4, 2014.

38. U.S. National Park Service. Triangle Shirtwaist Factory building. n.d. http://www.cr.nps.gov/nr/travel/pwwmh/ny30.htm. Accessed January 19, 2014.

39. Linder D. The Triangle Shirtwaist Factory fire trial. n.d. http://law2.umkc.edu/faculty/projects/ftrials/triangle/triangleaccount.html. Accessed January 19, 2014.

40. Kuschner WG. Introduction to the symposium. *Postgrad Med.* 2003;113(4). http://www.postgradmed.com/index.php?art=pgm_04_2003?article=1397. Accessed January 19, 2014.

41. Steenland K, Burnett C, Lalich N, et al. Dying for work: the magnitude of US mortality from selected causes of death associated with occupation. *Am J Ind Med.* 2003;43:461–482.

42. Ahonen EQ, Benavides FG, Benach J. Immigrant populations, work and health: a systematic literature review. *Scand J Work Environ Health.* 2007;33(2):96–104.

43. International Labour Organization. Hazardous work. n.d. http://www.ilo.org/safework/areasofwork/hazardous-work/lang--en/index.htm. Accessed August 13, 2013.

44. Driscoll T, Takala J, Steenland K, et al. Review of estimates of the global burden of injury and illness due to occupational exposures. *Am J Ind Med.* 2005;48:491–502.

45. Fingerhut M, Driscoll T, Nelson DI, et al. Contribution of occupational risk factors to the global burden of disease: a summary of findings. *SJWEH.* 2005;1(suppl):58–61.

46. Nelson DI, Concha-Barrientos M, Driscoll T, et al. The global burden of selected occupational diseases and injury risks: methodology and summary. *Am J Ind Med.* 2005;48:400–418.

47. Leigh JP. Economic burden of occupational injury and illness in the United States. *Milbank Qrtly.* 2011;89(4):728–772.

48. U.S. Department of Labor, Bureau of Labor Statistics. Employer-reported workplace injuries and illnesses—2012. n.d. http://www.bls.gov/news.release/pdf/osh.pdf. Accessed January 19, 2014.

49. Herbert R, Landrigan PJ. Work-related death: a continuing epidemic. *Am J Public Health.* 2000;90(4):541–545.

50. Schulte PA. Characterizing the burden of occupational injury and disease. *J Occup Environ Med.* 2005;47(6):607–622.

51. *Associated Press.* Investigators examining Arizona blaze that killed 19 firefighters looking at what went wrong. FoxNews.com. July 3, 2013. http://www.foxnews.com/us/2013/07/03/investigators-examining-arizona-blaze-that-killed-1-firefighters-looking-at/. Accessed August 16, 2013.

52. Hanna J, Hegeman R. Associated Press. Last victims of Kansas grain elevator blast found. *San Francisco Chronicle.* November 1, 2011. http://www.sfgate.com/nation/article/Last-victims-of-Kansas-grain-elevator-blast-found-2324654.php. Accessed August 16, 2013.

53. U. S. Department of Labor, Bureau of Labor Statistics. Fatal occupational injuries and Workers' Memorial Day. n.d. http://www.bls.gov/iif/oshwc/cfoi/worker_memorial.htm. Accessed August 16, 2013.

54. Wallick F. *The American worker: an endangered species.* New York, NY: Ballantine Books; 1972.

55. U. S. Department of Labor, Bureau of Labor Statistics. The employment situation—July 2013. USDL-13-1527. News release, August 2, 2013.

56. Clott CB. Perspectives on global outsourcing and the changing nature of work. *Bus Soc Rev.* 2004;109(2):153–170.

57. European Agency for Safety and Health at Work. *Promoting occupational safety and health through the supply chain.* Luxembourg: Publications Office of the European Union; 2012.

58. Slaughter MJ. Globalization and declining unionization in the United States. *Industrial Relations.* 2007;46(2):329–346.

59. Office of the United States Trade Representative. North American Free Trade Agreement (NAFTA). n.d. http://www.ustr.gov/trade-agreements/free-trade-agreements/north-american-free-trade-agreement-nafta. Accessed August 29, 2013.

60. *Huffington Post.* U.S. economy lost nearly 700,000 jobs because of NAFTA, EPI says. May 12, 2011. http://www.huffingtonpost.com/2011/05/12/nafta-job-loss-trade-deficit-epi_n_859983.html. Accessed December 23, 2013

61. Centers for Disease Control and Prevention, National Institute for Occupational Safety and Health (NIOSH). *General safe practices for working with engineered nano-materials in research laboratories.* DHHS (NIOSH) Pub. No. 2012-147. 2012.

62. Centers for Disease Control and Prevention. Workplace safety and health topics. Nanotechnology: overview. n.d. http://www.cdc.gov/niosh/topics/nanotech/. Accessed May 12, 2013.

63. Engeman CD, Baumgartner L, Carr BM, et al. The hierarchy of environmental health and safety practices in the U.S. nanotechnology workplace. *J Occup Environ Hyg.* 2013;10:487-495.

64. Centers for Disease Control and Prevention, National Institute for Occupational Safety and Health (NIOSH). Nanotechnology: 10 critical topic areas. n.d. http://www.cdc.gov/niosh/topics/nanotech/critical.html. Accessed May 12, 2013.

65. Schulte PA, Salamanca-Buentello F. Ethical and scientific issues of nanotechnology in the workplace. *Environ Health Perspect.* 2007;115(1):5–12.

66. United Nations Environment Programme (UNEP). *Green jobs: towards decent work in a sustainable, low carbon world.* Nairobi, Kenya: UNEP; 2008.

67. European Agency for Safety and Health at Work. *Green jobs and occupational safety and health.* Luxembourg: Publications Office of the European Union; 2013

68. Olsen L. What policies for a green economy that works for social progress? [Editorial]. *Int J Labour Res.* 2012;4(2):135–149.

69. Lundgren K. *The global impact of e-waste: addressing the challenge.* Geneva, Switzerland: International Labour Organization; 2012.

70. McCunnie T. Regulation and the health of child workers in the mid-Victorian silk industry. *Local Popul Stud.* 2005;74:54–74.

71. Gharaibeh M, Hoeman S. Health hazards and risks for abuse among child labor in Jordan. *J Pediatr Nurs.* 2003;18(2):140–147.

72. Rohlman DS, Nuwayhid I, Ismail A, Saddik B. Using epidemiology and neurotoxicology to reduce risks to young workers. *Neurotoxicology.* 2012;33(4):817–822.

73. Kane P, ed.; Dennerstein L, project director. *Women and occupational health.* Geneva, Switzerland: World Health Organization; 1999.

74. Hernandez DJ. Demographic change and the life circumstances of immigrant families. *Future Child.* 2004;14(2):16–47.

75. Azaroff LS, Levenstein C, Wegman DH. Occupational health of Southeast Asian immigrants in a US city: a comparison of data sources. *Am J Public Health.* 2003;93(4):593–598.

76. Arcury TA, Quandt SA. Delivery of health services to migrant and seasonal farmworkers. *Annu Rev Public Health.* 2007;28:345–363.

77. Hansen E, Donohoe M. Health issues of migrant and seasonal farmworkers. [Editorial]. *J Health Care Poor Underserved.* 2003;14(2):153–164.

78. Silverstein M. Meeting the challenges of an aging workforce. *Am J Ind Med.* 2008;51:269–280.

79. Loeppke RR, Schill AL, Chosewood C, et al. Advancing workplace health protection and promotion for an aging workforce. *JOEM*. 2013;55(5);500–506.
80. Winslow C-EA. The untilled fields of public health. *Science*. 1920;51(1306):23–33.
81. Guillemin MP. Occupational health: a very important component of public health. [Editorial]. *Soz Praventivmed*. 2006;51:1–2.
82. Moll SE, Gewurtz RE, Krupa TM, Law MC. Promoting an occupational perspective in public health. *Can J Occup Ther*. 2013;80(2):111–119.
83. Murray LR. Sick and tired of being sick and tired: scientific evidence, methods, and research implications for racial and ethnic disparities in occupational health. *Am J Public Health*. 2003;93(2):221–226.
84. Briggs NC, Levine RS, Hall I, et al. Occupational risk factors for selected cancers among African American and white men in the United States. *Am J Public Health*. 2003;93(10):1748–1752.
85. Quinn MM. Occupational health, public health, worker health. *Am J Public Health*. 2003;93(4):526.
86. Healey BJ, Walker KT. *Introduction to occupational health in public health practice*. San Francisco, CA: Jossey-Bass; 2009.
87. Institute of Medicine. *The future of public health*. Washington, DC; 1988.
88. Centers for Disease Control and Prevention, Environmental Health Services (EHS). Core functions of public health and how they relate to the 10 essential services. n.d. http://www.cdc.gov/nceh/ehs/ephli/core_ess.htm. Accessed August 17, 2013.

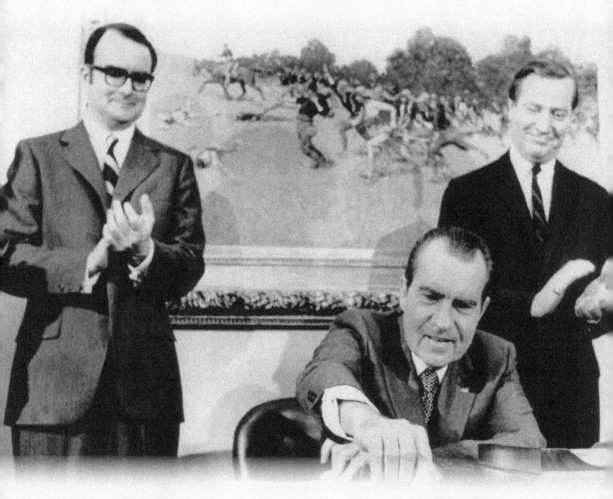

FIGURE 2.1   President Nixon signing the Occupational Safety and Health Act, December 29, 1970

© Everett Collection/Age Fotostock.

The 1970 Occupational Safety and Health Act, which reinforced safe working conditions for employees, was a landmark in the history of occupational health policy.

CHAPTER 2

Occupational Health Policy and the Regulatory Climate

Learning Objectives

By the end of this chapter, the reader will be able to:

- Describe the functions of international agencies in promoting occupational health and safety.
- Describe three historically significant occupational health laws.
- List at least four federal agencies responsible for the protection of workers' health and describe their functions.
- State the names of three current national laws designed to protect the health of workers.
- Describe the role of unions and other organizations in protecting workers' health.

Chapter Outline

- Introduction
- History of Legislation Protecting American Workers
- International Organizations Protecting Workers' Rights
- U.S. Federal Agencies for Occupational Health and Safety
- Current Federal Regulations Protecting Workers
- Private-Sector Organizations and Activities Supporting Workers' Health
- Union Participation in Protecting Workers' Health
- Summary
- Study Questions and Exercises

Introduction

In this chapter, we will learn about the crucial function of occupational health policies for protecting workers from job-related hazards. Policies define standards for a safe workplace and procedures for enforcement of regulations for worker safety. An occupational health policy is "a plan of action primarily concerned with protecting the health, safety, and welfare of persons at work. The policies typically are designed to protect workers from hazardous work environments by ensuring clean work areas, the use of protective equipment and assuring employees are properly trained."[1]

At the worldwide level, several international organizations have created policies for the protection of workers' health. International agencies for the protection of health and the workplace include the International Labour Organization (ILO) and the European Agency for Safety and Health at Work (EU-OSHA).

At the national level, in the United States, the movement to create occupational health policies began gathering momentum in the early 20th century. During this era, one of the major developments was the creation of programs for improving working conditions in the U.S. mining industry. Later, in 1970, legislators passed the groundbreaking Occupational Safety and Health Act, which reinforced safe working conditions for employees. This act created the Occupational Safety and Health Administration (OSHA), which enforces standards for a safe work environment. Private (nongovernmental) organizations and labor unions also are instrumental in protecting workers from occupational illnesses and injuries.

History of Legislation Protecting American Workers

In the United States, as a result of federalism, which allocates functions among levels of government, the U.S. Congress, and other branches of the federal government are key players in creating initiatives for protection of workers. Often advocacy organizations such as unions lobby members of Congress to introduce occupational health legislation. For example, unions were instrumental in the development of occupational health acts for the protection of miners. Political forces that tend to weaken governmental legislative efforts on behalf of workers include the public's concerns about the costs of government spending and the climate of deregulation. In sum, "[t]he primary responsibility for the provision of a healthy work environment rests with the employer. Government, however, provides education services and formulates minimum standards for the protection of workers. Although a large part of government's role is to promulgate and enforce these minimum standards, it can provide technical toxicological and clinical occupational medicine advice."[2(p. 580)]

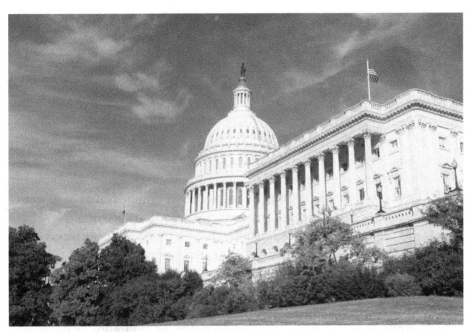

FIGURE 2.2 U.S. Capitol, the setting for federal occupational health legislation and policy development

© naureenrafiq/iStock/Thinkstock.

FIGURE 2.2 shows the U.S. Capitol, where occupational health legislation is enacted at the national level. Enforcement of legislation is often the responsibility of federal agencies as well. This section traces the history of the major occupational health legislative acts listed in **TABLE 2.1**.

TABLE 2.1   Dates and History of Major Occupational Health Legislation

Date Enacted	Name of Legislative Act
1908	Act of 1908 for Federal Employees' Compensation
1916	Federal Employees' Compensation Act of 1916 (FECA)
1938	Fair Labor Standards Act of 1938
1970	Occupational Safety and Health Act
Mine Safety and Health Legislation (1952–2006)	
1952	Federal Coal Mine Safety Act of 1952
1966	Metal and Nonmetallic Mine Safety Act of 1966
1969	Federal Coal Mine Health and Safety Act (Coal Act)
1977	Federal Mine Safety and Health Act (Mine Act)
2006	Mine Improvement and New Emergency Response Act (MINER Act)

Data from U.S. Department of Labor. History of Mine Safety and Health Legislation. Available at: http://www.msha.gov/MSHAINFO/MSHAINF2.HTM. Accessed September 5, 2013.

Federal Employees' Compensation Act of 1916

The Federal Employees' Compensation Act of 1916 (FECA) was enacted in recognition of traumatic injuries endured by some groups of federal workers. "All U.S. workers' compensation programs are the products of the Industrial Revolution. An intriguing legislative catharsis took place between roughly 1860 and 1920, with society recognizing that among the prices to be paid for the fruits of the Industrial Revolution was the injury or death of large numbers of workers."[3(p. 3)]

FECA superseded an earlier law that had been signed by President Theodore Roosevelt in 1908. The original law compensated a subset of federal employees who worked in especially hazardous occupations; FECA expanded the compensation to all federal employees. Compensation for lost wages, medical care, and survivors' benefits were made available to all federal employees, but the law did not provide retirement benefits. According to the Department of Labor, "the Federal Employees Compensation Act (FECA) ... establishes a comprehensive and exclusive workers' compensation program which pays compensation for the disability or death of a federal employee resulting from personal injury sustained while in the performance of duty. The FECA, administered by OWCP [Office of Workers' Compensation Programs], provides benefits for wage loss compensation for total or partial disability, schedule awards for permanent loss or loss of use of specified members of the body, related medical costs, and vocational rehabilitation.... . All civilian employees of the United States, except those paid from non-appropriated funds, are covered."[4]

Fair Labor Standards Act of 1938

The Fair Labor Standards Act of 1938 (FLSA) was an act of Congress designed "[t]o provide for the establishment of fair labor standards in employments in and affecting interstate commerce, and for other purposes."[5(p. 1)] The act sought to ban oppressive child labor practices, establish a minimum hourly wage of 25 cents, and limit the maximum work week to 44 hours.[6]

> [The FLSA] prescribes standards for the basic minimum wage and overtime pay, [and] affects most private and public employment. It requires employers to pay covered employees who are not otherwise exempt at least the federal minimum wage and overtime pay of one-and-one-half times the regular rate of pay. For non-agricultural operations, it restricts the hours that children under age 16 can work and forbids employment of children under age 18

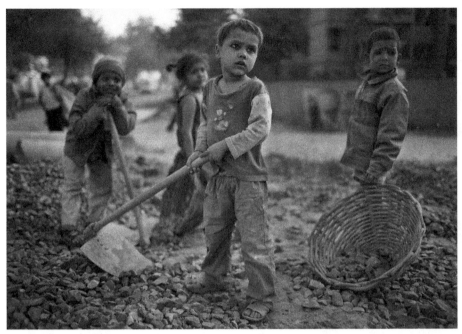

FIGURE 2.3   Child labor

© Daniel Berehulak/Getty Images News/Thinkstock.

in certain jobs deemed too dangerous. For agricultural operations, it prohibits the employment of children under age 16 during school hours and in certain jobs deemed too dangerous.[7]

In many developing countries, the practice of child labor continues. Children—even very young children—are forced to work under deplorable and hazardous conditions (**FIGURE 2.3**).

Mine Safety and Health Legislation, 1952–2006

At one time, U.S. miners worked under extremely unsafe conditions that exposed them to injuries and high levels of coal dust, the cause of coal worker's pneumoconiosis (**FIGURE 2.4**). As a result of improving working conditions, the death toll among miners in the United States has declined but remains at unacceptable levels. **EXHIBIT 2.1** summarizes injury trends in mining.

Concerns over mining hazards led to several major legislative acts that are noteworthy for their protections afforded to mine workers. **EXHIBIT 2.2** details the history of mine safety and health legislation. Two especially noteworthy legislative achievements were the Federal Coal Mine Health and Safety Act of 1969 (Coal Act) and the Federal Mine Safety and Health Act of 1977 (Mine Act).

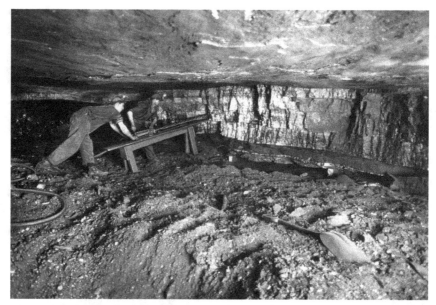

FIGURE 2.4   Historical picture of working conditions in a coal mine

Courtesy of Centers for Disease Control and Prevention, National Institute of Occupational Safety and Health, Public Health Image Library.

EXHIBIT 2.1   Injury Trends in Mining

Since the earliest days of mining, the job of digging coal and other useful minerals out of the earth has been considered one of the world's most dangerous occupations. During the 20th century, public concern about the toll of deaths, injuries, and destruction in mine accidents prompted passage of much-needed safety legislation and intensified the search for safer methods and improved training practices and technology.

Today, mine safety and health legislation and advances in technology and training have reduced mining deaths and injuries from the earlier high levels. However, any mining death or injury is still unacceptable.

The Tragic Early Toll

From 1880 to 1910, mine explosions and other accidents claimed thousands of victims. The deadliest year in U.S. coal mining history was 1907, when an estimated 3242 deaths occurred in this industry. That year, America's worst mine explosion ever killed 358 people near Monongah, West Virginia. While metal and nonmetal (non-coal) mining was less deadly than coal mining, available records for the era show that it, too, was highly hazardous. Fires, explosions, and roof collapses caused many deaths and injuries. One of the deadliest non-coal mining accidents involved a mine fire in Montana that killed 163 miners in 1917.

Decades of Difficult But Impressive Progress

Total deaths in all types of U.S. mining, which had averaged 1500 or more per year during earlier decades, decreased on average during the 1990s to fewer than 100 per year, and

(Continues)

EXHIBIT 2.1   Injury Trends in Mining (*Continued*)

reached historic lows of 35 total deaths in 2009 and 2012. The average annual injuries to miners in all segments of the mining industry have also decreased steadily.

While annual coal mining deaths numbered more than 1000 per year in the early part of the 20th century, they decreased to an average of about 451 annual fatalities in the 1950s, and to 141 in the 1970s. From 2006 to 2010, the yearly average number of fatalities in coal mining decreased to 35. In 2009, there were 18 recorded coal mining deaths, a record low number. Sadly, coal mining fatalities dramatically increased to 48 in 2010, with the tragedy at the Upper Big Branch Mine (West Virginia) claiming 29 lives and 19 other coal miners being killed that year. In 2011, 21 coal miners were killed in accidents. In 2012, 19 coal miners were killed in accidents.

Reprinted from Mine Safety and Health Administration. MSHA Fact Sheets—Injury trends in mining. http://www.msha.gov/MSHAINFO/FactSheets/MSHAFCT2.HTM

EXHIBIT 2.2   History of Mine Safety and Health Legislation

In 1891, Congress passed the first federal statute governing mine safety, marking the beginning of what was to be an extended evolution of increasingly comprehensive federal legislation regulating mining activities. The 1891 law was relatively modest legislation that applied only to mines in U.S. territories. Among other things, it established minimum ventilation requirements for underground coal mines and prohibited operators from employing children younger than 12 years of age.

* *Bureau of Mines.* The Bureau of Mines was established by Congress in 1910, becoming a new agency within the Department of the Interior. During the previous decade, the number of coal mine fatalities exceeded 2000 annually. The Bureau was charged with conducting research and reducing accidents in the coal mining industry but was given no inspection authority until 1941.

* *Federal Coal Mine Safety Act of 1952.* This federal legislation provided for annual inspections of certain underground coal mines and gave the Bureau of Mines limited enforcement authority, including the power to issue violation notices and imminent danger withdrawal orders. The 1952 act also authorized the assessment of civil penalties against mine operators for noncompliance with withdrawal orders and for refusing to give inspectors access to mine property, although no provision was made for monetary penalties for noncompliance with the safety provisions. In 1966, Congress extended the coverage of the 1952 Coal Act to all underground coal mines.

* *Federal Metal and Nonmetallic Mine Safety Act of 1966.* This act was the first federal statute directly regulating non-coal mines. The 1966 act provided for the promulgation of standards, many of which were advisory, and for inspections and investigations; however, its enforcement authority was minimal.

* *Federal Coal Mine Health and Safety Act of 1969 (Coal Act).* The Coal Act was more comprehensive and more stringent than any previous federal legislation governing the mining industry. It included surface as well as underground coal mines

(Continues)

EXHIBIT 2.2   History of Mine Safety and Health Legislation (*Continued*)

within its scope, required two annual inspections of every surface coal mine and four annual inspections of every underground coal mine, and dramatically increased federal enforcement powers in coal mines. The Coal Act also mandated monetary penalties for all violations and established criminal penalties for knowing and willful violations. The safety standards for all coal mines were strengthened, and health standards were adopted. The Coal Act included specific procedures for the development of improved mandatory health and safety standards and provided compensation for miners who were totally and permanently disabled by the progressive respiratory disease called pneumoconiosis or "black lung," caused by the inhalation of fine coal dust.

- *Mining Enforcement and Safety Administration (MESA).* In 1973, the Secretary of the Interior, through administrative action, created MESA as a new departmental agency separate from the Bureau of Mines. MESA assumed the safety and health enforcement functions formerly carried out by the Bureau of Mines so as to avoid any appearance of a conflict of interest between the enforcement of mine safety and health standards and the Bureau's responsibilities for mineral resource development.

- *Federal Mine Safety and Health Act of 1977 (Mine Act).* The Mine Act amended the 1969 Coal Act in a number of significant ways and consolidated all federal health and safety regulations governing the mining industry (i.e., coal as well as noncoal mining) under a single statutory scheme. It strengthened and expanded the rights of miners and enhanced the protection of miners from retaliation for exercising such rights. Mining fatalities dropped sharply under the Mine Act, from 272 in 1977 to 86 in 2000. This act also transferred responsibility for carrying out its mandates from the Department of the Interior to the Department of Labor, with the new agency being named the Mine Safety and Health Administration (MSHA). Additionally, the Mine Act established the independent Federal Mine Safety and Health Review Commission to provide for independent review of the majority of MSHA's enforcement actions.

- *Mine Improvement and New Emergency Response Act (MINER Act).* In 2006, Congress passed the MINER Act, which amended the Mine Act to require mine-specific emergency response plans in underground coal mines; added new regulations regarding mine rescue teams and sealing of abandoned areas; required prompt notification of mine accidents; and enhanced civil penalties.

Modified from U.S. Department of Labor. History of Mine Safety and Health Legislation. http://www.msha.gov/MSHAINFO/MSHAINF2.HTM. Accessed September 5, 2013.

Federal Coal Mine Health and Safety Act of 1969 (Coal Act)

In addition to strengthening previous legislation (see Exhibit 2.2), the Federal Coal Mine Health and Safety Act of 1969 (Title IV) established the federal black lung benefit program, which provides for coal mine workers' compensation for total disability from pneumoconiosis acquired from employment in mines.[8] Title IV was amended in 1972 with the enactment of the Black Lung Benefits Act of 1972:

> The Black Lung Benefits Act (BLBA) provides monthly payments and medical benefits to coal miners totally disabled from pneumoconiosis (black lung disease) arising from employment in or around the nation's coal mines. This Act also provides monthly benefits to a miner's dependent survivors if pneumoconiosis caused or hastened the miner's death. The Division of Coal Mine Workers' Compensation (DCMWC), within the U.S. Department of Labor Employment Standards Administration's Office of Workers' Compensation Programs (OWCP), adjudicates and processes claims filed by coal miners and their survivors under the BLBA.[9]

The act funds medical treatment for lung conditions associated with employment in coal mines.[10] As noted earlier, it is administered through the Division of Coal Mine Workers' Compensation, a unit of the Department of Labor.

Federal Mine Safety and Health Act of 1977 (Mine Act)

Following previous legislative acts, the Federal Mine Safety and Health Act of 1977 sought to further improve the working conditions of miners. Senator Tom Harkin of Iowa described the deplorable conditions that existed formerly in Iowa coal mines:

> At one time, Iowa was the third-largest coal-producing state in the nation, and my father—after many years of working in coal mines—was stricken with black lung that left him from prone to pneumonia and made it difficult for him to work. Although he stopped working in the mines before I was born, he told me stories of losing friends in the mines—in accidents that were frighteningly common. Generations of brave miners have risked their health and safety every day to provide for their families.[11]

According to Sen. Harkin, "Prior to the 1977 Act, an average of one miner was killed each day in a mining accident; ... In 2012, there were 35 fatalities in U.S. mines—a number that is still too high, but represents significant improvements in worker safety."[11]

The Federal Mine Safety and Health Act of 1977 applies to all workers employed on mine property. It is administered by the Mine Safety and Health Administration. In summary:

The Mine Act holds mine operators responsible for the safety and health of miners; provides for the setting of mandatory safety and health standards, mandates miners' training requirements; prescribes penalties for violations; and enables inspectors to close dangerous mines. The safety and health standards address numerous hazards including roof falls, flammable and explosive gases, fire, electricity, equipment rollovers and maintenance, airborne contaminants, noise, and respirable dust. MSHA enforces safety and health requirements at more than 13,000 mines, investigates mine accidents, and offers mine operators training, technical and compliance assistance.[12]

EXHIBIT 2.3 presents excerpts of the text from this important act.

Occupational Safety and Health Act of 1970

The Occupational Safety and Health Act of 1970 (OSH Act) was established by Congress "[t]o assure safe and healthful working conditions for working men and women; by authorizing enforcement of the standards developed under the Act; by assisting and encouraging the States in their efforts to assure safe and healthful working conditions; by providing for research, information, education, and training in the field of occupational safety and health; and for other purposes."[13] The OSH Act was an important breakthrough for U.S. workers in that it created important safeguards for the workplace. However, the act's declaration that all workers should be able to work in a safe and healthful environment has not been realized completely: "The persistence of preventable, life-threatening hazards at work is a failure to keep a national promise."[14(p. 416)] **EXHIBIT 2.4** summarizes congressional findings regarding the OSH Act and its purposes.

Provisions of the Occupational Safety and Health Act

The OSH Act created the Occupational Safety and Health Administration (OSHA), which is discussed elsewhere in this chapter. Coverage of employees under this legislation varies by type of employer and workplace. The OSH Act defines the role of OSHA in setting standards and sets forth the responsibilities of employers and employees. An important feature of the act is known as the General Duty Clause.

Almost all private-sector employees are covered under the OSH Act. However, the act does not cover "[t]he self-employed, immediate family members of farm employers; and workplace hazards regulated by another federal agency (for example, the Mine Safety and Health Administration,

EXHIBIT 2.3   The Federal Mine Safety and Health Act of 1977, Public Law 91-173, as Amended by Public Law 95-164

An Act
Be it enacted by the Senate and House of Representatives of the United States of America in Congress assembled.
That this Act may be cited as the "Federal Mine Safety and Health Act of 1977."

Findings and Purpose

SEC. 2. Congress declares that—
(a) The first priority and concern of all in the coal or other mining industry must be the health and safety of its most precious resource—the miner;
(b) Deaths and serious injuries from unsafe and unhealthful conditions and practices in the coal or other mines cause grief and suffering to the miners and to their families;
(c) There is an urgent need to provide more effective means and measures for improving the working conditions and practices in the Nation's coal or other mines in order to prevent death and serious physical harm, and in order to prevent occupational diseases originating in such mines;
(d) The existence of unsafe and unhealthful conditions and practices in the Nation's coal or other mines is a serious impediment to the future growth of the coal or other mining industry and cannot be tolerated;
(e) The operators of such mines with the assistance of the miners have the primary responsibility to prevent the existence of such conditions and practices in such mines;
(f) The disruption of production and the loss of income to operators and miners as a result of coal or other mine accidents or occupationally caused diseases unduly impedes and burdens commerce; and
(g) It is the purpose of this Act
   (1) To establish interim mandatory health and safety standards and to direct the Secretary of Health, Education, and Welfare and the Secretary of Labor to develop and promulgate improved mandatory health or safety standards to protect the health and safety of the Nation's coal or other miners;
   (2) To require that each operator of a coal or other mine and every miner in such mine comply with such standards;
   (3) To cooperate with, and provide assistance to, the States in the development and enforcement of effective State coal or other mine health and safety programs; and
   (4) To improve and expand, in cooperation with the States and the coal or other mining industry, research and development and training programs aimed at preventing coal or other mine accidents and occupationally caused diseases in the industry.

Reprinted from U.S. Department of Labor. Federal Mine Safety and Health Act of 1977; Public Law 91-173. http://www.msha.gov/REGS/ACT/ACT1.HTM. Accessed September 5, 2013.

the Department of Energy, Federal Aviation Administration, or Coast Guard)."[15(p. 5)] Protections afforded by this law also apply to federal agencies, although OSHA does not fine federal agencies.

The General Duty Clause of the OSH Act requires that "[e]ach employer shall furnish to each of his employees employment and a place of employment

EXHIBIT 2.4   Occupational Safety and Health Act of 1970

SEC. 2. Congressional Findings and Purpose

(a) The Congress finds that personal injuries and illnesses arising out of work situations impose a substantial burden upon, and are a hindrance to, interstate commerce in terms of lost production, wage loss, medical expenses, and disability compensation payments.

(b) The Congress declares it to be its purpose and policy, through the exercise of its powers to regulate commerce among the several States and with foreign nations and to provide for the general welfare, to assure so far as possible every working man and woman in the Nation safe and healthful working conditions and to preserve our human resources—

  (1) By encouraging employers and employees in their efforts to reduce the number of occupational safety and health hazards at their places of employment, and to stimulate employers and employees to institute new and to perfect existing programs for providing safe and healthful working conditions;

  (2) By providing that employers and employees have separate but dependent responsibilities and rights with respect to achieving safe and healthful working conditions;

  (3) By authorizing the Secretary of Labor to set mandatory occupational safety and health standards applicable to businesses affecting interstate commerce, and by creating an Occupational Safety and Health Review Commission for carrying out adjudicatory functions under the Act;

  (4) By building upon advances already made through employer and employee initiative for providing safe and healthful working conditions;

  (5) By providing for research in the field of occupational safety and health, including the psychological factors involved, and by developing innovative methods, techniques, and approaches for dealing with occupational safety and health problems;

  (6) By exploring ways to discover latent diseases, establishing causal connections between diseases and work in environmental conditions, and conducting other research relating to health problems, in recognition of the fact that occupational health standards present problems often different from those involved in occupational safety;

  (7) By providing medical criteria which will assure insofar as practicable that no employee will suffer diminished health, functional capacity, or life expectancy as a result of his work experience;

  (8) By providing for training programs to increase the number and competence of personnel engaged in the field of occupational safety and health, affecting the OSH Act since its passage in 1970 through January 1, 2004;

  (9) By providing for the development and promulgation of occupational safety and health standards;

  (10) By providing an effective enforcement program which shall include a prohibition against giving advance notice of any inspection and sanctions for any individual violating this prohibition;

(Continues)

EXHIBIT 2.4   Occupational Safety and Health Act of 1970 (*Continued*)

(11) By encouraging the States to assume the fullest responsibility for the adminis-tration and enforcement of their occupational safety and health laws by provid-ing grants to the States to assist in identifying their needs and responsibilities in the area of occupational safety and health, to develop plans in accordance with the provisions of this Act, to improve the administration and enforcement of State occupational safety and health laws, and to conduct experimental and demonstration projects in connection therewith;

(12) By providing for appropriate reporting procedures with respect to occupa-tional safety and health which procedures will help achieve the objectives of this Act and accurately describe the nature of the occupational safety and health problem;

(13) By encouraging joint labor–management efforts to reduce injuries and disease arising out of employment.

Reprinted from U.S. Department of Labor, Occupational Safety and Health Administration (OSHA). OSHA Content Document. http://www.osha.gov/pls/oshaweb/owadisp.show_document?p_table=OSHACT&p_id=2743. Accessed January 31, 2014.

---

which are free from recognized hazards that are causing or are likely to cause death or serious physical harm to his employees."[16] The OSH Act delineates rights and responsibilities for employers and employees, sets stan-dards, allows inspections to be initiated without advance notice, provides help for employees (e.g., consultation and assistance with compliance), and offers information and education (e.g., a training institute and informa-tion and publications).[17]

"OSHA standards are rules that describe the methods employers are legally required to follow to protect their workers from hazards. Before OSHA can issue a standard, it must go through a very extensive and lengthy process that includes substantial public engagement, notice and comment. The agency must show that a significant risk to workers exists and that there are feasible measures employers can take to protect their workers."[17] Some examples of OSHA standards are those directed at preventing falls, exposures to toxic substances, and contact with infectious disease agents. EXHIBIT 2.5 provides a statement of the rights and responsibilities of employ-ers and employees under the OSH Act.

OSHA Protections for Federal Employees

Occupational illnesses and injuries occur frequently among civilian federal employees—165,000 cases in fiscal year 2004 and workers' compensation bill-ings exceeding $2.3 billion.[18] Federal agencies are required to protect workers by providing "workplaces free from recognized health and safety hazards."[18]

EXHIBIT 2.5 Rights and Responsibilities for Employers and Employees under the OSH Act

Employers must:

* Follow all relevant OSHA safety and health standards.

* Find and correct safety and health hazards.

* Inform employees about chemical hazards through training, labels, alarms, color-coded systems, chemical information sheets, and other methods.

* Notify OSHA within 8 hours of a workplace fatality or when three or more workers are hospitalized (1-800-321-OSHA [6742]).

* Provide required personal protective equipment at no cost to workers. (Employers must pay for most types of required personal protective equipment.)

* Keep accurate records of work-related injuries and illnesses.

* Post OSHA citations, injury and illness summary data, and the OSHA "Job Safety and Health: It's The Law" poster in the workplace where workers will see them.

* Not discriminate or retaliate against any worker for using his or her rights under the law.

Employees have the right to:

* Working conditions that do not pose a risk of serious harm.

* Receive information and training (in a language workers can understand) about chemical and other hazards, methods to prevent harm, and OSHA standards that apply to their workplace.

* Review records of work-related injuries and illnesses.

* Get copies of the results of tests performed to find and measure hazards in the workplace.

* File a complaint asking OSHA to inspect their workplace if they believe there is a serious hazard or that their employer is not following OSHA rules. When requested, OSHA will keep all identities confidential.

* Use their rights under the law without retaliation or discrimination. If an employee is fired, demoted, transferred, or discriminated against in any way for exercising his or her rights under the law, the employee can file a complaint with OSHA. This complaint must be filed within 30 days of the alleged discrimination.

Reprinted from U.S. Department of Labor. Occupational Safety and Health Administration (OSHA). At-A-Glance OSHA. U.S. Department of Labor. 2011. OSHA 3439-06N.

This requirement is met by taking steps such as establishing "procedures for responding to workplace emergencies and reporting unsafe and unhealthful working conditions.... Federal employees must comply with agency policies, procedures, and directives concerning health and safety; use personal protective equipment and other safety equipment provided by the agency; and observe all agency safety and health rules, procedures, and standards."[18]

International Organizations Protecting Workers' Rights

This section highlights the work of the United Nations—specifically, the World Health Organization and the International Labour Organization—in occupational health. The principles advanced by the United Nations are instrumental in developing standards for individual countries throughout the world. Another prominent international group is the European Agency for Safety and Health at Work.

World Health Organization

The World Health Organization (WHO) is a major player in the international arena for the protection of workers' health. The organization's webpage declares that "the main functions of WHO (occupational health) … include promoting the improvement of working conditions and other aspects of environmental hygiene. Recognizing that occupational health is closely linked to public health and health systems development, WHO is addressing all determinants of workers' health, including risks for disease and injury in the occupational environment, social and individual factors, and access to health services."[19] The guiding tenet of WHO with respect to occupational health is as follows: "According to the principles of the United Nations, WHO and ILO, every citizen of the world has a right to healthy and safe work and to a work environment that enables him or her to live a socially and economically productive life."[20(p. 6)] WHO works collaboratively on occupational health issues with the International Labour Organization (an agency of the United Nations), the International Commission on Occupational Health, the International Occupational Hygiene Association, and the International Ergonomics Association.[21] Its programs for promotion of occupational health operate through six regional offices located throughout the world. A Network of Collaborating Centers on Occupational Health help to realize WHO's objectives for improving workers' health.[22]

Globally Harmonized System of Classification and Labelling of Chemicals

One of the United Nations' noteworthy achievements was the creation of the Globally Harmonized System of Classification and Labelling of Chemicals (GHS). The GHS provides for standardization of the manner in which chemicals are classified and labeled as well as for communication of risks associated with chemicals. Differences among countries in regulatory systems for chemicals can lead to inconsistent protections for persons who might be exposed to chemicals.[23]

The work [of the United Nations] began with the premise that existing systems should be harmonized in order to develop a single, globally harmonized system to address classification of chemicals, labels, and safety data sheets... . The international mandate that provided the impetus for completing this work was adopted at the 1992 United Nations Conference on Environment and Development (UNCED), as reflected in Agenda 21, para.19.27: ... "A globally harmonized hazard classification and compatible labelling system, including material safety data sheets and easily understandable symbols, should be available, if feasible, by the year 2000."[24(p. iii)]

International Labour Organization

The International Labour Organization (ILO) is a specialized United Nations agency devoted to the work setting; it was founded in 1919. "The main aims of the ILO are to promote rights at work, encourage decent employment opportunities, enhance social protection and strengthen dialogue on work-related issues."[25] The ILO has four strategic objectives:

1. "Promote and realize standards and fundamental principles and rights at work
2. Create greater opportunities for women and men to decent employment and income
3. Enhance the coverage and effectiveness of social protection for all
4. Strengthen tripartism [giving an equal voice to workers, employers, and governments] and social dialogue"[26]

The headquarters of the ILO, which is called the International Labour Office, is supported by regional offices in more than 40 countries.[27] The ILO maintains institutes and centers for conducting research, training, and support in the field of occupational health. It is an excellent resource for occupational safety and health information, especially from an international perspective. "The International Labour Organization (ILO) is devoted to promoting social justice and internationally recognized human and labour rights, pursuing its founding mission that labour peace is essential to prosperity."[26]

European Agency for Safety and Health at Work

The European Agency for Safety and Health at Work (EU-OSHA) focuses on the work environment in Europe; it is "committed to making Europe a safer, healthier and more productive place to work. We promote a culture of risk prevention to improve working conditions in Europe."[28] The agency seeks to increase awareness of occupational health and safety, design instruments for assessing workplace risks, collaborate with governments and other organizations on occupational safety and health issues, and conduct research germane to the work environment. A director oversees the management of the agency. The director is appointed by a governing board composed of representatives from European Union member states, representatives of the European Commission, and other relevant stakeholders. Advisory groups provide additional input into the European Risk Observatory and other units affiliated with EU-OSHA. The agency is staffed by specialists drawn from various European countries who have expertise in the field of occupational safety and health as well as communication and public administration.

U.S. Federal Agencies for Occupational Health and Safety

TABLE 2.2 lists selected U.S. federal agencies that are involved with regulation, research, and training in occupational health. This list is not exhaustive, as other branches of government make important contributions to occupational health in the United States, either directly or indirectly.

U.S. Department of Labor

The U.S. Department of Labor (US DOL) is the federal government agency charged with administration and enforcement of federal laws that pertain to workplace activities for approximately 10 million employers and 125 million workers (FIGURE 2.5).[12] TABLE 2.3 summarizes the major laws enforced by the Department of Labor.

TABLE 2.2   Examples of U.S. Federal Agencies Germane to Occupational Health

U.S. Department of Labor (US DOL)
National Institute of Environmental Health Sciences (NIEHS)
National Institute for Occupational Safety and Health (NIOSH)
Occupational Safety and Health Administration (OSHA)
Environmental Protection Agency (EPA)
Agency for Toxic Substances and Disease Registry (ATSDR)

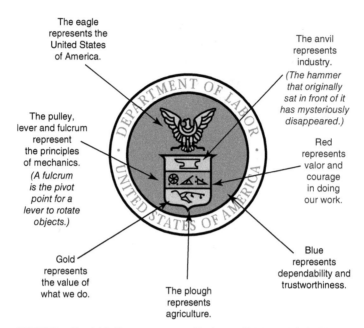

The eagle represents the United States of America.

The anvil represents industry. *(The hammer that originally sat in front of it has mysteriously disappeared.)*

The pulley, lever and fulcrum represent the principles of mechanics. *(A fulcrum is the pivot point for a lever to rotate objects.)*

Red represents valor and courage in doing our work.

Gold represents the value of what we do.

The plough represents agriculture.

Blue represents dependability and trustworthiness.

FIGURE 2.5   U.S. Department of Labor official seal (1913) with legend

Courtesy of the U.S. Department of Labor.

TABLE 2.3   Summary of the Major Laws of the Department of Labor

Wages and hours	Fair Labor Standards Act (FLSA)
Workplace safety and health	Occupational Safety and Health (OSH) Act
Workers' compensation	Longshore and Harbor Workers' Compensation Act (LHWCA)
	Energy Employees Occupational Illness Compensation Program Act (EEOICPA)
	Federal Employees' Compensation Act (FECA)
	Black Lung Benefits Act (BLBA)
Employment benefits security	Employee Retirement Income Security Act (ERISA): a law that sets minimum standards for pension and health plans in private industry
Unions and their members	Labor–Management Reporting and Disclosure Act (LMRDA; also known as the Landrum-Griffin Act): deals with the relationship between a union and its members
Family and Medical Leave Act	Family and Medical Leave Act (FMLA): provides up to 12 weeks of unpaid leave in companies with 50 or more employees
Migrant and seasonal agricultural workers	Migrant and Seasonal Agricultural Worker Protection Act (MSPA): affords protections such as disclosure of conditions of employment, prompt and accurate payment of wages, and assurance that any housing, if supplied, meets standards for health and safety
Mine safety and health	Federal Mine Safety and Health Act of 1977 (Mine Act)

Modified from U. S. Department of Labor. Summary of the major laws of the Department of Labor. http://www.dol.gov/opa/aboutdol/lawsprog.htm. Accessed September 14, 2013.

National Institute of Environmental Health Sciences

The National Institute of Environmental Health Sciences (NIEHS) is "one of 27 Institutes and Centers of the National Institutes of Health (NIH).... The NIEHS supports a wide variety of research programs directed toward preventing health problems caused by our environment."[29(p. 1)] Research activities supported by NIEHS include the National Toxicology Program (described elsewhere in this chapter), in-house environmental research laboratories at NIEHS facilities, grants programs, and publication of the journal *Environmental Health Perspectives*. Other activities of NIEHS include training and education of workers and members of the community—for example, on health and safety issues for workers in handling hazardous wastes and restoration of the environment.[30]

National Institute for Occupational Safety and Health

The National Institute for Occupational Safety and Health (NIOSH) is the federal agency responsible for conducting research and making recommendations for the prevention of work-related illness and injury.[31] Established in 1970 under the Occupational Safety and Health Act of 1970, NIOSH is part of the U.S. Centers for Disease Control and Prevention (CDC) and the U.S. Department of Health and Human Services (DHHS). EXHIBIT 2.6 describes the mission of NIOSH. FIGURE 2.6 shows the locations of NIOSH offices and research laboratories.

EXHIBIT 2.6   NIOSH Mission

NIOSH produces new scientific knowledge and provides practical solutions vital to reducing risks of injury and death in traditional industries, such as agriculture, construction, and mining. NIOSH also supports research to predict, prevent, and address emerging problems that arise from dramatic changes in the 21st-century workplace and workforce. NIOSH partners with diverse stakeholders to study how worker injuries, illnesses, and deaths occur. NIOSH scientists design, conduct, and support targeted research, both inside and outside the institute, and support the training of occupational health and safety professionals to build capacity and meet increasing needs for a new generation of skilled practitioners. NIOSH and its partners support U.S. economic strength and growth by moving research into practice through concrete and practical solutions, recommendations, and interventions for the building of a healthy, safe and capable workforce.

Reprinted from National Institute for Occupational Safety and Health (NIOSH). NIOSH fact sheet. April 2013. DHHS (NIOSH) Publication No. 2013-140. http://www.cdc.gov/niosh/docs/2013-140/pdfs/2013-140.pdf. Accessed December 26, 2013.

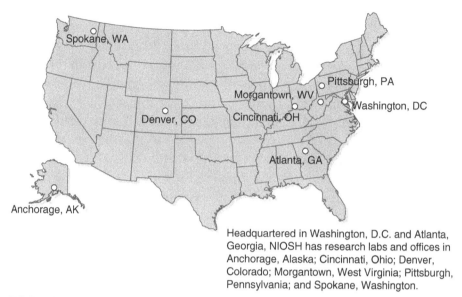

FIGURE 2.6 NIOSH offices and research laboratories

Reproduced from Centers for Disease Control and Prevention, Publication No. 2013-140, April 2013, http://www.cdc.gov/niosh/docs/2013-140/pdfs/2013-140.pdf

Occupational Safety and Health Administration

The Occupational Safety and Health Administration (OSHA) was established by Congress "to assure safe and healthful conditions for working men and women by setting and enforcing standards and providing training, outreach, education and compliance assistance... . Under the OSHA law, employers are responsible for providing a safe and healthful workplace for their workers."[15(p. 4)] **FIGURE 2.7** summarizes the history of OSHA; **FIGURE 2.8** depicts its organizational chart. A regulatory agency, OSHA is part of the U.S. Department of Labor and, therefore, is distinct organizationally from NIOSH, which is part of the U.S. Centers for Disease Control and Prevention and the U.S. Department of Health and Human Services. **FIGURE 2.9** shows the differing roles of NIOSH and OSHA.

History of OSHA

- OSHA stands for the Occupational Safety and Health Administration, an agency of the U.S. Department of Labor
- OSHA's responsibility is worker safety and health protection
- On December 29, 1970, President Nixon signed the OSH Act
- This Act created OSHA, the agency, which formally came into being on April 28, 1971

FIGURE 2.7 History of OSHA

Reproduced from U.S. Department of Labor, Occupational Safety & Health Administration, History of OSHA, https://www.osha.gov/dte/outreach/intro_osha/intro_to_osha_english/slide6.html.

OSHA Inspections

OSHA conducts inspections of worksites to ensure that health and safety requirements

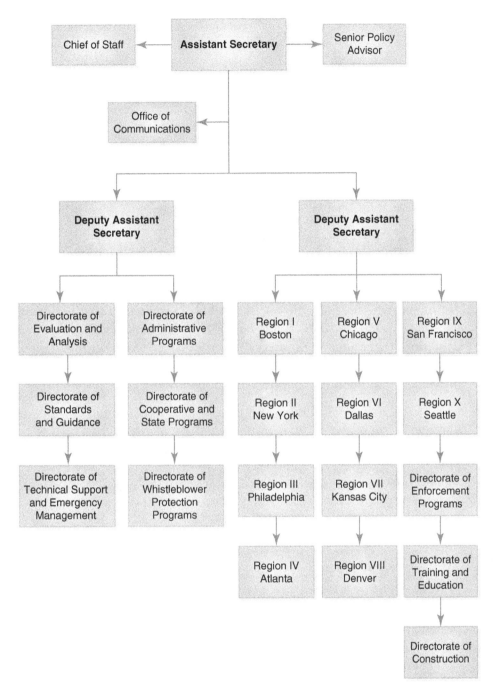

FIGURE 2.8 OSHA organizational chart

Reproduced from U.S. Department of Labor, Occupational Safety & Health Administration, OSHA Organizational Chart, December 2014, http://www.osha.gov/html/OSHAorgchart.pdf.

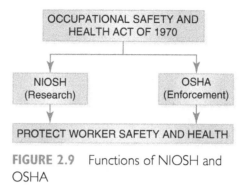

FIGURE 2.9   Functions of NIOSH and OSHA

Reproduced from National Institute for Occupational Safety and Healt, Stress at work. DHHS (NIOSH) Publication No. 99-101 http://www.cdc.gov/niosh/docs/99-101/pdfs/99-101.pdf Accessed February 1, 2014.

are being met there. In most cases, OSHA inspections are performed without advance notice to employers. OSHA has established six priority conditions for conducting inspections (**TABLE 2.4**): "OSHA cannot inspect all 7 million workplaces it covers each year. The agency seeks to focus its inspection resources on the most hazardous workplaces."[32(p. 1)]

TABLE 2.4   OSHA Inspection Priorities

1. **Imminent danger situations**—hazards that could cause death or serious physical harm—receive top priority. Compliance officers ask employers to correct these hazards immediately—or remove endangered employees.

2. **Fatalities and catastrophes**—incidents that involve a death or the hospitalization of three or more employees—come next. Employers must report such catastrophes to OSHA within 8 hours.

3. **Complaints**—allegations of hazards or violations—also receive a high priority. Employees may request anonymity when they file complaints.

4. **Referrals** of hazard information from other federal, state, or local agencies; individuals; organizations; or the media receive consideration for inspection.

5. **Follow-ups**—checks for abatement of violations cited during previous inspections—are also conducted by the agency in certain circumstances.

6. **Planned or programmed investigations**—inspections aimed at specific high-hazard industries or individual workplaces that have experienced high rates of injuries and illnesses—also receive priority.

Reprinted from U.S. Department of Labor. Occupational Safety and Health Administration (OSHA). OSHA Fact Sheet. OSHA Inspections. https://www.osha.gov/OshDoc/data_General_Facts/factsheet-inspections.pdf. Accessed January 27, 2014.

Most Frequently Cited Standards

OSHA publishes a list of the top 10 most frequently cited standards following inspections of worksites. The publication of this list enables employers to identify and rectify hazardous conditions and thereby prevent occupational illnesses and injuries. TABLE 2.5 lists the most-cited standards for fiscal year 2013 (October 1, 2012–September 30, 2013). In 2013, the most frequently cited standard was fall protection—OSHA's standard that requires safeguards against falls in the workplace.

U.S. Environmental Protection Agency

Two important functions of the U.S. Environmental Protection Agency (EPA) are oversight of pesticides and oversight of chemicals.[33] The EPA regulates pesticides as well as new and existing chemicals to make sure they are being used safely. The Toxic Substances Control Act (TSCA) of 1976 allows "EPA to regulate new commercial chemicals before they enter the market, to regulate existing chemicals ... when they pose an unreasonable risk to health or to the environment, and to regulate their distribution and use."[34] However, the agency does not intervene directly in the workplace environment with respect to occupationally associated chemical exposures. EXHIBIT 2.7 describes the activities of the EPA. The headquarters of the EPA are housed in the Clinton Federal Building, a vast office complex located in Washington, D.C. (FIGURE 2.11).

Agency for Toxic Substances and Disease Registry

An independent federal organization, the Agency for Toxic Substances and Disease Registry (ATSDR) is based in Atlanta, Georgia.[35] It is one of 11 federal agencies within the U.S. Department of Health and Human Services.[36] The CDC performs many of ATSDR's administrative functions; the director of the CDC also serves as the administrator of the ATSDR.

The ATSDR was established by Congress in 1980 under the Comprehensive Environmental Response, Compensation, and Liability Act (CERCLA),[37] also known as the Superfund Law. This agency "determines public health implications associated with hazardous waste sites and other environmental releases."[38] TABLE 2.6 provides more examples of ATSDR's specific functions.

The ATSDR forms partnerships with other federal agencies (e.g., CDC and EPA), state agencies, and universities in researching the health effects of chemical exposures and communicating public health information to healthcare providers and communities.[36] With respect to occupational health concerns, the ATSDR created the World Trade Center Registry to

TABLE 2.5   Top 10 Standards Most Frequently Cited by OSHA, 2013

1. **Fall Protection**: The employer shall determine if the walking/working surfaces on which its employees are to work have the strength and structural integrity to support employees safely. Each employee on a walking/working surface (horizontal and vertical surface) with an unprotected side or edge which is 6 feet (1.8 m) or more above a lower level shall be protected from falling by the use of guardrail systems, safety net systems, or personal fall arrest systems.

2. **Hazard Communication**: The hazards of all chemicals produced or imported are classified, and that information concerning the classified hazards is transmitted to employers and employees. The transmittal of information is to be accomplished by means of comprehensive hazard communication programs, which are to include container labeling and other forms of warning, safety data sheets, and employee training. (Refer to **FIGURE 2.10**.)

3. **Scaffolding**: Each scaffold and scaffold component shall be capable of supporting, without failure, its own weight and at least 4 times the maximum intended load applied or transmitted to it.

4. **Respiratory Protection**: In the control of those occupational diseases caused by breathing air contaminated with harmful dusts, fogs, fumes, mists, gases, smokes, sprays, or vapors, the primary objective shall be to prevent atmospheric contamination. This shall be accomplished as far as feasible by accepted engineering control measures (for example, enclosure or confinement of the operation, general and local ventilation, and substitution of less toxic materials). When effective engineering controls are not feasible, or while they are being instituted, appropriate respirators shall be used pursuant to this section.

5. **Electrical—Wiring Methods**: Metal raceways, cable trays, cable armor, cable sheaths, enclosures, frames, fittings, and other metal non-current-carrying parts that are to serve as grounding conductors, with or without the use of supplementary equipment grounding conductors, shall be effectively bonded where necessary to ensure electrical continuity and the capacity to conduct safely any fault current likely to be imposed on them. Any nonconductive paint, enamel, or similar coating shall be removed at threads, contact points, and contact surfaces or be connected by means of fittings designed so as to make such removal unnecessary.

6. **Powered Industrial Trucks**: This section contains safety requirements relating to fire protection, design, maintenance, and use of fork trucks, tractors, platform lift trucks, motorized hand trucks, and other specialized industrial trucks powered by electric motors or internal combustion engines.

7. **Ladders**: This category of citation pertains to requirements that apply to all ladders, including job-made ladders.

8. **Lockout/Tagout**: This standard covers the servicing and maintenance of machines and equipment in which the unexpected energization or start-up of the machines or equipment, or release of stored energy, could harm employees.

9. **Electrical—General Requirements**: Electric equipment shall be free from recognized hazards that are likely to cause death or serious physical harm to employees.

10. **Machine Guarding**: One or more methods of machine guarding shall be provided to protect the operator and other employees in the machine area from hazards such as those created by point of operation, ingoing nip points, rotating parts, flying chips and sparks. Examples of guarding methods include barrier guards, two-hand tripping devices, and electronic safety devices.

Data from U.S. Department of Labor. Occupational Safety and Health Administration (OSHA). Top 10 most frequently cited standards for fiscal 2013. https://www.osha.gov/Top_Ten_Standards.html. Accessed January 28, 2014.

Hazard Communication

Workers have the right to *know* and *understand* the hazardous chemicals they use and how to work with them safely.

www.osha.gov/hazcom   800-321-OSHA (6742)   TTY 1-877-889-5627

FIGURE 2.10 Hazard communication—OSHA

Reproduced from Occupational Safety & Health Administration, https://www.osha.gov/Publications/OSHA3658.pdf. Accessed February 1, 2014.

EXHIBIT 2.7   Functions of the U.S. Environmental Protection Agency (EPA)

The U.S. Environmental Protection Agency (EPA) implements federal laws designed to promote public health by protecting our nation's air, water, and soil from harmful pollution. [This agency] accomplishes its mission by a variety of research, monitoring, standard-setting, and enforcement activities. EPA also coordinates and supports research and anti-pollution activities of state and local and tribal governments, private and public groups, individuals, and educational institutions.... Problems with the environment inside the workplace, such as presence or handling of chemicals or noxious fumes, are under the jurisdiction of the Occupational Safety and Health Administration, an arm of the U.S. Department of Labor.... The EPA is responsible for the safe use of pesticides in controlling insects, rodents, fungus, and sanitizers that are used on surfaces.

Modified from "Does EPA Handle All Environmetal Concerns." http://publicaccess.supportportal.com/link/portal/23002/23012/Article/15450/Does-EPA-handle-all-environmental-concerns.

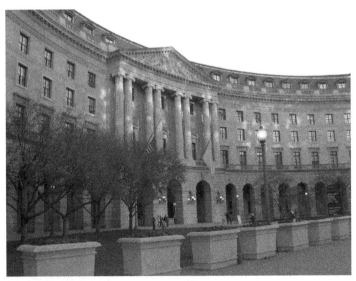

FIGURE 2.11 William Jefferson Clinton Federal Building, headquarters for the U.S. Environmental Protection Agency

© Jason Maehl/ShutterStock, Inc.

TABLE 2.6 Examples of Functions of the Agency for Toxic Substances and Disease Registry (ATSDR)

Public health assessments of waste sites

Health consultations concerning specific hazardous substances

Health surveillance and registries

Response to emergency releases of hazardous substances

Applied research in support of public health assessments

Information development and dissemination

Education and training concerning hazardous substances

Reprinted from Agency for Toxic Substances and Disease Registry (ATSDR). About ATSDR. http://www.atsdr.cdc.gov/about/index.html. Accessed June 21, 2014.

monitor the health effects of first responders, recovery workers, and others exposed to hazards from the September 11, 2001, terrorist attacks. The ATSDR also developed the Tremolite Asbestos Registry to track the health of workers and family members exposed to asbestos in Libby, Montana.

One way in which the ATSDR informs occupational health and safety is through research in the field of environmental science and translation of research findings into practice. Scientists affiliated with this agency are available to respond to questions about environmental exposures and supply evidence-based guidance to those who work in the environmental health field and need to cope with such exposures.[38] When concerns about occupational health issues arise, the ATSDR can help employees locate occupational health clinics.[39]

To support professionals regarding these activities, the ATSDR publishes 172 toxicological profiles called ToxProfiles, which occupational health specialists, workers, and employers can consult as references for information about toxic materials used in the workplace. Shorter versions of ToxProfiles are provided as ToxFAQs, as discussed in EXHIBIT 2.8.

EXHIBIT 2.8   About ToxFAQs™

The ATSDR's ToxFAQs is a series of summaries about hazardous substances developed by the agency's Division of Toxicology. Information for this series is excerpted from the ATSDR Toxicological Profiles and Public Health Statements. Each fact sheet serves as a quick and easy-to-understand guide. Answers are provided to the most frequently asked questions (FAQs) about exposure to hazardous substances found around hazardous waste sites and the effects of exposure on human health.

Reprinted from Agency for Toxic Substances and Disease Registry (ATSDR). Toxic substances portal. ToxFAQs.™ http://www.atsdr.cdc.gov/toxfaqs/index.asp#bookmark01. Accessed December 24, 2013.

Current Federal Regulations Protecting Workers

The OSH Act specifies employers' rights and responsibilities with respect to workers. In addition, the current regulations for protecting U.S. workers identify compensation programs and disability payments for employees who incur job-related illnesses and injuries. The U.S. Equal Employment Opportunity Commission (EEOC) enforces regulations that prohibit illegal discrimination against employees.

Freedom from Discrimination in the Workplace

Achievement of fair employment practices has been a continuing goal of the U.S. civil rights movement.[40] Congress's adoption of Title VII of the Civil Rights Act of 1964 led to the creation of the EEOC. In addition to making it illegal for private employers to discriminate against job applicants and workers on the basis of race, Title VII "prohibit[ed] employment discrimination based on race, color, religion, sex, and national origin."[41]

"[The EEOC] is responsible for enforcing federal laws that make it illegal to discriminate against a job applicant or an employee because of the person's race, color, religion, sex (including pregnancy), national origin, age (40 or older), disability, or genetic information."[42] EEOC laws regarding workplace discrimination apply to most workplaces that employ at least 15 persons, to most labor unions, and to most employment agencies. At least 20 individuals must be in a workplace for age discrimination cases to be filed. The EEOC is authorized to conduct investigations of discrimination when an allegation has been made and to provide educational programs to prevent the occurrence of discrimination.

The passage of the Civil Rights Act of 1964 led to improvements in economic and other opportunities for workers from minority groups and for women.[43] These achievements include higher wages, increased participation of women in business leadership positions, and growing numbers of female and minority professional workers. Speaking on the 50th anniversary of the Civil Rights Act on July 2, 2014, President Barack Obama noted that the act had increased opportunities for all Americans irrespective of race and ethnicity as well as sexual orientation and disability status.[44] Nevertheless, despite the improved status of these groups in the workplace, the U.S. Department of Labor asserts that continuing efforts will be required to eliminate discrimination in the workplace.[43] FIGURE 2.12 highlights the theme of equal opportunity in employment.

Whistleblowing

Whistleblowing is defined as "the disclosure by a person, usually an employee in a government agency or private enterprise, to the public or to

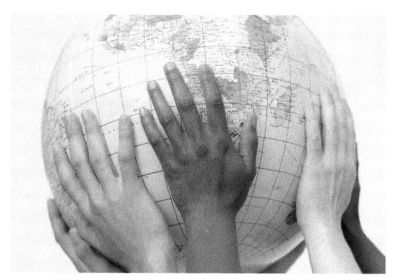

FIGURE 2.12　Equal opportunity in employment

© Zoonar RF/Zoonar/Thinkstock.

those in authority, of mismanagement, corruption, illegality, or some other wrongdoing."[45] The Occupational Safety and Health Act protects the rights of employees to file a health or safety complaint with OSHA.

> OSHA's Whistleblower Protection Program enforces the whistleblower provision of more than twenty whistleblower statutes protecting employees who report violations of various workplace safety, airline, commercial motor carrier, consumer product, environmental, financial reform, food safety, health insurance reform, motor vehicle safety, nuclear, pipeline, public transportation agency, railroad, maritime, and securities laws. Rights afforded by these whistleblower acts include, but are not limited to, worker participation in safety and health activities, reporting a work-related injury, illness or fatality, or reporting a violation of the statutes.[46]

The OSH Act prohibits retaliation by employers against workers who have filed a whistleblower complaint with OSHA.

Workers' Compensation Programs/Laws

The first modern workers' compensation laws originated in Germany with the 1884 Sickness and Accident Laws, followed by enactment of such laws in England in 1897.[47] Workers' compensation programs "provide cash benefits, medical care, and rehabilitation services to workers who experience work-related injuries."[48(p. 3)] **FIGURE 2.13** portrays an injured worker who is receiving medical treatment.

All states in the United States have workers' compensation statutes; several federal government programs also provide workers' compensation benefits. These programs have the common feature of legal tests to ascertain whether an injury is "work-related" and, therefore, the injured employee is entitled to the payment of benefits. The oldest continuous U.S. workers' compensation program is the Wisconsin workers' compensation law of 1911.

In the United States, workers' compensation programs developed early in the 20th century to help workers overcome the challenges associated with filing a negligence suit. Before the adoption of such programs, the only recourse for an injured employee was to file a negligence suit—in which the employer usually prevailed.

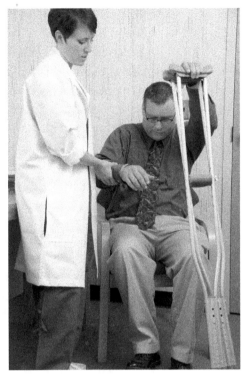

FIGURE 2.13   Injured worker receiving treatment
© Jupiterimages/liquidlibrary/Thinkstock.

Workers' compensation was designed to overcome some of the deficiencies of the negligence suit approach. All workers' compensation statutes incorporate the "workers' compensation principle," which has two elements. Workers' compensation is a no-fault system, which means that in order to receive benefits, a worker does not need to demonstrate the employer is negligent and the employer cannot use the special defenses, such as contributory negligence [meaning that injuries sustained were due to employee negligence]. The employee only has to prove the injury is "work-related."[48(p. 3)]

Workers' compensation programs in the 50 states and the District of Columbia as well as federal programs paid $57.5 billion in benefits in 2010.[47]

Disability Benefits/Permanent Disability

The federal Social Security Administration (SSA) provides disability benefits to people who have become disabled and are unable to work. Its two major programs are the Social Security disability insurance program and the Supplemental Security Income (SSI) program. According to the SSA, "Social Security pays benefits to people who cannot work because they have a medical condition that is expected to last at least one year or result in death. Federal law requires this very strict definition of disability. While some programs give money to people with partial disability or short-term disability, Social Security does not."[49(p. 4)] To receive benefits, the disabled worker needs to meet the "recent work" test, which is based on the worker's age at time of disability, and the "duration of work" test, which is based on the worker's length of employment.

State Programs: State of California

An example of a state workers' compensation program is California's program, which is operated by the state's Division of Workers' Compensation. This program, by law, requires employers to pay benefits to injured workers. These injuries might involve an acute event, such as a fall, or an injury from a continuing and repeated exposure, such as an exposure to repeated motions or loud noises. State benefits include paid medical care, temporary disability benefits, permanent disability benefits, supplemental job displacement benefits, and death benefits. To workers, the Division of Workers' Compensation emphasizes, "[It is] illegal for your employer to punish or fire you for having a job injury, or for filing a workers' compensation claim when you believe your injury was caused by your job."[50] **FIGURE 2.14** shows a simplified flowchart of California's claims process, which requires immediate notification of a supervisor and then a series of additional steps until a benefit can be awarded.

Private-Sector Organizations and Activities Supporting Workers' Health

Examples of nongovernmental organizations that support workers' health include professional associations, advocacy groups, and employee assistance programs offered by individual employers. The following list gives examples of three key organizations that provide service, research, or education in occupational safety and health:

- *American Public Health Association (APHA)*—Occupational Health and Safety Section: "The Section provides leadership and expertise on occupational health matters, recognizing the intrinsic link between the work environment, and the health and safety of families, communities and the environment at large."[51]
- *American College of Occupational and Environmental Medicine (ACOEM)*: "ACOEM is a professional association that represents the

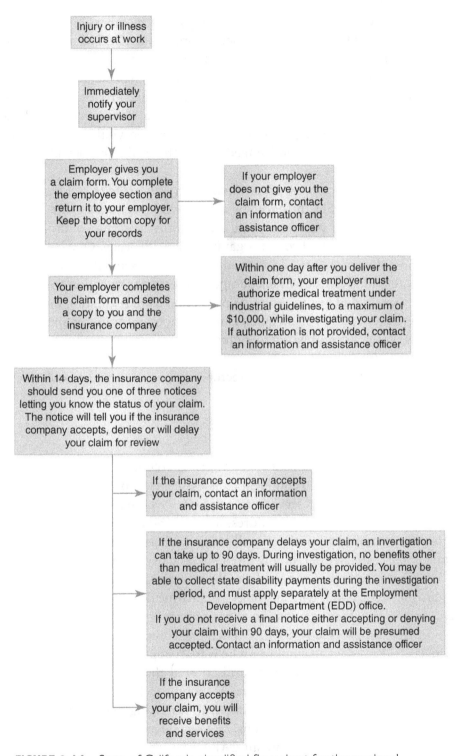

FIGURE 2.14   State of California, simplified flow chart for the workers' compensation claims process

Courtesy of State of California Department of Industrial Relations.

interests of its company-employed physician members."[52] The website for the college (http://www.acoem.org/aboutACOEM.aspx) states: "Founded in 1916, ACOEM is the nation's largest medical society dedicated to promoting the health of workers through preventive medicine, clinical care, research, and education. A dynamic group of physicians encompassing specialists in a variety of medical practices is united via the College to develop positions and policies on vital issues relevant to the practice of preventive medicine both within and outside of the workplace."[53]

- *National Council for Occupational Safety and Health (COSH)*: The website for COSH (http://www.coshnetwork.org) states that COSH "is dedicated to promoting safe and healthy working conditions for all working people through organizing and advocacy. Our belief that almost all work-related deaths and serious injuries and illnesses are preventable motivates us to encourage workers to take action to protect their safety and health, promote protection from retaliation under job safety laws, and provide quality information and training about hazards on the job and workers' rights."[54]

TABLE 2.7 lists other private-sector occupational health and safety organizations.

Employer-Sponsored Employee Assistance Programs

An employee assistance program (EAP) is "a voluntary, work-based program that offers free and confidential assessments, short-term counseling, referrals, and follow-up services to employees who have personal and/or work-related problems. EAPs address a broad and complex body of issues affecting mental and emotional well-being, such as alcohol and other substance abuse, stress, grief, family problems, and psychological disorders."[55] EAPs benefit employees and employers by increasing organizational morale, improving interactions with customers, improving the performance of workers, and helping the organization to attain business goals.[56]

In an example of how its EAP aided one company, a major hurricane and flash flood killed an employee who was attempting to report to work.[56] The EAP assisted a manager who discovered the deceased employee in overcoming the manager's emotional responses to this incident. Also, the EAP acted as a counselor and facilitator in restarting the facility after the hurricane interrupted its operations. In a second example, a multinational company was able to integrate an EAP with a disease management program that helps to improve the overall wellness of its employees.

TABLE 2.7   Private-Sector Occupational Health and Safety Organizations

American Association of Safety Councils: Professional association of independent, nonprofit, community-based health and safety organizations. It provides organization news, membership information, and links to local affiliates.

American Board of Industrial Hygiene: Professional organization working to improve the practice and educational standards of the industrial hygiene profession through an accredited certification system. Its website includes program details, code of ethics, and related information.

Construction Safety: The premier host for construction safety resources around the world.

International Sharps Injury Prevention Society (ISIPS): International group of medical device manufacturers, pharmaceutical companies, healthcare institutions, and industry professionals that have joined forces to reduce medical sharps injuries worldwide.

International Institute of Risk and Safety Management (IIRSM): A professional body for health and safety practitioners, based in the United Kingdom. Its mission is "to advance professional standards in accident prevention and occupational health throughout the world."

National Safety Council (NSC): Site provides information on many safety, health, and environmental topics; training resources; products; publications; news; programs; and home safety. NSC is a U.S.-based membership organization.

NEBOSH Exam Board: National Examination Board in Occupational Safety and Health (NEBOSH). It is an independent accreditation-awarding body that was founded in 1979.

OSH.NET: Occupational Safety and Health Network. It provides occupational safety and health information.

Occupational Knowledge International: An organization that facilitates the exchange of volunteers and donated equipment to environmental programs in developing countries, and offers a certification to facilities that meet environmental performance goals.

Semiconductor Safety Association: An organization dedicated to the prevention of workplace injuries and accidents through the sharing of safety and health information and the promotion of technological advances in high technology, safety, and health.

Board of Certified Safety Professionals (BCSP): A group that administers testing for individuals to become Certified Safety Professionals.

Institution of Occupational Safety and Health (IOSH): Europe's leading body for individuals with a professional involvement in occupational safety and health. The Chat Forum of this U.K.-based organization focuses on the issue of the day.

National Association of Safety Professionals: Provides information about membership and offers workplace safety resources and training aids.

Wellness Councils of America: A North American resource for worksite wellness. The Councils are dedicated to building world-class corporate and hospital wellness programs.

Workplace Safety North: A health and safety association in forestry under the Workplace Safety and Insurance Board (WSIB). It provides training, consulting, and publications.

Union Participation in Protecting Workers' Health

Labor unions perform an important function in articulating the rights of workers and introducing protections for their health. The federal government protects the formation of workers' unions and similar organizations. The National Labor Relations Act (NLRA) maintains the rights of employees and employers. "Congress enacted the National Labor Relations Act ('NLRA') to protect the rights of employees and employers, to encourage collective bargaining, and to curtail certain private sector labor and management practices, which can harm the general welfare of workers, businesses and the U.S. economy."[57] Further, the National Labor Relations Board operates as an independent federal agency with the mission of protecting the rights of employees to organize.[58] "The National Labor Relations Board protects the rights of most private-sector employees to join together, with or without a union, to improve their wages and working conditions."[59]

Maintenance of health and safety standards—for example, through implementation of regulations such as the OSH Act—is more likely to occur in unionized than in non-unionized places of employment.[60] Former Harvard epidemiology professor and School of Public Health dean at the University of North Carolina–Chapel Hill, Milton J. Rosenau[61] wrote that organized labor has contributed to the protection of employees' well-being "in limiting the avarice of the employer, in shortening the hours of work, in obtaining a better wage, in improving sanitary conditions, and in exacting a modicum of human consideration."[62(p. 34)]

An example of labor unions' leadership in spearheading the introduction of health and safety protections comes from the United Mine Workers of America (UMWA). Beginning in the early 20th century, the UMWA called public attention to lung diseases among coal workers. Shortly thereafter, the union advocated for workers' compensation for coal miners.[63] Later, the UMWA argued the need for epidemiologic research on this topic. Eventually, its efforts led to the development of the Federal Coal Mine Health and Safety Act of 1969.

The American Federation of Labor and Congress of Industrial Organizations (AFL-CIO) is another labor organization devoted to the protection of the welfare of workers. The AFL-CIO is an umbrella organization of 57 unions that cover approximately 12 million U.S. workers. According to the AFL-CIO's mission statement, "We work to ensure that all people who work receive the rewards of their work—decent paychecks and benefits, safe jobs, respect and fair treatment."[64] Unions such as the AFL-CIO advocate for the rights of workers in the halls of federal and state governments and among corporate leaders.

Starting during the 1950s, membership in unions has declined, with an accelerating trend becoming evident in recent years.[65] One of the factors driving this trend is the increasing globalization of the U.S. economy.[66] A possible effect of declining union membership over the past several decades is an exacerbation of wage inequality, such as that between whites and minority groups, including African Americans.[65] Also, the decline has reduced the representation of unions in hazardous workplaces.[64] This decline could reduce the effectiveness of government policies designed to lower the rates of occupational illnesses and injuries should health and safety regulations not be enforced adequately when the collective voice of workers is not being heard.

SUMMARY

Occupational health policies are plans for actions to protect the health and safety of workers. Examples of key occupational laws include the Occupational Safety and Health of 1970 and the Federal Mine Safety and Health Act of 1977. Other occupational laws provide for fair standards in the compensation of employees and prohibit discrimination against workers. In the past, workers who experienced discrimination in employment often were members of minority groups, older individuals, and women. Workers' compensation laws ensure income for employees who are temporarily sidelined or who have become permanently disabled from occupational illnesses or injuries.

In the United States, federal agencies such as OSHA, NIOSH, and the Department of Labor administer and enforce occupational health and safety laws and, in some instances, conduct research on the health of the workforce. Private organizations such as unions and occupational health associations make additional contributions to worker safety. From the international perspective, the World Health Organization and the International Labour Organization support initiatives for improvement of workers' health and safety.

STUDY QUESTIONS AND EXERCISES

1. Describe what is meant by "occupational health policy," and give some examples of such policies.
2. Which provisions for worker health emanate from international organizations such as the World Health Organization and the International Labour Organization?
3. Discuss the functions of the following U.S. governmental agencies regarding occupational health and safety.
   A. US DOL
   B. OSHA
   C. NIEHS
   D. NIOSH
   E. EPA
4. Which historical developments led to the creation of health and safety laws for workers? Which trends inspired the creation of the Occupational Safety and Health Act of 1970? Which types of policies and assurances did the OSH Act provide?

5. What was the impetus for the enactment of the Federal Employees' Compensation Act of 1916? What was the purpose of the Fair Labor Standards Act of 1938? What are the main provisions of both acts?
6. Compare and contrast the functions of OSHA and NIOSH with respect to workers' health and safety.
7. Which policies are in place for the prevention of discrimination in U.S. workplaces?
8. Define the term "whistleblower" and discuss protections for whistleblowers.
9. Describe the activities of two private-sector organizations in protecting workers' health.
10. Describe at least two ways in which unions support workers' health. How does the role of labor organizations differ from that of governmental agencies?

REFERENCES

1. Wisegeek.com. What is occupational health policy? n.d. http://www.wisegeek.com/what-is-occupational-health-policy.htm. Accessed September 13, 2013.
2. Wade R. The evolution of occupational health and the role of government. *West J Med.* 1982;137(6):577–580.
3. Nordlund WJ. The Federal Employees' Compensation Act. *Monthly Labor Rev.* September 1991:3–14.
4. U.S. Department of Labor. Federal Employees Compensation Act (FECA): summary. n.d. http://www.oig.dol.gov/public/feca/fecasummary.pdf. Accessed September 17, 2013.
5. U.S. Department of Labor, Wage and Hour Division. *The Fair Labor Standards Act of 1938, As Amended.* WH publication 1318. Revised May 2011.
6. Grossman J. Fair Labor Standards Act of 1938: maximum struggle for a minimum wage. n.d. http://www.dol.gov/osam/programs/history/flsa1938.htm. Accessed September 13, 2013.
7. U.S. Department of Labor. The Fair Labor Standards Act (FLSA). n.d. http://www.dol.gov/compliance/laws/comp/flsa.htm. Accessed September 13, 2013.
8. U.S. Social Security Administration. Black lung benefits program. n.d. http://www.dol.gov/brb/References/reference_works/bla/bldesk/BD01-A.pdf. Accessed January 26, 2014.
9. U.S. Department of Labor. The Black Lung Benefits Act (BLBA). n.d. http://www.dol.gov/compliance/laws/comp-blba.htm. Accessed January 26, 2014.
10. U.S. Department of Labor, Division of Coal Mine Workers' Compensation (DCMWC). About the black lung program. n.d. http://www.dol.gov/owcp/dcmwc. Accessed September 5, 2013.
11. Harkin T. On 35th anniversary of Mine Safety and Health Act, still more work to do. n.d. http://www.huffingtonpost.com/sen-tom-harkin/on-35th-anniversary-of-mi_b_2859793.html. Accessed September 5, 2013.
12. U.S. Department of Labor. Summary of the major laws of the Department of Labor. n.d. http://www.dol.gov/opa/aboutdol/lawsprog.htm. Accessed September 14, 2013.
13. U.S. Department of Labor, Occupational Safety and Health Administration (OSHA). OSH Act of 1970. n.d. http://www.osha.gov/pls/oshaweb/owadisp.show_document?p_table=OSHACT&p_id=2743, Accessed January 31, 2014.

14. Silverstein M. Getting home safe and sound: Occupational Safety and Health Administration at 38. *Am J Public Health*. 2008;98(3):416–423.

15. U.S. Department of Labor, Occupational Safety and Health Administration. *All about OSHA*. Washington, DC: U.S. Department of Labor (OSHA); 2013.

16. National Council for Occupational Safety and Health (COSH). Using OSHA's General Duty Clause. n.d. http://www.coshnetwork.org/node/353. Accessed September 13, 2013.

17. U.S. Department of Labor, Occupational Safety and Health Administration). *At-a-glance OSHA*. OSHA 3439-06N. Washington, DC: U.S. Department of Labor (OSHA); 2011.

18. U.S. Department of Labor. Occupational Safety and Health Administration. OSHA fact sheet: occupational safety and health for federal employees. n.d. https://www.osha.gov/OshDoc/data_General_Facts/federal-employee-factsheet.pdf. Accessed January 26, 2014.

19. World Health Organization. About occupational health. n.d. http://www.who.int/occupational_health/about/en/index.html. Accessed December 28, 2013.

20. World Health Organization. *Global strategy on occupational health for all*. Geneva, Switzerland: WHO; 1995.

21. World Health Organization. WHO regions and partners. n.d. http://www.who.int/occupational_health/regions/en/. Accessed December 28, 2013.

22. World Health Organization. Network of WHO Collaborating Centres in Occupational Health. n.d. http://www.who.int/occupational_health/network/en/. Accessed December 28, 2013.

23. U.S. Department of Labor, Occupational Safety and Health Administration. A guide to the Globally Harmonized System of Classification and Labelling of Chemicals (GHS). n.d. https://www.osha.gov/dsg/hazcom/ghs.html. Accessed June 11, 2014.

24. United Nations. *Globally Harmonized System of Classification and Labelling of Chemicals (GHS)*. 5th ed. New York, NY/Geneva, Switzerland: United Nations; 2013.

25. International Labour Organization. About the ILO. n.d. http://www.ilo.org/global/about-the-ilo/lang--en/index.htm. Accessed August 13, 2013.

26. International Labour Organization. Mission and objectives. n.d. http://www.ilo.org/global/mission-and objectives/lang--en/index.htm. December 26, 2013.

27. International Labour Organization. Structure. n.d. http://ilo.org/global/about-the-ilo/who-we-are/lang--en/index.htm. Accessed December 26, 2013.

28. EU-OSHA. About us. n.d. http://osha.europa.eu/en/about. Accessed October 24, 2013.

29. National Institute of Environmental Health Sciences. *Your environment—your health*. Research Triangle Park, NC: NIEHS; November 2012.

30. National Institute of Environmental Health Sciences. Occupational health. n.d. http://www.niehs.nih.gov/health/topics/population/occupational/index.cfm. Accessed September 13, 2013.

31. National Institute for Occupational Safety and Health. NIOSH fact sheet. DHHS (NIOSH) Publication No. 2013-140. April 2013. http://www.cdc.gov/niosh/docs/2013-140/pdfs/2013-140.pdf. Accessed December 26, 2013.

32. U.S. Department of Labor, Occupational Safety and Health Administration. OSHA fact sheet: OSHA inspections. n.d. https://www.osha.gov/OshDoc/data_General_Facts/factsheet-inspections.pdf. Accessed January 27, 2014.

33. U.S. Environmental Protection Agency. Frequently asked questions about EPA and Region 8. n.d. http://www.epa.gov/region 8/about/faqsr8.htm. Accessed September 14, 2013.

34. U.S. Environmental Protection Agency. Toxic Substances Control Act (TSCA). n.d. http://www.epa.gov/agriculture/tsca.htm. Accessed September 13, 2013.

35. Agency for Toxic Substances and Disease Registry. Agency for Toxic Substances and Disease Registry [Homepage]. n.d. http://www.atsdr.cdc.gov. Accessed September 13, 2013.

36. Agency for Toxic Substances and Disease Registry. *Safeguarding communities from chemical exposures.* Atlanta, GA: U.S. DHHS, ATSDR, n.d.

37. Agency for Toxic Substances and Disease Registry. *Public health assessment guidance manual (update).* Atlanta, GA: U.S. DHHS, PHS, ATSDR; 2005.

38. Agency for Toxic Substances and Disease Registry. *Agency for Toxic Substances and Disease Registry.* CS232362. Atlanta, GA: ATSDR, n.d.

39. Agency for Toxic Substances and Disease Registry. Toxic substances portal: ToxFAQs.™ n.d. http://www.atsdr.cdc.gov/toxfaqs/index.asp#bookmark01. Accessed December 24, 2013.

40. Santoro WA. The civil rights movement's struggle for fair employment: a "dramatic events—conventional politics" model. *Soc Forces.* 2002;81(1):177–206.

41. U.S. Equal Employment Opportunity Commission. Title VII of the Civil Rights Act of 1964. n.d. http://www.eeoc.gov/laws/statutes/titlevii.cfm. Accessed July 1, 2014.

42. U.S. Equal Employment Opportunity Commission. About EEOC. Overview. n.d. http://www1.eeoc.gov/eeoc/index.cfm. Accessed May 13, 2013.

43. U.S. Department of Labor, Office of the Secretary. *Futurework.* Washington, DC: U.S. Department of Labor, Office of the Secretary; 1999.

44. Muskal M. Civil Rights Act at 50: why race still matters. *Los Angeles Times.* July 3, 2014, A12.

45. *Free Online Dictionary.* Definition of whistleblowing. n.d. http://legal dictionary .thefreedictionary.com/Whistleblowing. Accessed October 13, 2014.

46. U.S. Department of Labor, Occupational Safety and Health Administration. The whistleblower protection programs. n.d. http://www.whistleblowers.gov/. Accessed January 26, 2014.

47. Sengupta I, Reno V, Burton JF, Baldwin M. *Workers' compensation: benefits, coverage, and costs, 2010.* Washington, DC: National Academy of Social Insurance; August 2012.

48. Burton JF. An overview of workers' compensation. *Workers' Compens Policy Rev.* 2007;7(3):3–27.

49. U.S. Social Security Administration. *Disability benefits.* SSA Publication No. 05-10029. Woodlawn, MD: Social Security Administration; June 2012.

50. State of California, Division of Workers' Compensation, Department of Industrial Relations. Fact Sheet. *What is workers' compensation?* San Francisco, CA: DWC, Department of Industrial Relations; July 2010. n.d. http://www.dir.ca.gov/dwc /FactSheets/Employee_FactSheet.pdf. Accessed January 31, 2014.

51. American Public Health Association. Occupational health and safety. n.d. http:// www.apha.org/membergroups/sections/aphasections/occupational/. Accessed December 26, 2013.

52. Ladou J, Teitelbaum DT, Egilman DS, et al. American College of Occupational and Environmental Medicine (ACOEM). *Int J Occup Environ Health.* 2007;13:404–426.

53. American College of Occupational and Environmental Medicine. ACOEM overview. n.d. http://www.acoem.org/aboutACOEM.aspx. Accessed January 31, 2014.

54. National Council for Occupational Safety and Health. Our mission. n.d. http://www.coshnetwork.org. Accessed September 13, 2013.

55. U.S. Office of Personnel Management. What is an employee assistance program (EAP)? n.d. http://www.opm.gov/faqs. Accessed December 27, 2013.

56. Center for Prevention and Health Services. An employer's guide to employee assistance programs. December 2008. http://www.businessgrouphealth.org/pub/f31372a2-2354-d714-51e4-ae4127ced552. Accessed December 27, 2013.

57. National Labor Relations Board. National Labor Relations Act. n.d. http://www.nlrb.gov/resources/national-labor-relations-act. Accessed December 27, 2013.

58. National Labor Relations Board. What we do. n.d. http://www.nlrb.gov/what-we-do. Accessed December 27, 2013.

59. National Labor Relations Board. Rights we protect. n.d. http://www.nlrb.gov/resources/rights-we-protect. Accessed December 27, 2013.

60. Weil D. Enforcing OSHA: The role of labor unions. *Industrial Relations.* 1991;30(1):20–36.

61. Centers for Disease Control and Prevention. Milton J. Rosenau, M.D. *MMWR.* 1999;48(40):907.

62. Abrams HK. A short history of occupational health. *J Public Health Policy.* 2001;22(1):34–80.

63. Derickson A. The United Mine Workers of America and the recognition of occupational expiratory diseases, 1902–1968. *Am J Public Health.* 1991;81(6):782–790.

64. AFL-CIO. About the AFL-CIO. n.d. http://www.aflcio.org/About. Accessed September 5, 2013.

65. Robinson JC. Labor union involvement in occupational safety and health, 1957–1987. *J Health Polit Policy Law.* 1988;13(3):453–468.

66. Slaughter MJ. Globalization and declining unionization in the United States. *Industrial Relations.* 2007;46(2):329–346.

67. Rosenfeld J, Kleykamp M. Organized labor and racial wage inequality in the United States. *AJS.* 2012;117(5):1460–1502.

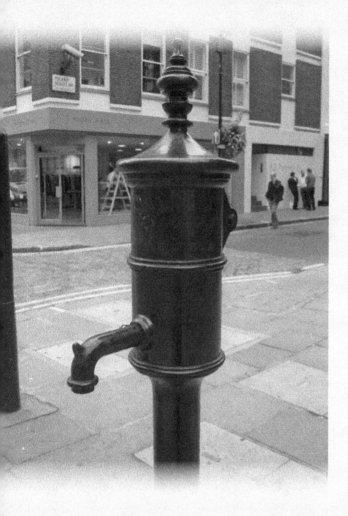

FIGURE 3.1 Replica of the Broad Street pump located in the Soho district of London

The following passage was taken from *Snow on Cholera*, authored by John Snow, a mid-19th-century pioneer in the development of epidemiologic methods:

> The most terrible outbreak of cholera [August 1849] which ever occurred in this kingdom, is probably that which took place in Broad Street, Golden Square, and the adjoining streets, a few weeks ago. Within two hundred and fifty yards of the spot where Cambridge Street joins Broad Street, there were upwards of five hundred fatal attacks of cholera in ten days.... There were a few cases of cholera in the neighbourhood of Broad Street, Golden Square, in the latter part of August; and the so-called outbreak, which commenced in the night between the 31st August and the 1st September, was, as in all similar instances, only a violent increase of the malady. As soon as I became acquainted with the situation and extent of this irruption of cholera, I suspected some contamination of the water of the much-frequented street-pump in Broad Street, near the end of Cambridge Street.[1](pp. 38–39)

CHAPTER 3

Epidemiologic and Toxicologic Aspects of Occupational Health and Safety

Learning Objectives

By the end of this chapter you will be able to:

- Describe the applications of epidemiology and toxicology in occupational health.
- Define the term *occupational epidemiology*.
- Define and calculate basic epidemiologic measures used in occupational health.
- Compare and contrast the strengths and weaknesses of three epidemiologic research designs used in occupational health.
- Define the term *occupational toxicology*.
- Describe toxicological concepts used in occupational health.

Chapter Outline

- Introduction
- Epidemiology
- Basic Measures Used in Epidemiology
- The Epidemiologic Triangle
- Epidemiologic Research Methods Used in Occupational Health and Safety
- Toxicology
- Summary
- Study Questions and Exercises

Introduction

Which occupations are dangerous for workers? Which adverse health effects are related to exposure to toxic chemicals on the job site? What are safe levels of workers' exposures to hazardous agents? How effective are interventions to prevent occupational illnesses? Epidemiology and toxicology are the fields that enable occupational health specialists to answer these questions. Occupational epidemiology examines the distribution and determinants of work-related health outcomes in employed populations. Occupational toxicology investigates the extent to which workplace chemicals used are poisonous.[2]

Epidemiology and toxicology provide a body of methods for assessing hazards and risks from occupational exposures. These methods identify associations between exposures and adverse health outcomes from work-related factors, support development of standards for permissible levels of exposures, and suggest preventive interventions for protecting workers from occupational hazards.

Occupational epidemiology and toxicology are complementary disciplines. Epidemiology supplies the methods—measures of morbidity, mortality, and risk—used to portray the distribution of health outcomes in worker populations and in the evaluation of exposure–disease associations. Toxicology is a sophisticated science for examining the toxic effects of the various agents and exposures that may impact the work environment. Both epidemiologic and toxicologic findings are useful for defining the exposure limits needed to protect workers from potentially hazardous agents.

The goals of occupational and environmental medicine have evolved over time, and these changes are reflected in the current activities of occupational epidemiology and occupational toxicology. "As we look toward the future, classical occupational and environmental hazards such as overexposure to lead, asbestos, and mercury are waning and being replaced by concerns around sustainable development, toxicology testing, and exposure information for high-production volume chemicals, [and] development of better approaches for setting workplace and community exposure limits."[3(p. 217)]

Epidemiology

Epidemiology is defined as "[t]he study of the occurrence and distribution of health-related states or events in specified populations, including the study of the determinants influencing such states, and the application of this knowledge to control the health problems."[4] By taking the perspective of the population, the field of epidemiology veers away from clinical medicine and other clinical disciplines, which focus on the health of individuals.

The study designs most commonly used in epidemiologic research are purely observational in nature, as in the historically important example of John Snow's investigation of a cholera epidemic in London in the mid-1800s. (Snow's work is discussed later in this section.) However, some epidemiologic study designs make use of experimental methods, which manipulate an independent variable (called an exposure variable)—for example, administration of a new medication. These so-called intervention designs include clinical trials (also known as randomized controlled trials) directed toward individuals and community trials that focus on interventions at the community level. A clinical trial is further differentiated from a community trial in that the former relies on random assignment of study subjects to the conditions of the experiment.

Epidemiology, as the basic science underlying public health and preventive medicine, has a plethora of applications in occupational health, including pinpointing groups at high risk of work-related morbidity, demonstrating associations between work exposures and adverse health outcomes, and controlling job-related illnesses. For example, Tager asserted, "Epidemiologic methods have played an important role in the identification of environmental and occupational causes of lung diseases and respiratory morbidity/mortality in populations."[5(p. 615)] When applied to the work environment, epidemiologic research examines associations between exposures and adverse health outcomes. Once these associations are known, methods for the control of occupationally related diseases can move forward. In addition, epidemiologic findings contribute much of the basic data used for developing occupational health policies and for monitoring the effectiveness of interventions for occupational illnesses.

Occupational epidemiologic studies are used to identify groups at high risk for occupational illnesses. Risk can be defined as the probability of experiencing an adverse effect. The basic premise of epidemiology is that disease does not occur randomly in populations, but rather follows systematic patterns that can reflect different levels of risk. These patterns can be ascertained by comparing the occurrence of disease among subgroups of populations subdivided by demographic characteristics such as age, sex, and race. For example, many chronic and infectious disorders, ranging from HIV infection to heart disease to cancer, are more common in some subgroups of the population than in others. These varying patterns of health outcomes may reflect the effects of different types and levels of exposures to risk factors that occur in population subgroups.

Three important epidemiologic concepts are epidemics, endemic disease, and pandemics. An epidemic is "[t]he occurrence in a community or region of cases of an illness, specific health-related behavior, or other health-related events clearly in excess of normal expectancy."[4] The periodic outbreaks of foodborne illness—for example, salmonellosis linked to *Salmonella* bacteria in chicken—represent the epidemic concept. The term pandemic denotes "[a]n epidemic occurring worldwide or over a very wide area, crossing international boundaries, and usually affecting a large number of people."[4] As an example, the World Health Organization (WHO) declared the global occurrence of H1N1 influenza (swine-origin influenza) in 2009 to be a pandemic. One of the implications of epidemics and pandemics for occupational health is that they could endanger first responders and healthcare personnel. This situation happened in Texas during 2014 when a patient from Africa became infected with the Ebola virus. Another potential impact of epidemic disease in the workplace is high levels of absenteeism that can disrupt work settings.

The epidemiologic concept endemic refers to an infectious disease (or condition) that is habitually present in a geographic area. Endemic diseases are found in various geographic areas of the United States and are associated with local environmental factors including the presence of vectors—that is, certain species of insects (e.g., mosquitoes and ticks) and rodents involved with the transmission of infectious diseases. A case in point is Lyme disease, which poses a hazard to outdoor workers in endemic regions of the United States such as the Northeast, Mid-Atlantic states, North-Central states, and the West Coast during the time of the year when the ticks that carry the bacteria causing Lyme disease are active.

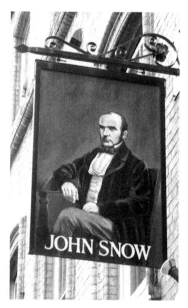

An example of a historically significant epidemiologic study was John Snow's pioneering investigation of a cholera outbreak in the Soho district of London during the mid-19th century. Snow (FIGURE 3.2) theorized that there was an association between the supply of polluted drinking water and cholera. He confirmed his theory by mapping cholera deaths in relation to the source of water supplies. The deaths tended to be more concentrated around one water pump—the Broad Street pump; Snow had the handle removed from the pump to limit further cholera cases. For his work demonstrating this association between impure water and cholera, Snow is regarded as the father of epidemiology.

FIGURE 3.2   John Snow

Overview of Epidemiologic Inference

FIGURE 3.3 diagrams the process of making epidemiologic inferences. As shown in the figure, descriptive epidemiology and analytic epidemiology are the two broad approaches employed in this field. The former—which

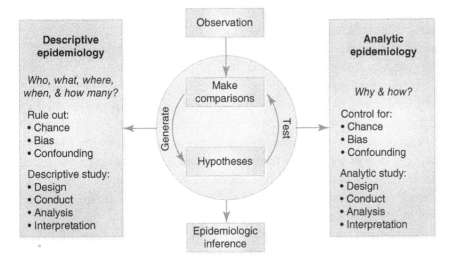

FIGURE 3.3   Process of epidemiologic inference

Reproduced from Aragón T. Descriptive epidemiology: Describing findings and generating hypotheses, Center for Infectious Disease Preparedness, UC Berkeley School of Public Health.

focuses on the questions of who, what, where, when, and how many—is aligned with the process of making comparisons among subgroups in the population and developing hypotheses. Analytic epidemiology is concerned with testing hypotheses.

Descriptive Epidemiology

A descriptive epidemiologic study is one that characterizes the amount and distribution of disease within a population. A descriptive study is "concerned with and designed only to describe the existing distribution of variables without much regard to causal relationships or other hypotheses."[4] An example of a descriptive epidemiologic study is an investigation that shows how the occurrence of lung cancer varies among different occupational categories. As indicated in Figure 3.3, a descriptive epidemiologic study would specify how many cases of occupationally associated lung cancer exist, where and when they occur, and who is affected.

Clustering

Clustering refers to "[a] closely grouped series of events or cases of a disease or other health-related phenomena with well-defined distribution patterns in relation to time or place or both. The term is normally used to describe aggregation of relatively uncommon events or diseases (e.g., leukemia, multiple sclerosis)."[4] Often clustering means spatial clustering—that is, concentration of disease cases in a particular geographic area. Another type of clustering is temporal clustering; an example of this type is a postvaccination reaction (e.g., arm soreness) that may occur after a time interval following administration of a vaccine.

Clustering (also called a disease cluster) is one of the observations that might be derived from descriptive epidemiologic studies of reported cases and may suggest common exposure to an environmental hazard; an alternative explanation is that the cluster is a chance occurrence. Most of the time, case clustering is an extremely unusual event. Examples of clustering include the cholera epidemic that occurred in London in the 1850s and the outbreak of Legionnaires' disease that took place at the Bellevue-Stratford Hotel in Philadelphia in 1976.

Clustering is a very noteworthy indicator for occupational health studies. For example, analyses of case clusters revealed the occurrence of angiosarcoma of the liver among workers exposed to vinyl chloride and the presence of neurotoxicity among pesticide applicators exposed to kepone.[6] Investigations of clusters can be used, for example, to explore potential associations among workers' exposure to ionizing radiation and the development of cancer. Such exposures could occur during nuclear weapons manufacture or while medical tests (e.g., X-rays) are conducted.

Cancer Clusters

The National Cancer Institute (NCI) defines a cancer cluster as "the occurrence of a greater than expected number of cancer cases among a group of people in a defined geographic area over a specific time period. A cancer cluster may be suspected when people report that several family members, friends, neighbors, or coworkers have been diagnosed with the same or related types of cancer."[7] Often the local or state health department is the agency that receives the first reports of a cancer cluster and responds to residents' concerns. To investigate cancer clusters, the NCI recommends the systematic procedures described later in this section.

The Centers for Disease Control and Prevention (CDC) provided the following example of a cancer cluster: "Three members of the staff of an elementary school were diagnosed with cancer over a two-year period; one person each with brain, liver, and ovarian cancer. Further inquiries led to the realization that four cases of breast cancer had also been recently diagnosed. Increased concern among employees regarding the potential association between the workplace and the cancers prompted a request for an investigation."[8] The CDC concluded that because cancer is a prevalent condition, the observed distribution of cases was not unusual in view of the ages and genders of the affected persons and the fact that no biologically significant exposures to cancer-causing agents had been identified in the school.

Two additional examples of cancer clustering are from Washington state in the United States and northern Germany. Ross and Davis studied a cluster of Hodgkin's disease cases in Washington using a case-control design. In the first investigation, statistical analyses suggested that patients with Hodgkin's disease who were older than age 40 had lived in closer residential proximity to one another as children and teenagers than would be predicted by chance. In the second example, German investigators reported a cluster of six childhood leukemia cases among residents who lived in close proximity to a nuclear reactor situated in the northern region of the country.

According to the NCI lists, an investigating agency should employ the procedures listed in **EXHIBIT 3.1** to check out suspected cancer clusters.

Analytic Epidemiology

The second major approach of epidemiology is known as analytic epidemiology. An analytic (analytical) epidemiologic study explores the determinants

---

EXHIBIT 3.1   How Are Suspected Cancer Clusters Investigated?

1. The investigating agency gathers information from the person who reported the suspected cancer cluster. The investigators ask for details about the suspected cluster, such as the types of cancer and the number of cases of each type, the ages of the people with cancer, and the area and time period over which the cancers were diagnosed. They also ask about specific environmental hazards or concerns in the affected area.
2. If the review of the findings from this initial investigation suggests the need for further evaluation, investigators compare information about cases in the suspected cluster with records in the state cancer registry and census data.
3. If the second step reveals a statistically significant excess of cancer cases, the investigators determine the feasibility of an epidemiologic study. This study would explore the possible association of the cluster with risk factors in the local environment. Sometimes, even if there is a clear excess of cancer cases, it may not be feasible to carry out further study—for example, if the total number of cases is very small.
4. If an epidemiologic study is feasible, the investigators determine whether the cluster of cancer cases is associated with a suspected contaminant in the environment. Even if a possible association with an environmental contaminant is found, however, further studies would be needed to confirm that the environmental contaminant did cause the cluster.

Modified from National Cancer Institute. Cancer clusters. n.d. http://www.cancergov /cancertopics/factsheet/Risk/clusters. Accessed July 9, 2014.

of diseases—that is, the causes of relatively high or low frequencies of diseases in specific populations. Analytic studies are "designed to examine putative or hypothesized causal relationships; hence, most such studies can be conceptualized as etiological studies."[4] Figure 3.3 shows that analytic studies test hypotheses obtained in descriptive studies. For example, a descriptive study might generate the hypothesis that exposures to chemicals used in the manufacture of plastics are associated with lung cancer. An analytic study might test this hypothesis by examining risks of lung cancer among workers who have different levels of exposure to these types of chemicals.

Occupational Epidemiology

Occupational epidemiology is defined as "[t]he study of the effects of workplace exposures on the frequency and distribution of diseases and injuries in the population."[4] Thus, occupational epidemiology extends epidemiology to the investigation of occupational health issues and uses methods that are analogous to those employed more generally in epidemiology. "The occupational epidemiologic approach to a particular disease is intended to identify high risk subgroups within the population and determine the effectiveness of subsequent preventive measures."[9(p. 381)]

In differentiating occupational epidemiology from occupational medicine, one should note that the clinical skills of an occupational physician (or other clinical provider) are helpful in the diagnosis and treatment of patients with conditions that occur in the occupational environment. However, occupational epidemiology provides the methods needed to link job-related exposures with health outcomes that occur in the work environment at the population level.

Objectives and Uses of Occupational Epidemiology

Merletti et al.[10] describe two objectives for occupational epidemiology: (1) "prevention through identifying the consequences of workplace exposures on health" and (2) "[use of] results from specific settings to reduce or to eliminate hazards in the population at large." Usually exposures to occupational hazards occur at much higher levels than exposures in the general population. Findings from the occupational environment can, therefore, be used to estimate the effects of lower-level exposures in the population.

Among the uses of occupational epidemiology is the study of the health effects of exposure to hazardous agents that occur in the workplace. Another application is to investigate and quantify health risks associated with such exposures. Finally, descriptive occupational epidemiologic studies can show the patterning of risks in different occupations and contribute to the development of hypotheses about how these risks may be related to adverse health outcomes. Ultimately, these applications of occupational epidemiology can lead to methods for preventing and controlling work-related health risks.

Basic Measures Used in Epidemiology

Epidemiologic measures are used for several purposes, including those that relate to occupational health. One application is for portraying the occurrence of health outcomes in descriptive epidemiologic research. Another is analytic (etiologic) studies to measure the associations between risk factors (exposures) and of adverse health outcomes. Epidemiologic measures can be adjusted to control for the influence of demographic variables such as age and sex. Two fundamental measures of disease occurrence used in epidemiology and specifically occupational epidemiology are prevalence (prevalence proportion) and incidence. A more complex measure is a rate, such as an incidence rate.

Counts, Ratios, and Proportions

Counts, ratios, and proportions are among the basic epidemiologic measures. The definitions of these terms are as follows:

- *Count*: the number of cases of disease (or other health outcome). Example: 20 cases of asbestosis among World War II shipyard workers.
- *Ratio*: a general term for a fraction having a numerator and denominator. Examples: a proportion, rate, and the standardized mortality ratio.
- *Proportion*: a type of ratio in which the numerator is part of the denominator. Example: prevalence proportion.

Prevalence/Prevalence Proportion

Prevalence refers to "the number of affected persons present in the population at a specific time divided by the number of persons in the population at that time—that is, what proportion of the population is affected by the disease at that time?"[11] Note that prevalence is not a rate.[4] As indicated by the foregoing definition, prevalence can be expressed as a proportion and can refer to point prevalence (the proportion of cases at a particular point in time) or period prevalence (the proportion of cases in a population during a particular time period such as a week, month, or other time period). A prevalence study examines the frequency of a condition in a population;

these data provide an indication of the extent of a health problem in that population. An occupational health example is the prevalence of unintentional injuries from needle sticks among microbiologists in hospital clinical laboratories.

Another example of a prevalence study is research on latent tuberculosis among healthcare workers in South Korea.[12] The rationale for this investigation was that healthcare workers could acquire latent tuberculosis infection from occupational exposure. Latent tuberculosis infection is a form of the disease wherein the infected person does not feel ill or have symptoms and is not infectious to others, but nonetheless is infected with tuberculosis bacteria. In the Korean study, researchers used a questionnaire to collect information on baseline demographics and risk factors for latent tuberculosis infection; they also performed medical tests to assess healthcare workers for tuberculosis. Information was collected between April 2012 and May 2012 among employees at eight tertiary referral hospitals in South Korea. The participants for this study totaled 493 persons (152 doctors and 341 nurses). A high prevalence of latent tuberculosis infection as suggested by the tuberculin skin test (36.7%) was found among the study participants.

When comparisons of prevalence data are made among populations that differ in size, a convenient measure to use is point prevalence, calculated as a prevalence proportion. Recall that prevalence refers frequently to point prevalence, which is prevalence at a specific point in time. The formula for point prevalence is

$$\text{Point prevalence} = \frac{\text{Number of persons ill (or with a characteristic)}}{\text{Total number in the group}} \text{ at a point in time}$$

Note that point prevalence can be expressed as a percentage by multiplying the equation result by 100. You can also use some other multiplier (e.g., 1000, 10,000, or 1,000,000).

Calculation Example

A community interview survey was used to determine the prevalence of smoking among Cambodian American residents of Long Beach, California. A total of 1414 respondents were identified (by a stratified random sample). Among the participants, 165 current smokers were found at the time of interview. The prevalence of smoking (point prevalence) was $165/1414 \times 100 = 11.7\%$.

In this example, prevalence was expressed as a percentage (11.7%). Prevalence may also be expressed in terms of cases per 1000 or some other convenient multiplier; the choice of a multiplier may be affected by consid-erations such as how frequently the condition (e.g., disease or other char-acteristic) occurs in the population.

Incidence

Incidence is defined as "[t]he number of instances of illnesses commencing, or of persons falling ill, during a given period in a specified population. More generally, the number of new health-related events in a defined population within a specified period of time. It may be measured as a frequency count, a rate, or a proportion."[4] Incidence is used as a measure of the risk of a speci-fied health-related event associated with a specific exposure. An example of incidence measured as a frequency count is the number of new cases of coal workers' pneumoconiosis diagnosed in a population of miners in a given year.

Rate

A rate is a measure with a numerator and a denominator, in which the denominator involves a measure of time. The numerator consists of the frequency of a disease over a specified period of time; the denominator is a unit size of population. One needs to know the beginning and the end of the time periods during which the disease occurred to estimate the time period. This definition will become clearer when the formulas for two types of rates—an incidence rate and a death rate—are defined.

Incidence Rate

An incidence rate is formed by dividing the number of new cases that occur during a time period by the number of individuals in the population at risk. (Several variations of incidence rates exist, but a discussion of all of them is beyond the scope of this chapter.) Statistically speaking, the incidence rate is a rate because of the specification of a time period during which the new cases occur. It is expressed using a multiplier, which can be any form that is convenient (e.g., per 1000, per 100,000, or per 1,000,000). The for-mula for an incidence rate is as follows:

$$\text{Incidence rate} = \frac{\text{Number of new cases}}{\text{Total population at risk}} \text{ over a time period} \times \text{multiplier (e.g., 1000)}$$

Calculation Example

During the calendar year 2016, a bakery that employed 978 bakers and pastry makers reported 5 new cases of diagnosed work-related asthma. The incidence rate (per 1000 bakers and pastry workers) was $(5/978) \times 1000 = 5.1$ per 1000.

The *cumulative incidence rate* refers to "[t]he number or proportion of a group (cohort) of people who experience the onset of a health-related event during a specified time interval."[4] The incidence rate in the foregoing calculation example is a cumulative incidence rate. Incidence measures are central to the study of causal mechanisms that explain how exposures affect health outcomes and are used to describe the risks associated with certain exposures. "The cumulative incidence (incidence proportion) or average risk in a base population is the probability of someone in that population developing the disease during a specified period, conditional on not dying first from another disease."[13(p. 23)] For example, the incidence rates of work-related asthma could be compared among workers in different occupations, such as bakers, healthcare workers, painters, and office workers, to ascertain which occupation has the greatest risk of this condition.

Death Rate (Mortality Rate)

The death rate is "[a]n estimate of the proportion of a population that dies during a specified period."[4] One of the commonly used measures of the death rate is the crude death rate (also known as the crude mortality rate). For example, in calculating the annual crude death rate in the United States, one would count all the deaths that occurred in the country during a certain year and assign this value to the numerator. The value for the denominator would be the size of the population of the country during that same year. The best estimate of the population would probably be the population around the midpoint of the year, if such information could be obtained. The formula for the crude death rate is as follows:

$$\text{Crude death rate} = \frac{\text{Number of deaths in a given year}}{\text{Reference population (during midpoint of the year)}} \times 100,000$$

Calculation Example

In 2010, a total of 2,468,435 deaths were reported in the United States. The population was estimated to be 308,745,538. The crude death rate per 100,000 was (2,468,435/308,745,538) × 100,000 = 799.5.

When applied to occupational health, the death rate is useful for comparing the mortality experiences of different occupations and for comparing the mortality within a particular occupation with the overall mortality that occurs in the United States. This type of death rate (shown in the calculation) is called a crude rate because it has not been adjusted in any way. A caveat regarding comparisons made with crude rates is that they do not take into account differences in populations with respect to age structures and other demographic characteristics. In this respect, crude rates may be misleading if, for example, comparisons are made among populations that have very different age distributions.

Age-Specific and Cause-Specific Rates

Although crude rates are important and useful summary measures of the occurrence of disease, they are not without limitations. A crude rate should be used with caution in making comparative statements about disease frequencies in populations. Observed differences between populations in crude rates of disease may be the result of systematic factors within the populations rather than true variations in rates. Systematic differences in sex or age distributions would affect observed rates. To correct for factors that may influence the make-up of populations and in turn influence crude rates, one may construct specific and adjusted rates.

Specific rates are a type of rate based on a particular subgroup of the population defined, for example, in terms of race, age, or sex; alternatively, they may refer to the entire population but be specific for some single cause of death or illness. Examples of specific rates are cause-specific rates and age-specific rates.

A cause-specific rate is "[a] rate that specifies events, such as deaths, according to their cause."[4] An example of a cause-specific rate is the cause-specific mortality rate. As the name implies, it is the death rate associated with a specific cause of death.

$$\text{Cause-specific rate} = \frac{\text{Mortality (or frequency of a give disease)}}{\text{Population size at midpoint of a time period}} \times 100{,}000$$

Calculation Example

The number of deaths in the United States (population 308,745, 538) due to malignant neoplasms (cancer) was 574,743 during 2010. The cause-specific mortality rate due to malignant neoplasms was $(574{,}743/308{,}745{,}538) \times 100{,}000$, or 186.2 per 100,000.

An age-specific rate is the number of events (e.g., deaths) during a specified time period that occur within an age group of the population divided by the number of persons in that age group times a multiplier. Because they involve a delimited age group in the population, age-specific rates are helpful in making comparisons across populations with respect to a particular cause of morbidity or mortality. An age-specific rate can be calculated for an age stratum of interest. Here is the formula for the age-specific death rate among persons aged 15 to 24 years:

$$\text{Age-specific death rate} = \frac{\text{Number of deaths among those aged 15--24 years}}{\substack{\text{Number of persons who are aged 15--24 year} \\ \text{(during a time period)}}} \times 100{,}000$$

Calculation Example

In the United States during 2010, there were 1604 deaths from malignant neoplasms among persons aged 15 to 24 years; the population size in this age stratum was 43,625,676. The age-specific mortality rate (persons aged 15 to 24 years) due to malignant neoplasms was (1604/43,625,676) × 100,000, or 3.7 per 100,000.

Rate Adjustment and Standardization

Adjusted rates are summary measures of the rate of morbidity or mortality in populations; statistical procedures have been applied to remove the effect of differences in composition of the various populations. A measure that has not been adjusted is termed a crude rate. For example, the cause-specific death rate described in the previous example for cancer was a crude rate. Mortality comparisons of populations that have very different age or demographic structures might produce misleading conclusions, and the process of rate adjustment helps to overcome these problems inherent in the crude rates. The two methods for rate adjustment are the direct method and the indirect method.

Age Standardization Using the Direct Method

Age standardization is a statistical procedure that removes the influence of age from a measure (e.g., death rate). Age is a factor commonly used for rate adjustment and is probably the most important variable in the risk of morbidity and mortality, although rates can be adjusted for other variables. Crude rates mask differences between populations that differ in age and, therefore, are not satisfactory for comparing health outcomes in such populations.[14] Members of older populations have a much greater risk of mortality than those in younger populations. Consequently, the crude mortality rate will be higher when a population is older than when the population is younger.

A full discussion of the direct method of age standardization is beyond the scope of this text. However, here are a few hints regarding the procedure for age standardization of death rates. The direct method requires a suitable standard population, which is used for standardizing some other population. Also, the age-specific death rates in the population for standardization must be known. In the case of standardization of mortality rates for the general U.S. population, the standard population is the U.S. population in the year 2000. The U.S. population for a later year—say, 2010—can be standardized by using the standard population. For example, the crude death rate in 2010 was 799.5 per 100,000 population.

After age standardization, the age-adjusted death rate was 747.0 deaths per 100,000. The age-adjusted death rate was lower than the crude rate as a result of demographic changes such as the aging of the country's residents. The U.S. population is changing substantially in age and demographic composition over time. The age-adjusted death rate is thought to provide an improved measure of the risk of death in light of this changing demographic composition.

In many occupational health studies, a suitable standard population and age-specific death rates in the population for standardization are not available. In this situation, occupational health investigators often rely on the indirect method of standardization—called the standardized mortality ratio—which is more appropriate for use in occupational studies than the direct method.

Standardized Mortality Ratio

The standardized mortality ratio (SMR) is the ratio of the observed mortality in a population to the expected mortality. The SMR can be multiplied by 100 to express it as a percentage. If the observed and expected numbers are the same, the SMR would be 100% (1.0), indicating that the observed mortality in the study population is not unusual. An SMR of 200% (2.0) is interpreted to mean that the death (or disease) rate in the study population is two times greater than expected. An SMR is calculated from the following formula:

$$SMR = \frac{\text{Observed deaths}}{\text{Expected deaths}} \times 100$$

Calculation Example

The number of observed deaths due to heart disease was 600 in a cohort of bus drivers during year 2014. The expected number of deaths was 1000. The SMR = (600/1000) × 100 = 60.0%; that is, the SMR is 60% of the expectation. When the SMR exceeds 100%, the number of deaths exceeds expectations.

As an example of this use of the standardized mortality ratio in occupational health, Rockette found that the overall SMR for miners covered for 1959 through 1971 by the United Mine Workers Health and Retirement plan was 102.1 (%).[15] Thus the overall mortality experience of the miners was close to the expected mortality. In the same study, the SMRs for asthma (165.0 [%]), tuberculosis (154.4 [%]), and unintentional injuries "accidents" (143.4 [%]) were higher than expected.

The Epidemiologic Triangle

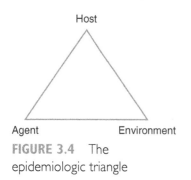

FIGURE 3.4   The epidemiologic triangle

The epidemiologic triangle, shown in **FIGURE 3.4**, is helpful for explaining the occurrence of work-related adverse health outcomes. The epidemiologic triangle recognizes three major factors—agent, environment, and host—in the pathogenesis of disease. Epidemiologists refer frequently to this venerable model, which has been used for many decades. The epidemiologic triangle provides one of the fundamental public health conceptions of disease causality.

Agent

The first component of the epidemiologic triangle is an agent, which in the occupational setting includes hazardous microbes (blood-borne, foodborne, and zoonotic), physical hazards (e.g., noise, ionizing and nonionizing radiation, and vibration), and potentially dangerous chemicals (toxic industrial chemicals, heavy metals, and pesticides). Other agent factors in a work setting include psychosocial influences such as stress that emanate from interpersonal interactions and the mode of configuration of the work setting.

Environment

The environment refers to the domain in which the disease-causing agent may exist, survive, or originate. Is this text we focus on the importance of the work environment for occupational health. The external environment is the sum total of influences that are not part of the host and comprises physical, climatologic, biologic, social, and economic components. The physical environment includes temperature and humidity in the work setting as well as weather, which is a salient factor for people who work outdoors. The social environment is the totality of the behavioral, personality, attitudinal, and cultural characteristics of a group of people. Both of these facets of the external environment have an impact on agents of disease and potential hosts because the environment may either enhance or diminish the survival of disease agents and may serve to bring agent and host into contact.

Host

The host is the third component of the epidemiologic triangle. In the work setting, the host is an individual worker, but it also can include family members of the worker (when an agent is transported home) and the larger community (when hazardous materials from a factory are emitted into the environment). This section provides a brief description of host defenses against occupational disease agents (occupational exposures), portals of entry for occupational agents, and host responses to exposures.

Host Defenses

The first type of defense against occupational agents is known as nonspecific defense mechanisms, which reduce the likelihood that an agent will enter the body and cause disease. Our skin provides a barrier against many environmental agents. Similarly, the mucosal surfaces of the body also afford protection against foreign invaders. Tears and saliva can be thought of as means to wash away infectious and chemical agents. The high pH of the human body's gastric juices is lethal to many infectious agents that manage to enter the body via ingestion. The immune system is also highly developed to ingest, via phagocytes and macrophages, infectious agents.

Although the foregoing examples of nonspecific mechanisms are important in determining host susceptibility, several other factors influence host responses to infectious agents. As we age, the ability of our nonspecific defense mechanisms to fend off agents may decrease (e.g., through reduced immune function). The nutritional status of the host also may be critical because, compared to those who have adequate nutrition, malnourished individuals—who include many workers in the developing world—may be less able to fight off infections. Genetic factors are involved as well, as illustrated by the clear differences in individuals' reactions to a mosquito bite, for example: Some people may demonstrate little or no reaction, whereas others may develop a large welt at the site. Disease-specific defenses include immunity against a particular infectious agent. Immunity refers to the resistance of the host to a disease agent.

Portals of Entry for Occupational Agents

For an agent to cause a response (i.e., an occupational disease or other health effect) in a human host, a means of contact and access to a portal of entry must be present. The agent must be able to overcome host defense mechanisms such as the barrier provided by the skin. Because the skin is one of the most common points of contact for toxic chemicals, dermatitis is a frequent manifestation of occupational exposures. When the skin is cut or abraded, toxic materials can enter the body more easily. Microbes can be introduced directly into the body by injection from sharp objects. Also, exposed surfaces of the skin are vulnerable to burns.

The lungs are a site of exposure to airborne agents—dust particles, chemicals, and microbes—through inhalation. The surface area of the lungs is huge and can facilitate the rapid absorption of inhaled materials into the body via the circulatory system. Long-term exposure to dusts can cause allergic reactions and chronic lung diseases such as fibrosis.

The mouth is a portal of entry of toxic materials via ingestion, as might occur through inadvertent hand-to-mouth transfer; another possibility is that food for consumption might lie around in the workplace and become unintentionally contaminated with chemicals. Chemicals, microbes, and other dangerous substances can splash onto the face of workers who are not wearing safety glasses and damage the sensitive tissues of the eyes.

Host Responses to Occupational Exposures

Host outcomes in response to exposure to agents used at work can encompass both acute and chronic effects. How quickly a chemical produces acute or other effects depends on the site and route of exposure. Among possible sites and routes, contact with the skin generally produces the slowest response, whereas direct injection into the bloodstream typically yields the fastest and strongest effects. Acute responses to occupational exposures—sometimes are called fulminant reactions—occur "suddenly, rapidly, and with great severity or intensity."[16] Examples of acute responses include sudden allergic reactions, poisoning, asphyxiation, and coughing. Other potential impacts (both acute and chronic) of occupational exposures are the following:

- Nervous system effects (e.g., central nervous system depression, brain injury, and nerve function disorders)
- Cardiovascular system effects (short and long term)
- Blood disorders (e.g., damage to the red blood cells)
- Liver damage (e.g., cirrhosis of the liver and ascites)
- Kidney disease (acute and chronic)
- Respiratory diseases and pulmonary fibrosis
- Musculoskeletal disorders

The effects of occupational exposures can be transitory and recede when the worker is removed from the work environment and contact with an offending agent, or their impacts can become chronic. Various forms of cancer (e.g., lung cancer) are examples of possible long-term effects of occupational exposures.

Epidemiologic Research Methods Used in Occupational Health and Safety

Considerations in the application of epidemiologic research methods to occupational health and safety include the selection of appropriate data sources, choice of study design, factors needed to ascertain causal linkages between exposures and outcomes, and the potential influence of bias. Generally speaking, most epidemiologic study designs are observational in nature, which makes it more difficult to verify associations between exposures and outcomes. Although clinical trials are regarded as the gold standard for evidence-based practice in occupational health research, they tend to be infeasible due to their impracticality and expense.

Occupational Health Data Sources

A variety of data sources are used in occupational health research: surveillance data, surveys, worker exposure data, information from employment records, and vital statistics data. These data may be used as information for specific epidemiologic research designs:

- *Public health surveillance data taken from surveillance systems.* "Public health surveillance is the ongoing systematic collection, analysis, and interpretation of health data essential to the planning, implementation, and evaluation of public health practices, closely integrated with the timely dissemination of these data to those who need to know."[17(p. 2)]
- *Population surveys.* Information from workers in a single company or a larger population can include self-reported demographic characteristics, type of occupation, health outcomes, duration of employment, and types of exposure.
- *Exposure measurements.* Sources of exposure information include data that have been collected by monitoring instruments placed in the work environment and by personal monitors (e.g., film badges used to measure radiation exposure) worn by employees.
- *Employment records.* This data source is useful for verifying duration of employment and exposures on the job site.
- *Vital statistics data.* An example of vital statistics data is death certificate records, in which the cause of death is examined in relation to occupational factors.

Study Designs

Cross-sectional, ecologic, case-control, and cohort study designs are the principal observational approaches used in occupational epidemiology.

These types of studies can be subdivided into hypothesis-generating designs (cross-sectional, ecologic) and hypothesis-testing research (case-control, cohort). Historically, much epidemiologic research was inspired by case reports and case series (groups of case reports). "Several of the classic advances in our understanding of occupational disease have begun with a report on a case series, including the observations of soot-related occupational scrotal cancer, aromatic amine-related bladder cancer, and vinyl chloride-related angiosarcoma of the liver."[18(p. 404)] The discussion here presents a simplified view of the extremely complex topic of study design.

Cross-Sectional Studies

A cross-sectional study is a study "that examines the relationship between diseases (or other health-related characteristics) and other variables of interest as they exist in a defined population at one particular time. The presence or absence of disease and the presence or absence of the other variables ... are determined in each member of the study population or in a representative sample at one particular time."[4] Thus, a cross-sectional study is a type of prevalence study in which the distributions of disease and exposure are determined, although it is not imperative for the study to include both exposure and disease—a cross-sectional study may focus only on the latter.[19] Cross-sectional designs make a one-time assessment of the prevalence of disease in a sample that, in most situations, has been selected randomly from the parent population of interest.[13] Cross-sectional studies may be used to formulate hypotheses that can be followed up in analytic studies.

Consider the following example of a cross-sectional study related to occupational health. Researchers in Goa, India, studied noise-induced hearing loss among shipbuilders, an employment setting affected by high noise levels.[20] The study sample consisted of 552 workers (276 shipbuilders and 276 office staff members). Respondents were interviewed by means of a questionnaire used to elicit information about hearing loss, use of drugs that might affect hearing, ear disease, smoking, and use of earplugs. This information was combined with hearing tests and examination of the respondents' ears. The researchers found noise-induced hearing loss in 6% of shipbuilders and none of the office workers. Consistent use of earplugs helped to protect the shipbuilders from hearing loss.

Ecologic Studies

An ecologic study (also called an ecological study) is " a study in which the units of analysis are populations or groups of people rather than individuals."[4]

In occupational health studies, the unit of analysis might be the type of occupation. Mortality rates for a hypothesized occupational exposure could then be compared according to type of occupation. An example would be an ecologic study that compares rates of mesothelioma (a form of asbestos-associated lung cancer) among different occupations[21]—for example, asbestos mining and insulation installing. Other ecologic studies might compare disease rates between blue- and white-collar occupations or between occupations that involve sedentary work versus physically active tasks.

To reiterate, ecologic studies differ from most other types of epidemiologic research in regard to the unit of analysis. For example, the occurrence of an outcome of interest (e.g., a disease, mortality, health effect) might be assessed over different geographic areas—states, census tracts, or counties. To illustrate, one could study the "relationship between the distribution of income and mortality rates in states or provinces."[4] The assumption is made that outcome rates would be comparable in exposed and nonexposed groups if the exposure did not take place in the exposed group. For example, if the outcome were mortality from cancer, researchers might hypothesize that persons living in lower-income areas have greater exposure to environmental carcinogens than those who live in higher-income areas, with this factor then producing differences in cancer mortality.

Ecologic analyses have been used to correlate air pollution with adverse health effects such as mortality. Instead of correlating individual exposure to air pollution with mortality, the researcher measures the association between average exposure to air pollution within a census tract (a geographic subdivision of a city defined by the U.S. Bureau of the Census) and the average mortality in that census tract. This type of study attempts to demonstrate that mortality is higher in more polluted census tracts than in less polluted census tracts.

In the past, ecologic studies have examined the association between water quality and both stroke and coronary diseases. One group of studies has demonstrated that the "hardness" (mineral content) of the domestic water supply is associated inversely with risk of cerebrovascular mortality and cardiovascular diseases. However, a Japanese investigation did not support a relationship between water hardness and cerebrovascular diseases. In the latter ecologic study, the unit of analysis was municipalities (population subdivisions in Japan that consisted of from 6000 to 3 million inhabitants). In analyzing the 1995 death rates from strokes in relationship to water hardness values, the researchers did not find statistically significant associations across municipalities.[22]

Other ecologic studies have examined the possible association between use of agricultural pesticides and childhood cancer incidence. For example, a total of 7143 incident cases of invasive cancer diagnosed among children younger than age 15 were reported to the California Cancer Registry during the years 1988–1994. In this ecologic study, the unit of analysis was census blocks, with average annual pesticide exposure estimated per square mile. The study showed no overall association between pesticide exposure determined by this method and childhood cancer incidence rates. However, a significant increase in childhood leukemia rates was linked to census block groups that had the highest exposure to propargite, a type of pesticide.[23]

Ecologic studies have both advantages and disadvantages. An advantage of these studies is that often they make use of data (e.g., mortality data and census data) that have been collected routinely. These types of data may be the best available sources of quantitative information on exposures and health outcomes for some environmental and occupational health research.

In contrast, a major problem of the ecologic technique is the difficulty of assessing the impacts of unmeasured exposures that may be related to the study outcome. For example, ecologic investigations of air pollution (and virtually all ecologic studies) might be affected by uncontrolled factors such as individual levels of smoking and smoking habits, occupational exposures to respiratory hazards and air pollution, differences in social class and other demographic factors, genetic background, and length of residence in the area. The term ecologic fallacy refers to "[a]n erroneous inference that may occur because an association observed between variables on an aggregate level does not necessarily represent or reflect the association that exists at an individual level."[4]

Despite these drawbacks, ecologic studies are one of the types of hypothesis-generating studies that have played an important role in occupational health by advancing occupational health research. Often researchers are able to perform hypothesis-generating studies such as ecologic studies quickly by using existing data sources. Despite their inability to demonstrate etiologic relationships, ecologic studies may pave the way for the next generation of investigations; the interesting observations and hypotheses gathered in ecologic research may provide the impetus for more carefully designed inquiries. The next wave of explorations that build on ecologic studies then may attempt to take advantage of more rigorous analytic study designs.

Case-Control Studies

In a case-control study (FIGURE 3.5), subjects who participate in the study are defined on the basis of the presence or absence of an outcome of interest. The cases are those who have the outcome or disease of interest, and

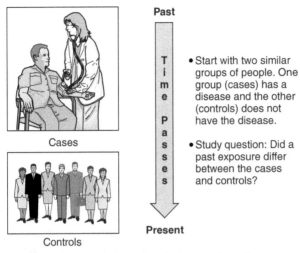

Past

T
i
m
e
P
a
s
s
e
s

- Start with two similar groups of people. One group (cases) has a disease and the other (controls) does not have the disease.

- Study question: Did a past exposure differ between the cases and controls?

Present

Cases

Controls

FIGURE 3.5   Diagram of a case-control study

Modified from Cahn MA, Auston I, Selden CR, Pomerantz KL. Introduction to HSR, May 23, 1998. National Information Center on Health Services Research and Health Care Technology (NICHSR), National Library of Medicine. 1998. Available at: http://www.nlm.nih.gov/nichsr/pres/mla98/cahn/sld034.htm. Accessed July 30, 2008.

the controls are those who do not. In a case-control study, cases and controls generally are matched according to criteria such as sex, age, race, or other variables. Exposure to a factor is determined retrospectively, meaning that the exposure has already occurred. One method to determine past exposure is for the investigator to interview cases and controls regarding their exposure history. An advantage of case-control studies is that they can examine many potential exposures. For example, subjects may be queried about one or more exposures that they may have had in the past; in some variations of this approach, it may be possible to conduct direct measurements of the environment for various types of exposures. A disadvantage of case-control studies is that, in most circumstances, they can examine only one or a few outcomes.[18]

Researchers have a variety of sources available for the selection of cases and controls. For example, they may use patients from hospitals, specialized clinics, or medical practices. Sometimes, advertisements are placed in various media outlets to solicit cases. Cases may also be selected from disease registries such as cancer registries. Controls can be either healthy persons or those affected by a disease that is etiologically unrelated to the outcome of interest. For example, investigators may identify as controls patients from hospitals or clinics; however, these control patients must not have been affected by the outcome of interest. In other studies, controls may be friends or relatives of the cases or be from the community.

The measure of association between exposure and outcome used in case-control studies is known as the odds ratio (OR). One form of OR, the exposure-odds ratio, refers to "the ratio of the odds in favor of exposure among the cases [A/C] to the odds in favor of exposure among noncases [the controls, B/D]."[4]

TABLE 3.1 illustrates the method for labeling cells in a case-control study: the so-called 2 × 2 table.

The OR is defined as $\dfrac{\frac{A}{C}}{\frac{B}{D}}$, which can be expressed as $\dfrac{AD}{BC}$

An odds ratio greater than 1 suggests a positive association between the exposure and the disease or other outcome (provided that the results are statistically significant—a concept that will not be discussed here).

Calculation Example

Suppose we have the following data from a case-control study: A = 9, B = 4, C = 95, D = 88. The OR is calculated as follows:

$$OR = \frac{AD}{BC} = \frac{(9)(88)}{(4)(95)} = 2.08$$

In this calculation, the OR is greater than 1, suggesting that the odds of the disease are higher among the exposed persons than among the nonexposed persons.

Case-control studies are very common in environmental and occupational epidemiologic research. For example, environmental health researchers have been concerned about the possible health effects of exposure to electromagnetic fields (EMFs). A case-control study among female residents of Long Island, New York, examined the possible association between exposure to EMFs and breast cancer.[24] Eligible subjects were women who were younger than 75 years of age and had lived in the study area for 15 years or longer. Cases (n = 576) consisted of women diagnosed with in

TABLE 3.1   Table for a Case-Control Study

		Disease Status—Outcome of Interest	
		Yes (Cases)	No (Controls)
Exposure Status	Yes	A	B
	No	C	D
	Total	A + C	B + D

situ or invasive breast cancer. Controls ($n = 585$) were selected from the same community by random-digit dialing procedures. Several types of measurement of EMFs were taken in the subjects' homes and by mapping overhead power lines. The investigators reported that the odds ratio between EMF exposure and breast cancer was not statistically significantly different from 1; thus the results suggested that there was no association between breast cancer and residential EMF exposure.

In comparison with cross-sectional study designs, case-control studies may provide more complete exposure data, especially when the exposure information is collected from the friends and relatives of cases who died of a particular cause. Nevertheless, some unmeasured exposure variables as well as methodological biases may remain in case-control studies. For example, in studies of health and air pollution, exposure levels are difficult to quantify precisely. Also, it may be difficult to measure unknown and unobserved factors, including smoking habits and occupational exposures to air pollution, which affect the lungs.[18]

Cohort Studies

A cohort study design (**FIGURE 3.6**) classifies subjects according to their exposure to a factor of interest and then observes them over time to document the occurrence of new cases (incidence) of disease or other health events. Cohort studies are a type of longitudinal design, meaning that subjects are followed over an extended period of time. Using cohort studies, epidemiologists are able to evaluate many different outcomes (causes of death) but few exposures.[18]

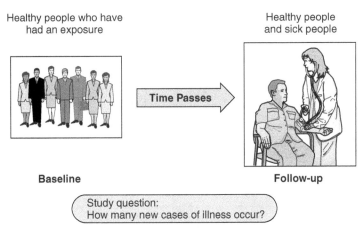

Healthy people who have had an exposure

Healthy people and sick people

Time Passes

Baseline

Follow-up

Study question:
How many new cases of illness occur?

FIGURE 3.6   Diagram of a prospective cohort study

Modified from Cahn MA, Auston I, Selden CR, Pomerantz KL. Introduction to HSR, May 23, 1998. National Information Center on Health Services Research and Health Care Technology (NICHSR), National Library of Medicine. 1998. Available at: http://www.nlm.nih.gov/nichsr/pres/mla98/cahn/sld034.htm. Accessed July 30, 2008.

Cohort studies may be either prospective or retrospective. At the inception of a prospective cohort study, participating individuals must be certified as being free from the outcome of interest. As these individuals are followed into the future, the occurrence of new cases of the disease is noted. A retrospective cohort study (historical cohort study) is "conducted by reconstructing data about persons at a time or times in the past. This method uses existing records about the health or other relevant aspects of a population as it was at some time in the past and determines the current (or subsequent) status of members of this population with respect to the condition of interest."[4] An example of a retrospective cohort study would be one that examined mortality among an occupational cohort such as shipyard workers who were employed at a specific naval yard during a defined time interval (e.g., during World War II).

The measure of association used in cohort studies is called relative risk (RR), the ratio of the incidence rate of a disease or health outcome in an exposed group to the incidence rate of the disease or condition in a nonexposed group. An incidence rate may be interpreted as the risk of occurrence of an outcome that is associated with a particular exposure. Thus the RR provides a ratio of two risks—the risk associated with an exposure in comparison with the risk associated with nonexposure.

Mathematically, the term *relative risk* is defined as A/(A + B) (the rate [incidence] of the disease or condition in the exposed group) divided by C/(C + D) (the rate [incidence] of the disease or condition in the nonexposed group):

$$RR = \frac{\dfrac{A}{A+B}}{\dfrac{C}{C+D}}$$

TABLE 3.2 shows a 2 × 2 table for the elements used in the calculation of a relative risk.

Calculation Example

Suppose that we are researching whether exposure to solvents is associated with risk of liver cancer. From a cohort study of industrial workers, we find

TABLE 3.2   Table for a Cohort Study

		Disease Status		
		Yes	No	Total
Exposure Status	Yes	A	B	A + B
	No	C	D	C + D

that three persons who worked with solvents developed liver cancer (cell A of Table 3.2) and 104 did not (cell B). Two cases of liver cancer occurred among nonexposed workers (cell C) in the same type of industry. The remaining 601 nonexposed workers (cell D) did not develop liver cancer. The RR is

$$RR = \frac{\dfrac{3}{3+104}}{\dfrac{2}{2+601}} = 8.45$$

We may interpret relative risk in a manner similar to the way we interpret the odds ratio. For example, a relative risk greater than 1 (and statistically significant) indicates that the risk of disease is greater in the exposed group than in the nonexposed group. In other words, there is a positive association between exposure and the outcome under study. In the calculation example, the risk of developing liver cancer is eight times greater among workers who were exposed to solvents than among those who were not exposed to solvents.

Sometimes a relative risk calculation yields a value that is less than 1. If the relative risk is less than 1 (and statistically significant), the risk is lower among the exposed group. This level of risk (i.e., less than 1) may be called a protective effect.

Accurate disease verification is necessary to optimize measures of relative risk; disease misclassification affects estimates of relative risk. In particular, the type of disease and method of diagnosis affect the accuracy of the diagnosis.[18] To illustrate, death certificates are often used as a source of information about the diagnosis of a disease. Information from death certificates regarding cancer as the underlying cause of death is believed to be more accurate than the information for other diagnoses such as those for nonmalignant conditions. Nevertheless, the accuracy of diagnoses of cancer as a cause of death varies according to the particular form of cancer.

Cohort studies are applied widely in environmental health. For example, they have been undertaken to examine the effects of environmental and work-related exposures to potentially toxic agents. One notable concern addressed by cohort studies has been the relationship between exposure of female workers to occupationally related reproductive hazards and adverse pregnancy outcomes.[25]

In another example, an Australian study examined the health impacts of occupational exposure of male outdoor workers to insecticides.[26] The investigators selected a cohort of 1999 outdoor workers exposed to pesticides and known to be employed as field officers or laboratory staff for the New South Wales Board of Tick Control between 1935 and 1996. The control cohort consisted of 1984 men who were not occupationally exposed to pesticides and who had worked as outdoor field officers at any time since 1935. Occupational monitoring programs demonstrated that members of the exposure cohort had worked with pesticides, including DDT. The investigators carefully evaluated all of the study participants' exposure status and health outcomes such as mortality from various chronic diseases and cancer. They reported an association between exposure to pesticides and adverse health effects, particularly for asthma, diabetes, and some forms of cancer including pancreatic cancer.

Experimental Studies

An experimental study—also known as an intervention study—is one in which an investigator manipulates a factor, such as an exposure of interest, and randomizes study participants to the exposure or control conditions of the study. Experiments that involve toxic exposures of human subjects are rare in occupational health because of ethical considerations.[27] In contrast, an experimental study used in the health field may consist of a clinical trial that tests a new medication. An application of an experimental design in the occupational setting is an intervention study that is designed to reduce hazardous exposures and improve health in the occupational environment. Clinical trials are regarded as the gold standard for evidence-based practice in occupational health research, but in many instances they are difficult and expensive to perform in the work environment.

Epidemiologic Concepts of Causality

Analytic studies in the field of occupational epidemiology explore associations between exposures that occur on the job and health outcomes. These exposures may be thought of as agent factors in the occupational environment. One of the central concerns of epidemiology (including occupational epidemiology) is to be able to assert that a causal association exists between an agent (exposure) and a disease in the host. As Hill has pointed out, in the realm of occupational health, extreme conditions in the physical environment or exposure to known toxic chemicals are invariably injurious.[28] More commonly, weaker associations have been observed between certain aspects of the environment and the occurrence of health events—for example, with the development of lung diseases among persons exposed to dusts (e.g., miners who work in dusty, unventilated mines). Hill raised the question of how one moves from such an observed association to the verdict of causation (e.g., exposure to coal dust *causes* coal miner's pneumoconiosis). Another perplexing question is the extent to which studies reveal a causal association between a specific environmental exposure and a particular form of cancer.[29]

To verify causality, Hill proposed a situation in which there is a clear association between two variables and in which statistical tests have suggested that this association is not due to chance. For example, data have revealed that smoking is associated with lung cancer in humans and that chance can be ruled out as being responsible for this observed association. The 1964 U.S. government report *Smoking and Health* stated that the evaluation of a causal association does not depend solely upon evidence from a probabilistic statement derived from statistics, but rather is a matter of judgment that depends upon several criteria.[30] Similarly, Hill listed nine causal criteria that need to be taken into account in the assessment of a causal association between factor A and disease B. For our purposes, we will consider seven of these criteria, which are listed in TABLE 3.3.

Strength

Strong associations support a causal relationship between a factor and a disease. Hill gives the example of the very large increase in scrotal cancer (by a factor of 200 times) among chimney sweeps in comparison with workers who were not exposed occupationally to tars and mineral oils. Another example arises from the steeply elevated lung cancer mortality rates noted among heavy cigarette smokers (20 to 30 times higher) in comparison with nonsmokers. Hill also cautioned that we should not be too ready to dismiss causal associations when the strength of the association is small, because many causal relationships are characterized by weak associations. For example, exposure to an infectious agent such as meningococcus produces relatively few clinical cases of meningococcal meningitis.

Consistency

According to Hill, a consistent association is one that has been observed repeatedly "by different persons, in different places, circumstances and times."[28(p. 296)] An example of consistency comes from research on the relationship between smoking and lung cancer, with this relationship having been found repeatedly in many retrospective and prospective studies.

TABLE 3.3 Hill's Criteria of Causality

Strength	Biological gradient
Consistency	Plausibility
Specificity	Coherence
Temporality	

Data from Hill AB, The environment and disease: association or causation? *Proc R Soc Med,* 1965;58:295–300.

Specificity

A specific association is one that is constrained to a particular disease–exposure relationship. In a specific association, a given disease results from a given exposure and not from other types of exposures. Hill gave the example of an association that "is limited to specific workers and to particular sites and types of disease and there is no association between the work and other modes of dying."[28(p. 297)] Returning to the smoking–lung cancer example, one might argue that the association is not specific, because "the death rate among smokers is higher than the death rate of non-smokers from many causes of death."[28(p. 297)] Nevertheless, Hill argued that one-to-one causation is unusual, because many diseases have more than one causal factor.

Temporality

The temporality criterion specifies that we must observe the cause before the effect; Hill states that we cannot "put the cart before the horse." For example, if we assert that air pollution causes lung cancer, we first must exclude persons who have lung cancer from our study; then we must follow those who are exposed to air pollution to determine whether lung cancer develops.

Biological Gradient

A biological gradient, also known as a dose–response curve (refer to the section on toxicology), shows a linear trend in the association between exposure and disease. For example, a linear association exists between the number of cigarettes smoked and the lung cancer death rate.

Plausibility

The plausibility criterion states that an association must be biologically plausible from the standpoint of contemporary biological knowledge. The association between exposure to tars and oils and the development of scrotal cancer is plausible in view of current knowledge about carcinogenesis. However, this knowledge was not available when Pott made his observations during the 18th century.

Coherence

The coherence criterion suggests that "the cause-and-effect interpretation of our data should not seriously conflict with the generally known facts of the natural history and biology of the disease."[28(p. 298)] Examples related to cigarette smoking and lung cancer include the rise in the number of lung cancer deaths associated with an increase in smoking, as well as lung cancer mortality differences between men (who smoke more and have higher lung cancer mortality rates) and women (who smoke less and have lower rates).

Bias in Occupational Health Research

Bias is defined as the "[s]ystematic deviation of results or inferences from truth. Processes leading to such deviation. An error in the conception and design of a study—or in the collection, analysis, interpretation, reporting, publication, or review of data—leading to results or conclusions that are systematically (as opposed to randomly) different from truth."[4] Examples of the many factors that can bias occupational health research include the study design, the method of data collection, the interpretation and review of findings, and the procedures used in data analysis. For example, in measurements of exposures and outcomes, faulty measurement devices may introduce bias into a study. Other types of bias include recall bias, selection bias, and sampling bias (healthy worker effect).

Recall Bias

Recall bias refers to the fact that cases may remember an exposure more clearly than controls.[31] Recall bias is particularly relevant to case-control studies. The consequence of recall bias is a reduction in the reliability of exposure information gathered from control groups in case-control studies.

Selection Bias

Selection bias is defined as "[d]istortions that result from procedures used to select subjects and from factors that influence participation in the study."[4] The effect of selection bias may be to cause systematic differences in characteristics between participants and nonparticipants in research.

Healthy Worker Effect

The healthy worker effect refers to the "observation that employed populations tend to have a lower mortality experience than the general population."[32(p. 114)] The healthy worker effect is a form of bias that may reduce the validity of exposure data when employed persons are chosen as research subjects in studies of occupational health.

The healthy worker effect may have an impact on occupational mortality studies in several ways. For instance, people whose life expectancy is shortened by disease are less likely to have been employed than healthy persons. One consequence of this phenomenon would be a reduced (or attenuated) measure of effect for an exposure that increases morbidity or mortality; that is, because the general population includes both employed and unemployed individuals, the mortality rate of that population may be somewhat elevated in comparison with a population in which everyone is healthy enough to work. As a result, any excess mortality associated with a given occupational exposure is more difficult to detect when the healthy worker effect is operative. The healthy worker effect is likely to be stronger for nonmalignant causes of mortality, which usually produce worker attrition during an earlier career phase, than for malignant causes of mortality, which typically have longer latency periods and occur later in life. In addition, healthier workers may have greater total exposure to occupational hazards than those who leave the workforce at an earlier age because of illness. Differentials in smoking levels between employed and comparison populations could be related to the healthy worker effect as well.[33]

Confounding

The term confounding denotes "the distortion of a measure of the effect of an exposure on an outcome due to the association of the exposure with other factors that influence the occurrence of the outcome."[4] Examples of confounding variables that could be relevant to occupational studies include age, smoking, and alcohol consumption. According to Axelson, "In occupational health epidemiology, general risk indicators of disease such as smoking, misuse of alcohol, etc., often attract considerable interest as an alternative or contributing explanation for excess morbidity associated with industrial exposure."[34(p. 98)]

By definition, confounding factors are associated with both exposures and disease risks and may produce a different distribution of outcomes in the exposure groups than in the comparison groups. The existence of confounding factors may lead researchers to draw invalid conclusions about the effects of an exposure. These factors may bias the findings of studies and add to the difficulty of making interpretations.[35] However, instances of major confounding in occupational epidemiology are believed to be rare.

An example of confounding arises from the possible association between exposure of workers to occupational dusts and development of lung cancer. One type of dust encountered in some workplaces is silica (e.g., from sand used in sandblasting). In a retrospective cohort study, researchers might compare the workers' mortality rates for lung cancer with those of the general population (by using SMRs). Suppose the researchers find that the SMR for lung cancer of workers exposed to silica is greater than

100% (i.e., exceeds the rate of the nonexposed population). One possible conclusion is that the workers have a higher risk of lung cancer than the nonexposed population. However, the issue of confounding also should be considered: Employees exposed to silica are usually blue-collar workers who, as a rule, have higher smoking rates than the general population (which might be used as a comparison population). When smoking rates are taken into account, the strength of the association between silica exposure and lung cancer is reduced—suggesting that smoking is a confounder that needs to be considered in the association.[36]

Weaknesses of Occupational Epidemiologic Research

Occupational epidemiology, as is true of other branches of epidemiology, is challenged by the need to obtain accurate exposure information. In the occupational environment, many exposures occur at higher levels than elsewhere. Low-level chemical exposures that involve a mixture of chemicals pose a particular challenge for exposure assessment. Another challenge is the difficulty of differentiating the effects of exposures that have long latency periods; an example would be a form of cancer that has a long latency period between exposure and development of the cancer. Finally, the effects of some exposures are nonspecific and could be a manifestation of any one of a number of possible exposures, making it difficult to isolate the effects of a particular type of exposure.

Toxicology

Toxicology, called "the science of poisons,"[37] is the parent discipline of occupational toxicology. According to the EPA, more than 80,000 chemicals have been registered for use in the United States, with hundreds more added to the list each year. Many of these chemicals have not been evaluated for their health risks.[38] Occupational toxicology can aid in assessing the safety of chemicals used in the workplace. FIGURES 3.7 and 3.8, respectively, illustrate technologies for rapid and automated toxicologic tests of chemicals.

Definition of Toxicology

Toxicology is defined as "the study of the adverse effects of chemicals on living organisms."[39] The science of toxicology concerns "the chemical and physical properties of poisons, their physiological or behavioral effects on living organisms, qualitative and quantitative methods for their analysis, and the development of procedures for the treatment

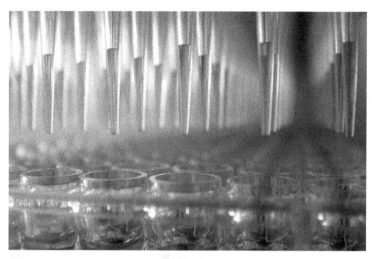

FIGURE 3.7   Rapid toxicology screening methods

© United States Environmental Protection Agency.

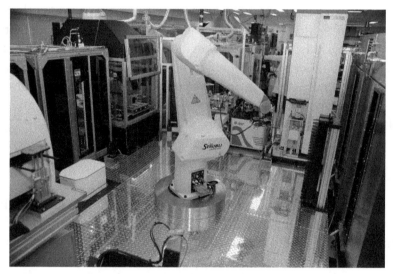

FIGURE 3.8   ToxCast robot used for automated tests of chemicals

Courtesy of the National Institute of Health.

of poisoning."[37(p. 498)] Modern toxicologists have developed sophisticated methods for understanding the effects of chemicals on human DNA (deoxyribonucleic acid) and at the molecular level.

Definition of Occupational Toxicology

The field of occupational toxicology "applies the principles and methodology of toxicology to chemical and biological hazards encountered at work."[40(p. 453)] According to the American Industrial Hygiene Association,

"Knowledge of the fundamentals of toxicology is critical to occupational health professionals tasked with evaluating the risks arising from exposure to chemicals in the workplace."[41] This discipline contributes to the prevention of disease caused by chemicals used in the workplace.[42]

Definitions of Terms Used in Toxicology

Examples of terms used in toxicology are *toxicity*, *toxicant*, and *toxin*. Toxic substances vary in the degree to which they are poisonous. They may be derived from human-made substances or from plants and animals.

Toxicity

Toxicity is defined as "[t]he degree to which a substance (a toxin or poison) can harm humans or animals. Acute toxicity involves harmful effects in an organism through a single or short-term exposure. Subchronic toxicity is the ability of a toxic substance to cause effects for more than one year but less than the lifetime of the exposed organism. Chronic toxicity is the ability of a substance or mixture of substances to cause harmful effects over an extended period, usually upon repeated or continuous exposure, sometimes lasting for the entire life of the exposed organism."[43] Toxicity is related to a material's physical and chemical properties. Some chemicals have low innate toxicity (e.g., ethyl alcohol, sodium chloride), whereas others have high toxicity (e.g., dioxin and botulinum toxin formed by the bacteria that cause botulism). Substances that have low toxicity must be ingested in large amounts for them to have toxic effects; the converse is true of chemicals that have high toxicity. For example, ingestion of large amounts of water (which has low toxicity) would be needed to produce water intoxication. In contrast, injection of only a small amount of highly toxic insect venom may be sufficient to cause severe damage to the body or even death. A black widow spider (FIGURE 3.9), for example, produces highly toxic venom that acts as a neurotoxin (poison that affects the neurological system).

A toxic effect may occur either directly or indirectly. For example, cyanide is highly toxic for humans.[44] In contrast, methanol, a form of alcohol (wood alcohol) that is not poisonous in itself, is indirectly toxic through the action of the liver, which converts it to formaldehyde.[45]

Toxicant

Toxicants are toxic substances that are human-made or result from human (anthropogenic) activity.[39] An example of a toxicant is the synthetic pesticide dichloro-diphenyl-trichloroethane (DDT), the first of the modern synthetic pesticides.

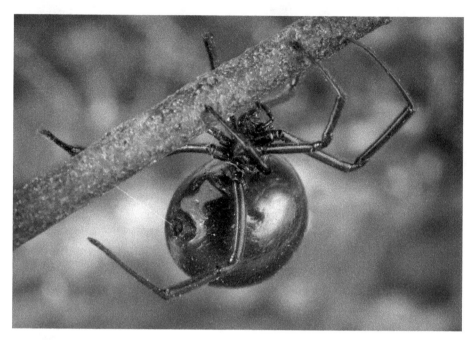

FIGURE 3.9   Black widow spider venom, a potent neurotoxin
Courtesy of James Gathany/CDC.

Toxin

The term toxin usually refers to a toxic substance made by living organisms, including reptiles, insects, plants, and microorganisms. To give one illustration, certain bacteria produce toxins that may act directly on the nervous or gastrointestinal system to produce symptoms of toxic effects. Foodborne botulism caused by *Clostridium botulinum* is an environmental hazard associated with improperly canned foods and other unsafe practices in food preparation. Toxin production by microorganisms differs from disease causation by actual invasion and multiplication of microorganisms and consequent organ and cell damage. *Systemic toxins* are those that affect the entire body or multiple organ systems; *target organ toxins* affect specific parts of the body.

Other toxins originate from plants. There are many examples of plants that are toxic:

- Some mushrooms (e.g., *Amanita phalloides*, "death cap")
- Poison hemlock
- Foxglove
- Poison oak/poison ivy
- Rhubarb, especially the leaves, which have high levels of oxalates
- Some houseplants such as dieffenbachia

Some Important Toxicologic Concepts

Important toxicologic concepts include dose, lethal dose 50 (LD$_{50}$), dose–response curve, threshold, latency, and synergism. These terms are used to describe the effects of toxic chemicals. One of the methodologic difficulties in evaluating the toxic effects of chemicals is that most occupational exposures involve mixtures of chemicals. Experts recognize "that human environmental exposures are not to single chemicals. Rather, humans are exposed, either concurrently or sequentially, to multiple chemicals."[46(p. 111)]

Dose

The term dose refers to "the amount of a substance administered at one time."[47] In practice, the dose often is expressed as a concentration of a substance in the body—for example, the concentration per milliliter (mL) of blood. **TABLE 3.4** lists several ways of describing a dose.

To describe the effects of a dose, toxicologists take into account the total dose, the frequency with which each individual dose occurs, and the time period during which the dosing occurs. When a dose is fractionated (broken up over a period of time), the effects may be different from those that transpire when a dose is administered all at one time. For example, poison that is fatal in a single, concentrated dose may no longer be lethal when the same dose is broken down into small units and given over time. Another consideration in the lethality or other effects of a dose relates to the body size of the subject. Young children, who have small body sizes, are more strongly affected by a specific dose than are large adults who are given the same dose. For this reason, environmental exotoxins (those originating from external sources, such as lead and mercury) at a given concentration may present a greater hazard to children than to adults.

TABLE 3.4 Ways to Describe a Dose

- *Exposure dose*: the amount of a chemical or substance encountered in the environment
- *Absorbed dose*: the actual amount of the exposed dose that enters the body
- *Administered dose*: the quantity administered usually orally or by injection
- *Total dose*: the sum of all individual doses

Reprinted from National Library of Medicine. Toxicology Tutor I. Basic principles: dose and dose response–dose. http://sis.nlm.nih.gov/enviro/toxtutor/Tox1/a21.htm. Accessed January 5, 2014.

Lethal Dose 50 (LD$_{50}$)

To describe toxic effects, toxicologists use the expression LD$_{50}$ (lethal dose 50), which is "the dosage (mg/kg body weight) causing death in 50 percent of exposed animals."[39(p. 8)] One application of the LD$_{50}$ concept is to compare the toxicities of chemicals (i.e., to describe whether one chemical is more or less toxic than another). Other variations of the lethal dose include LD$_{10}$ and LD$_{90}$ (the dosages causing 10% and 90% mortality in exposed animals, respectively). Lethality tests are becoming rare in research due to the availability of less destructive methods of study.

Dose–Response Relationship

A dose–response relationship refers to a type of correlative association between an exposure (e.g., a toxic chemical) and an effect (e.g., a biologic outcome such as cell death). Examples of other responses are intoxication, loss of consciousness, and death of an exposed organism.

Dose–Response Curve

A dose–response curve maps associations between exposures and effects. The curve is used to assess the effect of exposure to a chemical or toxic substance upon an organism (e.g., an experimental animal).

FIGURE 3.10 demonstrates a typical dose–response curve for a population of subjects (e.g., experimental animals). The x-axis and y-axis designate the dose and the response, respectively. The response could be measured as the percentage of exposed animals showing a particular effect, or it could

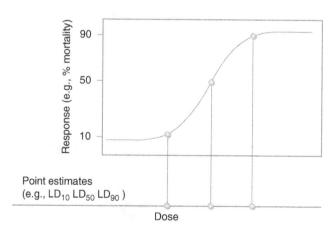

FIGURE 3.10   A population dose–response curve

Modified from Guidelines for Ecological Risk Assessment. U.S. Environmental Protection Agency, Risk Assessment Forum, Washington, DC, EPA/630/R095/002F, 1998, p. 81. Reprinted from *Essentials of Environmental Health*.

reflect the effect in an individual subject. The dose–response curve, which has a sigmoid shape, is also a cumulative percentage response curve. At the beginning of the curve, the flat portion suggests that at low levels, an increase in dosage produces no effect. This flat line is known as the sub-threshold phase. After the threshold is reached, the curve rises steeply and then progresses to a linear phase, where an increase in response is proportional to the increase in dose. When the maximal response is reached, the curve flattens out. A dose–response relationship is one of the indicators used to assess a causal effect of a suspected exposure on a health outcome.

Threshold

The threshold refers to the lowest dose at which a particular response may occur. It is unclear whether exposure (especially long-term exposure) to toxic chemicals at low (subthreshold) levels is sufficient to produce any health-related response. Nevertheless, some occupational health specialists have voiced increasing concerns about the long-term effects of low-level exposures to toxic substances in the workplace. FIGURE 3.11 depicts the threshold of a dose–response curve.

Latency

Latency refers to the time period between the initial exposure and a measurable response. The latency period can range from a few seconds (in the case of acutely toxic agents) to several decades. For example, mesothelioma (a rare form of cancer) has a latency period as long as 40 years between first exposure to asbestos and subsequent development of the condition. The long latency for many of the health events studied in environmental research makes detection of hazards a methodologically difficult problem.

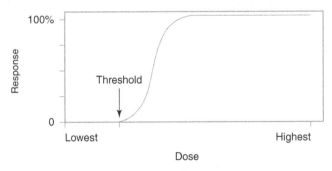

FIGURE 3.11   The threshold of a dose–response curve

Reproduced from National Institutes of Health, National Institute of Environmental Health Sciences, *Chemicals, the Environment and You: Explorations in Science and Human Health*, p. 63. Available at: http://science.education.nih.gov/supplements/nih2/chemicals/guide/pdfs/lesson3.pdf. Accessed October 10, 2013.

Because multiple exposures (often at low levels) may have occurred during the latency period, the epidemiologist may be unable to sort out which exposures are salient for a disease of interest and which are not important.

Effects of Chemical Mixtures

Often workers are exposed simultaneously to multiple substances. Terms from toxicology that describe the effects of combinations of chemicals, substances, and exposures are *additive*, *antagonistic*, and *synergistic*.

- Additive means that the combination of two or more chemicals produces an effect that is equal to their individual effects added together.
- Antagonistic denotes an instance in which one chemical cancels out the effect of another when the two are administered at the same time.
- Synergistic refers to a situation in which the combined effect of several exposures is greater than the sum of the individual effects. EXHIBIT 3.2 provides an example of a synergistic effect.

Workplace Exposure Limits

In most situations, workplace exposures to hazardous agents are higher than the exposures of the general public to the same agents. To protect workers from these higher exposure levels, organizations and government agencies have established guidelines and regulations intended to limit their exposures. The purpose of these so-called workplace exposure limits is to create a safe and healthful workplace.

Occupational Exposure Limits

One group of exposure limits, called occupational exposure limits (OELs), apply to acceptable levels of airborne hazardous agents. OELs are

---

EXHIBIT 3.2   Lung Cancer, Asbestos Exposure, and Smoking

A classic study of the relationship between asbestos exposure and smoking in association with lung cancer provides an example of synergism. Selikoff and colleagues reported lung cancer risk findings among asbestos insulation workers.[48] A total of 370 workers were studied between 1963 and 1967. The occurrence of lung cancer in this occupational group was seven to eight times greater than that expected for the general white population of the United States. It was apparent that exposure to asbestos was not the entire explanation, however. No lung cancer deaths were observed among the 87 workers who did not smoke, but 24 of 283 workers who smoked died of lung cancer, meaning they had a 92-fold greater risk than workers who did not smoke and were not exposed to asbestos as part of their occupation.

"expressed as acceptable ambient concentration levels for chemical and biologic agents."[40(p. 454)] Some workplace exposure standards make use of the terms *threshold limit values* (TLVs), *biological exposure indices* (BEIs), and *permissible exposure limits* (PELs) instead of OELs.

Threshold Limit Value

The term threshold limit value (TLV) refers to "airborne concentrations of substances and represents conditions under which it is believed that nearly all workers may be unaffected."[49] Guidelines for TLVs are published annually by the American Conference of Governmental Industrial Hygienists (ACGIH) for use by industrial hygienists to guide them in making decisions about safe levels of exposure to chemicals and other agents found in the occupational environment.[50]

Biological Exposure Indices

Biological exposure indices (BEIs) provide "[a] measure of the amount of chemical absorbed into the body."[49] "Based on the available information, ACGIH formulates a conclusion on the level of exposure that the typical worker can experience without adverse health effects. The TLVs and BEIs represent conditions under which ACGIH believes that nearly all workers may be repeatedly exposed without adverse health effects."[50] In addition to guidelines for TLVs, the ACGIH publishes information about BEIs on an annual basis.

Permissible Exposure Limits

The Occupational Safety and Health Administration (OSHA) sets standards for the permissible exposures to chemicals in the workplace. These enforceable standards are intended to protect workers against exposures to hazardous substances. Permissible exposure limits (PELs) are OSHA standards that are subject specific and that provide supporting documentation for promulgation and enforcement of occupational health regulations. PELs denote "[a]n allowable exposure level in the workplace air [that is] averaged over an eight-hour shift."[49] This type of average is called an 8-hour time weighted average (TWA). PELs refer to regulatory limits for airborne concentrations of substances, although they may refer also to dermatologic exposures.[51] Specific PELs are established for three occupational settings: construction, general industry, and shipyards.

Odor Threshold

Some workplace chemicals produce odors that can be smelled by workers. "The odor threshold is the lowest concentration of a chemical at which an odor can be detected."[52] This concentration varies from person to person as a result of individual sensitivity to odors. Some chemicals have odor threshold that exceeds their PELs. Hence, the odor threshold is not an appropriate indicator for exposure to potentially hazardous substances.

Toxicology and Risk Assessment

Toxicology is a complex field that makes a plethora of contributions to occupational health. It provides some of the basic data that are needed for assessments of risks associated with occupational exposures. Risk assessment is a multistep process that involves the following phases: (1) identification of hazards associated with chemicals and other toxic substances; (2) dose–response assessment; (3) exposure assessment; (4) risk characterization; and (5) risk management. Exposure assessment is one of the crucial and difficult issues for both toxicology and epidemiology; it includes defining populations that have been exposed to a toxicant, measuring the amounts of their exposures, and determining the lengths of their exposures. The process of exposure assessment is among the weakest aspects of risk assessment.

SUMMARY

Epidemiology and toxicology make fundamental contributions to research and policy development in occupational health and safety. Epidemiology contributes to the field by exploring the occurrence of work-associated adverse health outcomes in the population. Terms used to describe the occurrence of such adverse health outcomes include *prevalence*, *incidence*, *epidemic*, and *pandemic*. Examples of epidemiologic measures are incidence rates and mortality rates. To compare populations with respect to disease occurrence, procedures such as age standardization are performed on epidemiologic data. Age standardization is demonstrated in the standardized mortality ratio, for example.

The two categories of epidemiologic studies are descriptive and analytic studies. A cross-sectional study is an example of a descriptive study. Analytic epidemiologic studies specialize in the etiology (causes) of occupational illnesses and injuries. They include ecologic, case-control, and cohort studies. Results of occupational epidemiologic studies can be affected by bias (e.g., the healthy worker effect) and confounding.

Toxicology assesses the effects of potentially toxic exposures on living organisms; occupational toxicology specializes in exposures to toxic chemicals that may affect employees in their work environment. Among the concerns of toxicology are exposure assessment and examination of the dose–response relationship. Characteristics of exposure to toxic agents are latency and synergistic effects. The procedure of risk assessment helps occupational epidemiologists and toxicologists delineate the effects of exposures to hazards and provide input into policies for the protection of workers who are exposed to occupational hazards.

STUDY QUESTIONS AND EXERCISES

1. Define the following terms:
   A. Epidemiology
   B. Occupational epidemiology
   C. Risk factor
   D. Prevalence
   E. Incidence
2. Provide the formulas for the following measures: incidence rate, cause-specific rate, age-specific death rate, and standardized mortality ratio. Which types of inferences can be made from prevalence and incidence?
3. Three study designs used in occupational epidemiology are case-control, cohort, and experimental designs. Compare and contrast each of these designs and discuss their strengths and weaknesses.
4. Distinguish between descriptive and analytic approaches to occupational epidemiology. Using your own ideas, give an example of each approach.
5. Provide a scenario for how a descriptive epidemiologic study might lead to the prevention of an occupational illness.
6. Describe the key differences between associations and causes in the work environment, giving examples in your own words. Distinguish between risk factors and causal factors.
7. Define the following terms from the field of toxicology:
   A. Toxicology
   B. Toxin
   C. Dose–response relationship
   D. Threshold
   E. Latency
   F. Synergism
8. Compare and contrast the LD_{50} for a substance with a threshold effect.
9. What are some challenges to measuring exposures in the workplace? Describe methods for improving exposure assessment.
10. Using your own ideas, state how toxicology contributes to understanding the potential risks from toxic substances and aids in setting limits for exposures to such risks.

REFERENCES

1. Snow J. *Snow on cholera.* New York, NY: Hafner; 1965.
2. Johnson BL. Occupational toxicology: NIOSH perspective. *Int J Toxicol.* 1983;2(1):43–50.
3. Lewis PG. Occupational and environmental medicine: moving the factory fence or hedging our bets? *Occup Med (London).* 2000;50(4):217–220.
4. Porta M, ed. *A dictionary of epidemiology.* 5th ed. New York, NY: Oxford University Press; 2008.
5. Tager IB. Current view of epidemiologic study designs for occupational and environmental lung diseases. *Environ Health Perspect.* 2000;108(4):615–623.
6. Centers for Disease Control and Prevention. Guidelines for investigating clusters of health events. *MMWR.* 1990;39(RR-11):1–16.
7. National Cancer Institute. Cancer clusters. n.d. http://www.cancer.gov/cancertopics /factsheet/Risk/clusters. Accessed July 9, 2014.

8. Centers for Disease Control and Prevention. Cancer clusters. n.d. http://www.cdc.gov/niosh/topics/cancer/clusters.html. Accessed May 13, 2013.

9. Bang KM. Applications of occupational epidemiology. *Occup Med.* 1996;11(3):381–391.

10. Merletti F, Soskolne CL, Vineis P. Epidemiological method applied to occupational health and safety. n.d. http://www.ilo.org/safework_bookshelf/english?content&nd=857170307. Accessed December 29, 2013.

11. Gordis L. *Epidemiology.* 4th ed. Philadelphia, PA: Saunders Elsevier; 2009.

12. Jo K-W, Hong Y, Park JS, et al. Prevalence of latent tuberculosis infection among health care workers in South Korea: a multicenter study. *Tuberc Respir Dis.* 2013;75:18–24.

13. Morgenstern H, Thomas D. Principles of study design in environmental epidemiology. *Environ Health Perspect.* 1993;101(suppl 4):23–38.

14. Anderson RN, Rosenberg HM. Age standardization of death rates: Implementation of the year 2000 standard. *Natl Vital Stat Rep.* 1998;47(3). Hyattsville, MD: National Center for Health Statistics.

15. Rockette HE. Cause specific mortality of coal miners. *J Occup Med.* 1977;19(12):795–801.

16. *Free Online Dictionary.* Definition of fulminant. n.d. http://www.thefreedictionary.com/fulminant. Accessed December 30, 2013.

17. Centers for Disease Control and Prevention, National Institute for Occupational Safety and Health (NIOSH). *Tracking occupational injuries, illnesses, and hazards: the NIOSH surveillance strategic plan.* DHHS (NIOSH) Publication No 2001-118. Cincinnati, OH: NIOSH; 2001.

18. Blair A, Haves RB, Stewart PA, Zahm SH. Occupational epidemiologic study design and application. *Occup Med.* 1996;11:403–419.

19. Friis RH, Sellers TA. *Epidemiology for public health practice.* 5th ed. Burlington, MA: Jones & Bartlett Learning; 2014.

20. Bhumika N, Prabhu GV, Ferreira AM, Kulkarni MK. Noise-induced hearing loss still a problem in shipbuilders: a cross-sectional study in Goa, India. *Ann Med Health Sci Res.* 2013;3(1):1–6.

21. Hansell AL, Best NG, Rushton L. Lessons from ecological and spatial studies in relation to occupational lung disease. *Curr Opin Allergy Clin Immunol.* 2009;9:87–92.

22. Miyake Y, Iki M. Ecologic study of water hardness and cerebrovascular mortality in Japan. *Arch Environ Health.* 2003;58:163–166.

23. Reynolds P, Von Behren J, Gunier RB, et al. Childhood cancer and agricultural pesticide use: an ecologic study in California. *Environ Health Perspect.* 2002;110:319–324.

24. Schoenfeld ER, O'Leary ES, Henderson K, et al. Electromagnetic fields and breast cancer on Long Island: a case-control study. *Am J Epidemiol.* 2003;158:47–58.

25. Taskinen HK. Epidemiological studies in monitoring reproductive effects. *Environ Health Perspect.* 1993;101(suppl 3):279–283.

26. Beard J, Sladden T, Morgan G, et al. Health impacts of pesticide exposure in a cohort of outdoor workers. *Environ Health Perspect.* 2003;111:724–730.

27. Fleming LE, Bean JA. Epidemiologic issues in occupational and environmental health. In: Williams PL, James RC, Roberts SM, eds. *Principles of toxicology: environmental and industrial applications.* 2nd ed. New York, NY: Wiley; 2000:511–521.

28. Hill AB. The environment and disease: association or causation? *Proc R Soc Med.* 1965;58:295–300.

29. DeBaun MR, Gurney JG. Environmental exposure and cancer in children: a conceptual framework for the pediatrician. *Pediatr Clin North Am.* 2001;48:1215–1221.

30. U.S. Department of Health, Education, and Welfare, Public Health Service, Centers for Disease Control. *Smoking and health: report of the Advisory Committee to the*

Surgeon General of the Public Health Service. PHS Publication No. 1103. Washington, DC: U.S. Government Printing Office; 1964.

31. Prentice RL, Thomas D. Methodologic research needs in environmental epidemiology: data analysis. *Environ Health Perspect.* 1993;101(suppl 4):39–48.

32. Monson RR. *Occupational epidemiology.* Boca Raton, FL: CRC Press; 1990.

33. Burns CJ, Bodner KM, Jammer BL, Collins JJ, et al. The healthy worker effect in US chemical industry workers. *Occup Med.* 2011;61:40–44.

34. Axelson O. Aspects on confounding in occupational health epidemiology. *Scand J Work Environ Health.* 1978;4:98–102.

35. Blair A, Stewart P, Lubin JH, Forastiere F. Methodological issues regarding confounding and exposure misclassification in epidemiological studies of occupational exposures. *Am J Ind Med.* 2007;50:199–207.

36. Steenland K, Greenland S. Monte Carlo sensitivity analysis and Bayesian analysis of smoking as an unmeasured confounder in a study of silica and lung cancer. *Am J Epidemiol.* 2004;160:384–392.

37. Langman LJ, Kapur BM. Toxicology: Then and now. *Clin Biochem.* 2006;39(5):498–510.

38. U.S. Environmental Protection Agency. *Science and research at the U.S. Environmental Protection Agency.* EPA Progress Report, 2012. Washington, DC: EPA; 2012.

39. Eaton DL, Klassen CD. Principles of toxicology. In: Klassen CD, Watkins JB, eds. *Casarett and Doull's essentials of toxicology.* New York, NY: McGraw-Hill; 2003:6–20.

40. Thorne PS. Occupational toxicology. In: Klassen CD, Watkins JB, eds. *Casarett and Doull's essentials of toxicology.* New York, NY: McGraw-Hill; 2003:453–461.

41. American Industrial Hygiene Association. Fundamentals of occupational toxicology. n.d. http://aihce2013.org/chorus/fundamentals-of-occupational-toxicology/. Accessed September 19, 2013.

42. Carter JT. Occupational toxicology. *Hum Toxicol.* 1988;7(5):429–432.

43. MedicineNet.com. Definition of toxicity. n.d. http://www.medterms.com/script/main/art.asp?articlekey=34093. Accessed January 6, 2014.

44. U.S. Environmental Protection Agency. Cyanide compounds. n.d. http://www.epa.gov/ttn/atw/hlthef/cyanide.html. Accessed February 8, 2014.

45. WordIQ.com. Toxicology: definition. n.d. http://www.wordiq.com/definition/Toxicology. Accessed February 8, 2014.

46. Simmons JE. Chemical mixtures: challenge for toxicology and risk assessment. *Toxicology.* 1995;105(2–3):111–119.

47. National Library of Medicine. *Toxicology Tutor I.* Basic principles: dose and dose response. n.d. http://sis.nlm.nih.gov/enviro/toxtutor/Tox1/a21.htm. Accessed January 5, 2014.

48. Selikoff IJ, Hammond EC, Churg J. Asbestos exposure, smoking, and neoplasia. *JAMA.* 1968;204(2):104–110.

49. Extension Toxicology Network. Toxicology information briefs: standards. n.d. http://extoxnet.orst.edu/tibs/standard.htm. Accessed January 5, 2014.

50. American Conference of Governmental Industrial Hygienists. Statement of position regarding the TLVs and BEIs. n.d. http://www.acgih.org/tlv/PosStmt.htm. Accessed January 5, 2014.

51. U.S. Department of Labor, Occupational Safety and Health Administration. Permissible exposure limits (PELs). n.d. https://www.osha.gov/dsg/topics/pel/. Accessed January 5, 2014.

52. Fred Hutchinson Cancer Research Center. 10.0. Occupational toxicology. n.d. http://extranet.fherc.org/en/sections/ehs/hamm/chap3/section10.html. Accessed September 19, 2013.

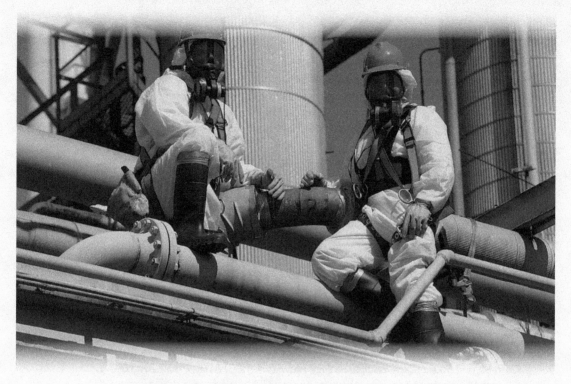

FIGURE 4.1 Workers in protective gear at a facility where they might be exposed to toxic chemicals

Courtesy of Agency for Toxic Substances and Disease Registry.

Many jobs might expose employees to hazardous materials, causing various health effects. Examples of workplace exposure can be found in factories, chemical plants, manufacturing, and automotive plants.

—Agency for Toxic Substances and Disease Registry

CHAPTER 4

Hazards from Chemicals and Toxic Metals

Learning Objectives

By the end of this chapter, you will be able to:

- State three occupations in which workers might be exposed to toxic chemicals.
- Describe potential adverse health effects of chemicals used in the workplace.
- Distinguish between dioxins and PCBs.
- Define the term *pesticide* and give examples of classes of pesticides.
- Describe hazards associated with the use of solvents in the workplace.

Chapter Outline

- Introduction
- Occupational Settings with Exposure to Chemicals
- Physiologic Properties of Chemicals and Metals
- Persistent Organic Pollutants in the Workplace
- Pesticides and Occupational Exposures to Pesticides
- Toxic Gases Encountered in the Work Setting
- Solvents Used in the Workplace
- Chemicals Used in the Manufacture of Plastics
- Metals
- Rubber, Petroleum, and Fossil Fuel–Based Products
- Other Chemicals and Substances
- Summary
- Study Questions and Exercises

Introduction

The chemical industry is a very significant component of the global and U.S. domestic economy as a creator of vital products and a major source of employment.[1] The U.S. chemical industry creates employment opportunities for as many as 800,000 workers.[2] Chemicals are essential to the modern way of life: Without them, contemporary society would grind to a halt.

Despite the vital importance of chemicals for society, the international toll among employees from chemically associated workplace illnesses due to the widespread and growing use of chemicals in industry is noteworthy. The International Labour Organization (ILO) estimates that industries use more than 50,000 chemicals, with 500 new chemicals added annually.[3]

Although many chemicals are entirely safe, especially when handled carefully, appropriate precautions must be taken with the application of others, or else serious or fatal injuries can occur. Some estimates place the annual global number of work-related injuries from use of chemicals at 35 million cases, including 430,000 fatalities.[3] Given the risks to health from improper use of chemicals, the ILO stresses the need to check the safety of newly introduced chemicals before they are marketed. Sometimes new chemicals that have been introduced without adequate vetting of their safety have produced severe adverse health effects among workers.

One problematic issue with respect to chemicals in the workplace is their potential for causing cancer. This topic merits much additional research, as the relationship between workplace exposures and cancer has not been established completely, with the exception of known carcinogens.

Employees of the chemical industry could be at increased risk of adverse health effects from exposures to cancer-causing chemicals. A meta-analysis examined a large number of studies that covered more than one million employees of the chemical industry in Europe and the United States. Interestingly, the authors reported lower cause-specific mortality and site-specific cancer incidence rates than those found in the general population. Mortality from all causes and many forms of chronic diseases was lower than expected. A possible explanation for these findings was the influence of the healthy worker effect.[4] However, weak to moderate excesses in mortality were found for lung and bladder cancer; these effects might have resulted from workers' exposures to cancer-causing chemicals.

The level of societal concern regarding the safety of chemicals for the environment and for occupational health was heightened by notorious historical incidents in which toxic chemicals were released unintentionally into the community. For example, on July 10, 1976, an explosion at a factory in Seveso, Italy (Lombardia region of Italy), dispersed the poisonous chemicals known as dioxins over an area of about 2.8 km^2. Residents of the zone of contamination had to be evacuated. The health effects believed to be associated with this episode included cases of chloracne (a potentially severe form of acne caused by dioxin) and the death of one resident from pancreatic cancer seven months after the explosion. Dioxins are highly toxic chemicals produced as the by-product of industrial activities.

Nearly a decade later, a runaway chemical reaction at a Union Carbide pesticide factory in Bhopal, India, released a different chemical (deadly methyl isocyanate) on the night of December 2, 1984. This industrial catastrophe killed at least 3800 residents of the Indian city.

Occupational exposures and the consequences of these exposures for workers are central topics for discourse in occupational health—especially in view of the wide range of suspected occupational illnesses that researchers have linked with chemical exposures. This chapter covers many types of chemical agents that are found in the workplace, sources of exposure, and health effects of such exposures. This compilation is not exhaustive, but rather provides selected examples of the major categories of chemicals used in work settings. The substances covered include the following categories:

- Toxic gases
- Industrial solvents/volatile organic compounds (VOCs)
- Heavy metals
- Rubber, petroleum, and fossil fuel–based products
- Persistent organic pollutants (POPs)
- Pesticides
- Other chemicals and substances (e.g., flavorings and pharmaceuticals)

Occupational Settings with Exposure to Chemicals

In addition to persons directly employed by the chemical industry, workers in many other fields have contact with potentially toxic chemicals. Some examples are healthcare providers and other workers in medical facilities, first responders to chemical disasters, and personnel involved with cleanup of toxic waste sites. FIGURE 4.2 shows hazardous materials (hazmat) technicians at work as they evaluate a toxic waste site. Such sites may be the legacy of the disposal of hazardous wastes or contamination from industrial plants where toxic materials were used or manufactured.

Another category of workers who may be exposed to chemicals includes persons in occupations such as cleaning and janitorial services, construction, pest control, recycling operations,[5] and cosmetology. For example, workers in nail salons may be exposed to a multitude of potentially injurious chemicals found in nail care products such as polishes and polish removers.[6] In addition to exposures via inhalation, they receive exposure to chemicals via

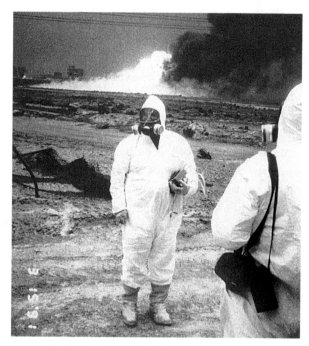

FIGURE 4.2   Hazmat technicians at a potentially toxic site

Courtesy of Centers for Disease Control and Prevention, Public Health Image Library.

skin contact. The workers in these low-paying and service fields may not have employment options other than occupations in which they must work under hazardous conditions and potentially be exposed to dangerous chemicals.

Another possibility for workplace exposure to chemicals is through inadvertent contamination of food brought to work by toxic chemicals (**FIGURE 4.3**). Foodstuffs intended for consumption at work should be isolated from hazardous materials that are present in many work settings. Before consuming foods, workers need to thoroughly wash off any chemicals that might be present on their hands.

A final example of exposure to workplace chemicals is known as take-home contamination of workers' homes. Employees who come into contact with hazardous materials can transport them home after their workday is complete; family members can then be exposed unknowingly. Incidents of such home transportation include exposures of family members to toxic heavy metals (e.g., lead and mercury) and other hazardous substances (e.g., arsenic, asbestos, pesticides, industrial chemicals, caustic farm products, estrogenic substances, and infectious agents). Family members and children, in particular, are at risk from exposures to such materials.

Hazardous materials might be present on workers' clothing (**FIGURE 4.4**), equipment stored in toolboxes and vehicles, and items such as rags and

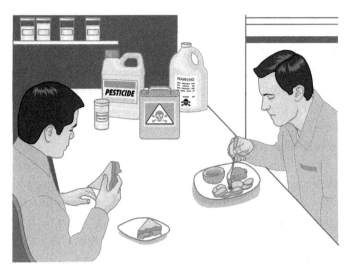

FIGURE 4.3   Workplace chemicals can contaminate foods consumed at work

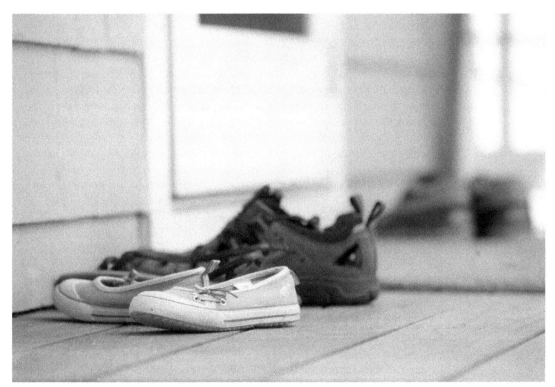

FIGURE 4.4   Chemicals used at work can be carried on clothing into one's home

Cade Martin, 2009. Courtesy of Centers for Disease Control and Prevention, Public Health Image Library.

scrap lumber brought home from work. Also, lead and other chemicals can be transported on workers' skin.[7] Employees who are exposed to hazardous materials can protect family members by showering and changing into clean clothing before returning home. At their residences, their work clothing should be washed separately from the rest of the family's wash load.[8] The problem of home contamination is especially difficult to control on farms and in other work environments where home and workplace have not been separated.

As an illustration of the potential for home contamination from workplace chemicals, the Centers for Disease Control and Prevention (CDC) screened children of employees who volunteered for a screening program at a lead acid battery recycling facility in Puerto Rico. As noted in EXHIBIT 4.1, almost one-fifth of screened children had dangerously elevated blood lead levels.[9]

EXHIBIT 4.1 Take-Home Lead Exposure among Children with Relatives Employed at a Battery Recycling Facility—Puerto Rico, 2011

The recycling of lead has increased during the past 20 years, with more workers and their families potentially being exposed to lead from recycling facilities, including facilities that recycle lead acid batteries. From November 2010 to May 2011, four voluntary blood lead screening clinics were conducted for children of employees of a battery recycling facility in Puerto Rico. A total of 227 persons from 78 families had blood lead tests. Among 68 children younger than 6 years of age, 11 (16%) had confirmed blood lead levels (BLLs) of 10 µg/dL or greater—the BLL at which CDC recommended individual intervention to reduce BLLs in 2010; 39 (57%) children aged 6 years or younger had venous or capillary BLLs of 5 µg/dL or greater—the reference value for elevated BLLs in children established by CDC in 2012. To determine whether take-home lead exposure contributed to the children's BLLs of 10 µg/dL or greater, vehicle and household environmental samples were collected and analyzed. Eighty-five percent of vehicle dust samples and 49% of home dust samples exceeded the U.S. Environmental Protection Agency's (EPA) level of concern.

In response to these findings, the EPA began clean-up of employee homes and vehicles, focusing first on homes with children with BLLs of 10 µg/dL or greater. The EPA also required that the company set up shower facilities, shoe washes, and clean changing areas at the battery recycling facility. Lastly, CDC assigned a case manager to provide education, environmental follow-up, and case management of all children with BLLs of 5 µg/dL or greater. On average, children's BLLs have decreased 9.9 µg/dL since being enrolled in case management.

Reproduced from Centers for Disease Control and Prevention (CDC). Take-home lead exposure among children with relatives employed at a battery recycling facility–Puerto Rico, 2011. *MMWR*. 2012;61(47):967.

Federal laws—for example, the Occupational Safety and Health Act, the Federal Mine Safety and Health Act, and the Toxic Substances Control Act—contain provisions for addressing home contamination with work-related materials. These provisions include making protective clothing, showering facilities, storage facilities, and technical assistance available.[9]

Physiologic Properties of Chemicals and Metals

A review of the physiologic properties of chemicals and metals aids in understanding their acute and chronic health effects. Chemicals may be classified in a number of ways—for example, as "systemic toxins, carcinogens, reproductive toxicants, neurological toxicants, sensitizers, immunological agents, dermatopathic agents, pneumoconiotic agents, or asthmagens."[10] TABLE 4.1 summarizes and defines these terms. For example, a carcinogen (FIGURE 4.5) is a cancer-causing substance for humans and other mammals.

The physical forms of chemicals include liquids, dusts and particles, and aerosols. The physical form of a chemical can influence its mode of exposure. For example, liquids can be absorbed through clothing and the skin and can splash into workers' eyes. Chemicals may become aerosolized and inhaled into the body. An aerosol consists of "small particles, usually in the range of 0.01 to 100 micrometers, dispersed in the air; [it] includes liquid (mist) and small particles (dust)."[11]

Persistent Organic Pollutants in the Workplace

Persistent organic pollutants (POPs) are a group of toxic chemicals that remain for long periods of time in the environment and can accumulate and pass from one species to the next through the food chain.[12] POPs have been used in industry, in agriculture, and for disease and pest control.[12] Among the familiar POPs are the dioxin/furan family, polychlorinated biphenyls (PCBs), and dichlorodiphenyltrichloroethane (DDT). Usually dioxins and furans are not made intentionally, but rather are by-products of combustion; that is, they are generated through burning of waste materials or as the result of certain industrial processes. In contrast, PCBs and DDT are manufactured intentionally. In 1991, the delegates to the international Stockholm Convention placed the aforementioned substances on the list of the most dangerous "dirty dozen" chemicals.

Dioxins and Furans

"Dioxins and furans is the abbreviated or short name for a family of toxic substances that all share a similar chemical structure."[13] "The term

TABLE 4.1   Physiologic Properties of Chemicals and Metals

Asphyxiant	"[A] substance that is capable of causing death from suffocation"—for example, by decreasing the capacity of the blood to carry oxygen.[1]
Asthmagen	"Asthmagens can be divided into two separate types, namely inducers and inciters. Inducers are substances which, on single or repeated exposure, cause a previously well individual to develop asthma. In contrast, inciters (or triggers) are substances which can cause symptoms in an individual with pre-existing abnormal airway responsiveness."[2]
Carcinogen	"A substance or agent that causes cancer in mammals, including humans."[3]
Dermatopathic agent	An agent that causes diseases of the skin.[4]
Immunologic agent	An agent that affects the immune system, which forms part of the body's natural defenses against disease.[5]
Neurological toxicant/ neurotoxin	A toxic substance that is "[a]ble to produce chemically an *adverse effect* on the nervous system: such effects may be subdivided into two types: central nervous system effects…and peripheral nervous system effects."[6]
Pneumonoconiotic agent	An agent (e. g., inorganic and organic dusts) etiologically associated with pneumoconiosis (fibrosis of the lung).[6]
Reproductive toxicant	"Substance or preparation that produces non-heritable adverse effects on male and female reproductive function or capacity and on resultant progeny."[6]
Sensitizer	A substance that causes sensitization, which is an "immune response whereby individuals become hypersensitive to substances, pollen, dandruff, or other agents that make them develop a potentially harmful allergy when they are subsequently exposed to the sensitizing material (allergen)."[6]
Systemic toxin	A toxin that affects the body as a whole.[6]
Teratogen	"Agent that, when administered prenatally (to the mother), induces permanent structural malformations or defects in the offspring."[6]

Definitions adapted from the following sources:

[1] Bert JL. *Occupational diseases.* Cincinnati, OH: CDC, National Institute for Occupational Safety and Health, 1991.

[2] Currie GP, Ayres JG. Occupational asthmagens. *Prim Care Respir J.* 2005;14:72–77.

[3] U.S. Department of Labor, Occupational Safety and Health Administration. Glossary of terms. https://www.osha.gov/doc/outreachtraining/HTMLfiles/hazglos.html. Accessed August 17, 2013.

[4] *The Free Dictionary.* http://medical-dictionary.the freedictionary.com. Accessed November 11, 2013.

[5] Biology-Online.org. http://www.biology-online.org/dictionary. Accessed November 11, 2013.

[6] U.S. Department of Health and Human Services, National Library of Medicine. IUPAC glossary of terms used in toxicology, 2nd edition. http://sis.nlm.nih.gov/enviro/iupacglossary/. Accessed November 11, 2013.

'dioxin' refers to a class of structurally and chemically related halogenated aromatic hydrocarbons that includes polychlorinated dibenzodioxins (PCDDs or dioxins), polychlorinated dibenzofurans (PCDFs or furans) and the 'dioxin-like' polychlorinated biphenyls (PCBs)."[14(p. 219)] The most toxic form of dioxin is thought to be 2,3,7,8-tetrachlorodibenzo-*p*-dioxin (TCDD). Regarded as human carcinogens, dioxins can affect hormonal regulation as well as cause a skin disease known as chloracne[13] (FIGURE 4.6). In a notorious European case, the Ukrainian presidential candidate Victor Yushenko was poisoned with TCDD dioxin, causing severe disfigurement.

As noted previously, the 1976 dioxin contamination in Seveso, Italy, resulted from an industrial explosion. Other sites in the United States where dioxins have been found are Times Beach, Missouri, and Love Canal, New York.[15]

As by-products of chemical manufacture, dioxins are found as contaminants in some herbicides, insecticides, fungicides, and the defoliant "Agent Orange" used during the Vietnam War.[15] Industrial processes such as those that involve incineration also produce dioxins as unwanted contaminants. Occupational exposures to dioxins and furans can occur during cement manufacture, production of ferrous and nonferrous metals, incineration of municipal waste, and even cremation of human remains.[14]

In one study, researchers studied the health of German workers who were exposed to dioxins that resulted from thermal oxygen cutting, welding,

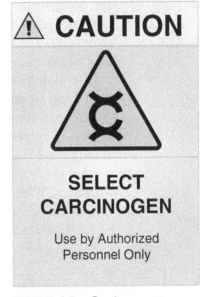

FIGURE 4.5 Carcinogen storage safety label

Reproduced from the University of North Carolina, Dept. of Environment, Health and Safety, http://ehs.unc.edu/ih/lab/labels/chem.shtml.

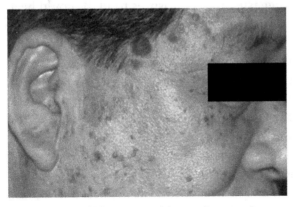

FIGURE 4.6 Chloracne and hyperpigmentation on the face of a Japanese incinerator worker

Reprinted from "Schecter A, Birnbaum L, Ryan JJ, JD. Dioxins: An overview. Environmental Research 101 (2006) 419–428 p 425.

and soldering of metals.[16] A positive correlation was found between duration and frequency of thermal oxygen cutting and workers' body burdens of dioxins. The workers were involved with cutting scrap metals; dioxins may be generated during the thermal cutting of such materials.

German researchers also conducted a review of mortality among more than 1500 workers exposed to dioxin at a chemical plant in Hamburg.[17] Dioxin exposure was associated with mortality from all forms of cancer, especially respiratory, esophageal, bladder, kidney, and rectal cancers, among these former chemical plant workers.

Another group studied 1615 workers exposed to dioxin at a plant in Michigan. With the exception of soft-tissue sarcoma, the evidence did not suggest an increased cancer or chronic disease mortality risk from exposure to 2,3,7,8-tetrachlorodibenzo-*p*-dioxin.[18]

Polychlorinated Biphenyls

Polychlorinated biphenyls (PCBs) "belong to a broad family of man-made organic chemicals known as chlorinated hydrocarbons. PCBs were domestically manufactured from 1929 until their manufacture was banned in 1979."[19] Prior to their discontinuation, PCBs were used as an insulating fluid in electrical components such as capacitors and transformers.

Several groups of scientists have examined the health effects among workers exposed to PCBs. For example, researchers conducted a cohort mortality study of manufacturing workers employed from 1944 to 1977 at an electrical capacitor factory where PCBs were used.[20] The workers were followed between 1944 and 2000. Elevated death rates (SMRs) were reported for some forms of cancer—for example, liver/biliary cancer among female workers who had been employed for 10 or more years. The findings suggested that exposures to PCBs could be associated with increased risks of liver/biliary as well as stomach, intestinal, and thyroid cancer.[20]

Other investigators tracked mortality among a cohort of workers believed to be highly exposed to polychlorinated biphenyls between 1939 and 1977 at two electrical capacitor manufacturing plants. Subsequently, researchers updated mortality data through 1998 for 2572 persons from this cohort. Excess mortality occurred for biliary, liver, and gallbladder cancer. Excess mortality for intestinal cancer was found among women, regardless of their duration of employment. Another cause of mortality among employees was myeloma, whose incidence was highest among workers employed for 10 years or more. Nevertheless, the small number of deaths reported for these forms of cancer made it difficult to reach definitive conclusions regarding the role of PCB exposure.[21]

Dichlorodiphenyltrichloroethane

Dichlorodiphenyltrichloroethane (DDT) is an organochloride pesticide. An organochloride pesticide contains chlorine, carbon, and, sometimes, several other elements. Developed as the first modern pesticide during World War II (FIGURE 4.7), DDT is one of the "dirty dozen" POPs. It was very effective for controlling malaria-carrying mosquitoes and was responsible for freeing much of the world from the scourge of malaria. In 1972, manufacture of DDT was banned following the discovery of its harmful effects on fish and birds, tendency to accumulate in human tissues, and persistence in the environment.

Pesticides and Occupational Exposures to Pesticides

This section describes types of pesticides and potential occupational exposures to them. "A pesticide is any substance or mixture of substances

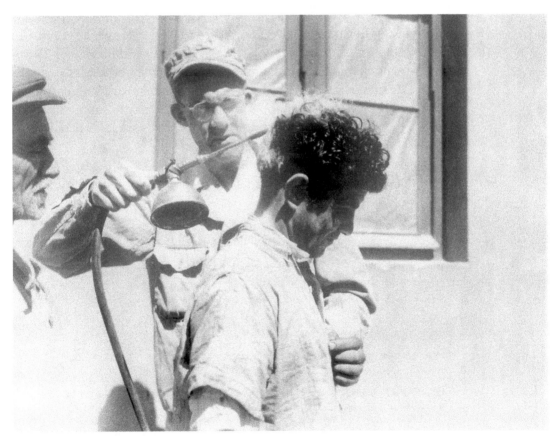

FIGURE 4.7   Soldier demonstrating use of DDT sprayer after WWII

Courtesy of Centers for Disease Control and Prevention, Public Health Image Library.

intended for preventing, destroying, repelling, or mitigating any pest. Though often misunderstood to refer only to insecticides, the term pesticide also applies to herbicides, fungicides, and various other substances used to control pests."[22]

More than 1 billion pounds of the active ingredients in pesticides is used in the United States annually.[23] Many benefits accrue to society from the use of pesticides—for example, in increasing agricultural productivity, helping to control exotic (introduced) plants and insects, and combatting disease-carrying vectors. However, pesticide use carries substantial risk, particularly in occupations such as farming, horticulture, veterinary services, and commercial pest control services. According to EPA, as many as 20,000 diagnosed pesticide poisonings happen each year among the approximately 2 million agricultural workers employed in the United States.[23] TABLE 4.2 provides information on occupations (both agricultural and non-agricultural) that may expose workers to pesticides. TABLE 4.3 lists categories, modes of action, and examples of chemical pesticides that may be encountered in a work setting.

One set of investigations has examined the adverse effects of pesticide use among agricultural employees (FIGURE 4.8). Pesticide-related exposures are associated with some forms of acute and chronic morbidity among farm workers. Among migrant farm workers in California, the main categories of pesticides associated with more than half of the cases of pesticide-associated illnesses are organophosphates, carbamates, inorganic compounds, and pyrethroids. Effects of exposure to pesticides include skin diseases, ocular effects, and systemic effects.[24]

The association between exposure to organochlorine pesticides and thyroid disease was examined in an analysis of data from the Agricultural

TABLE 4.2   Workers Involved with Pesticide Application

- *Mixer/Loaders*: Individuals who perform tasks in preparation for an application. For example, prior to application, mixer/loaders would mix a liquid pesticide concentrate with water and load it into the holding tank of the airplane.

- *Applicators*: Individuals who operate application equipment during the release of a pesticide product onto its target.

- *Mixer/Loader/Applicators*: Individuals who perform all aspects of the pesticide application process.

- *Flaggers*: Individuals who guide aerial applicators during the release of a pesticide product onto its target.

Reproduced from U.S. Environmental Protection Agency (EPA). Occupational pesticide handler exposure data. http://www.epa.gov/pesticides/science/handler-exposure-data.html. Accessed October 30, 2013.

TABLE 4.3   Categories, Modes of Action, and Examples of Chemical Pesticides

Category	Mode of Action	Examples
Organophosphates	Organophosphates affect the nervous system by disrupting the enzyme that regulates acetylcholine, a neurotransmitter. Most organophosphates are insecticides. They were developed during the early 19th century, but their effects on insects, which are similar to their effects on humans, were discovered in 1932. Some are very poisonous (they were used in World War II as nerve agents). However, they usually are not persistent in the environment.	Acephate Azinphos-methyl Bensulide Chlorethoxyfos Chlorpyrifos Chlorpyrifos-methy l Diazinon Dichlorvos (DDVP) Dicrotophos (For additional names, see http://www.epa.gov/pesticides/.)
Carbamate pesticides	Carbamate pesticides affect the nervous system by disrupting an enzyme that regulates acetylcholine, a neurotransmitter. The enzyme effects are usually reversible. There are several subgroups within the carbamates.	Aldicarb Carbaryl Carbofuran Formetanate HCl Methiocarb Methomyl Oxamyl Pirimicarb Propoxur Thiodicarb
Organochlorines	Organochlorines were commonly used in the past, but many have been since removed from the market due to their health and environmental effects and their persistence.	DDT Chlordane
Pyrethroids	Pyrethroids were developed as a synthetic version of the naturally occurring pesticide pyrethrin, which is found in chrysanthemums. They have been modified to increase their stability in the environment. Some synthetic pyrethroids are toxic to the nervous system.	Permethrin Bifenthrin Cyfluthrin Cypermethrin Telfluthrin

Modified from U.S. Environmental Protection Agency (EPA). Types of pesticides. http://www.epa.gov/pesticides/about/types.htm. Accessed October 30, 2013.

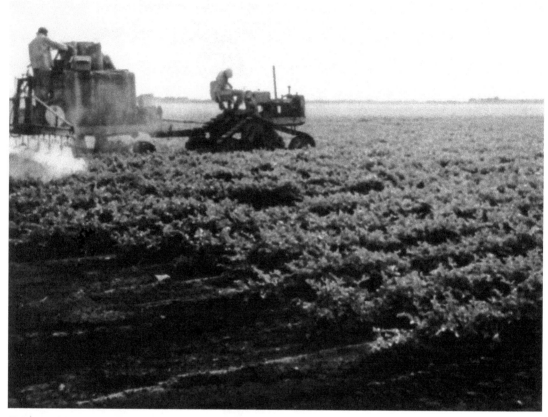

FIGURE 4.8   Agricultural workers applying pesticides

Dick Robbins, 1950. Courtesy of Centers for Disease Control and Prevention, Public Health Image Library/Barbara Jenkins, NIOSH.

Health Study. This prospective study, which was conducted in Iowa and North Carolina, enrolled licensed pesticide applicators and their spouses.[25] Focusing on the female spouses enrolled in the study from 1993 through 1997, researchers explored cross-sectional associations between pesticide exposures and thyroid disease. The results supported the relationship between exposures to organochlorines and fungicides in the etiology of thyroid disease in the study subjects.

Another group of researchers performed a cohort study of 310 agricultural workers (orchard workers) occupationally exposed to pesticides.[26] They found a possible association between Parkinsonism and long-term occupational exposure to pesticides. However, associations of the condition with specific pesticides could not be determined.

Another category of pesticides comprises the chemical herbicides, which are used to control unwanted plants. An example of a chemical herbicide is atrazine, classified as a member of the triazine group of herbicides. Approximately 75 million pounds of atrazine is used in the United States each year.[27] This herbicide targets weeds that grow in U.S. corn and sorghum fields. Atrazine is considered to be an endocrine disrupter that affects frogs and a potential risk factor for human breast cancer. Because of suspected adverse effects linked to atrazine, the European Union has banned its use since 2005.

Among the hypothesized effects of some herbicides are their possible impacts on the human neurological system. Weisskopf et al. reported that use of herbicides by French farmers was associated with psychological depression.[28] These results are consistent with the hypothesis that some types of pesticides have neurotoxic effects.

Reduction in pesticide-related illnesses and injuries may be accomplished through surveillance systems for high-risk episodes. A U.S. program called the Sentinel Event Notification System for Occupational Risk (SENSOR) collects national information on acute occupational pesticide-related illness and injury.[29] The state of California has implemented its own excellent surveillance system for work-related pesticide illnesses.[30] Surveillance systems can be instrumental in identifying risk factors for pesticide-related episodes and designing preventive interventions.

Toxic Gases Encountered in the Work Setting

Toxic gases are a hazard to workers in a variety of occupations—for example, construction workers, welders, persons involved with waste management and recycling, first responders to chemical spills, and gardeners. Some examples of toxic gases encountered in the work environment are the following:

- Carbon monoxide
- Hydrogen sulfide
- Phosphine gas
- Ozone
- Chlorine gas

Carbon Monoxide

The toxic gas carbon monoxide (CO) endangers workers in a broad spectrum of occupations. Carbon monoxide is a "colorless, odorless toxic gas produced by any process that involves the incomplete combustion of carbon-containing substances. It is emitted through the exhaust of gasoline powered vehicles."[31] Odorless, colorless, non-irritating, and poisonous, carbon monoxide is an example of a gas that acts as an asphyxiant.

Exhaust from small gasoline-powered engines can cause the build-up of hazardous levels of carbon monoxide in unventilated areas. Examples of

TABLE 4.4   Sources of Carbon Monoxide at the Worksite

• Internal combustion engines	• Forging, ceramic, petroleum, steel, and waste management industries
• Kilns, furnaces, and boilers	• Space heaters and improperly adjusted oil or gas burners
• Welding	• Fires and explosions
• Molding of plastics	• Cigarette smoking

Data from Government of Alberta, Carbon monoxide at the work site, Alberta, Canada: Government of Alberta, Human Resources and Employment, revised 2009.

tools that use gasoline-powered engines are pressure washers, compressors, and electrical generators. These sources can cause levels of carbon monoxide to accumulate to fatal concentrations within a few minutes. High-level exposures to carbon monoxide may result in illness, neurologic damage, and death.[32] **TABLE 4.4** lists examples of the numerous sources of carbon monoxide at worksites.

Carbon monoxide has a greater affinity than oxygen for red blood cell–containing hemoglobin, which normally transports oxygen throughout the body. The combination of carbon monoxide and hemoglobin is called carboxy hemoglobin (COHb). The formation of carboxy hemoglobin reduces the oxygen-carrying capacity of the blood. Carboxy hemoglobin levels in the blood greater than 25% are regarded as dangerous to one's health.

Workers who have inhaled carbon monoxide may not be immediately aware that they have been exposed to this extremely toxic gas. Certain work environments such as high temperatures, high altitudes, and physically demanding work may increase the harmful effects of carbon monoxide. People with heart conditions may be at greater risk of complications from exposure than other workers.[33]

Hydrogen Sulfide

Hydrogen sulfide (H_2S) is "a colorless, flammable, water-soluble, poisonous gas, ... having the odor of rotten eggs: used in the manufacture of chemicals, in metallurgy, and as a reagent."[34] It is produced by decaying organic matter such as sewage effluent. Poisonous hydrogen sulfide gas is dangerous to oil refinery workers and can result in severe illness and death. An episode of H_2S poisoning transpired at an oil refinery in Sri Lanka. Workers had been exposed to H_2S for approximately 10 minutes. Two of the exposed workers died soon after exposure and, of the remaining seven survivors, several experienced neurotoxicity, respiratory failure, breathing difficulties, and numbness.[35]

Phosphine Gas

Phosphine gas is yet another example of a toxic gas that can be encountered in the work environment. **EXHIBIT 4.2** provides more information about phosphine through case reports of phosphine gas poisoning among the staff of veterinary hospitals.

Ozone

Ozone—composed of three oxygen atoms—is a highly reactive, pungent, and irritating gas with industrial uses that include bleaching and disinfection. When electricity discharges in oxygen gas, ozone is formed.

Ozone, found in a range of commercial applications, can have deleterious health effects. For example, Ng et al. described a case in which workers were exposed to ozone and toxic gases following the installation of new processes that involved ultraviolet curing of print applied to electric motor casings.[36] Inadequate ventilation caused the build-up of toxic gases. Exposed workers reported various health symptoms such as eye and respiratory tract irritation.

Chlorine Gas

Chlorine gas has a greenish-yellow color and is extremely irritating and highly poisonous. It is used in occupational settings as a disinfectant and for purifying water and sewage. Exposure to chlorine gas can result in severe respiratory damage. In 2010, plant employees, nearby workers at other businesses, and customers were exposed to the toxic gas at a California metal recycling facility following the rupture of a metal pressure tank. The tank, which contained chlorine gas, was being recycled. A total of 23 persons were treated at nearby hospitals for chlorine gas exposure.[37]

Solvents Used in the Workplace

A solvent is a substance, usually a liquid, capable of dissolving another substance. By the late 20th century, numerous organic solvents had been adopted for industrial processes[38] and in the 21st century they continue to be used extensively in occupational settings. Consequently, workers in many job classifications have chronic exposure to solvents. Although numerous solvents are in use, this section covers only the following substances, which have major applications in occupational settings:

- Benzene
- Formaldehyde
- Toluene

EXHIBIT 4.2   Occupational Phosphine Gas Poisoning at Veterinary Hospitals from Dogs that Ingested Zinc Phosphide—Michigan, Iowa, and Washington, 2006–2011

Zinc phosphide (Zn_3P_2) is a rodenticide that interacts with stomach acid to release phosphine (PH_3) gas. A great potential for toxicity exists when Zn_3P_2 is ingested and PH_3 is inhaled. Four events of poisoning associated with Zn_3P_2 occurred in veterinary hospitals during 2006–2011. These events were the first reported cases of occupational PH_3 poisoning among veterinary hospital staff members treating dogs that had ingested Zn_3P_2.

* On May 3, 2006, a 70-pound (32-kg) dog that had consumed rodenticide containing Zn_3P_2 was brought into a veterinary hospital in Michigan. Vomiting was induced in the examination room using hydrogen peroxide, and two hospital workers were poisoned. The first worker was a female technical assistant, aged 53 years, with no noted comorbidities, who experienced shortness of breath, difficulty breathing, headache, and nausea. The second worker was a female office manager, aged 61 years, with a history of diabetes and congestive heart failure. She developed shortness of breath, difficulty breathing, headache, and lightheadedness. Both [victims] recovered completely and lost no time from work.

* On March 10, 2007, a convulsing dog, breed and weight unknown, was brought into an Iowa veterinary hospital after consuming an unknown brand of mole pellets containing Zn_3P_2. The dog had been sedated for lavage when it emitted PH_3, and one female staff member, aged 20 years, was poisoned.

* On August 21, 2008, a 62-pound (28-kg) dog was brought into a Michigan veterinary hospital after ingesting three Zn_3P_2 pellets. A female veterinarian, aged 42 years with a history of multiple sclerosis, induced the dog to vomit in a poorly ventilated room. She experienced multiple poisoning symptoms, including respiratory pain, headache, dizziness, chest pain, sore throat, and nausea (and was hospitalized briefly). She later reported that complete symptom resolution took approximately 2.5 weeks.

* On July 8, 2011, a female dachshund, weight unknown, was playing outdoors when she vomited behind some bushes and collapsed. Her owners rushed the limp dog to a Washington veterinary hospital. She was unresponsive and had diarrhea, a weak pulse, pinpoint pupils, and a temperature of 107°F (41.7°C). Subsequently, the semicomatose dog vomited onto paper towels. The owners initially reported no exposure of the dog to Zn_3P_2; however, later the same day, the owners brought in a package of gray pellets, recalling that the product had been applied in their yard 2 weeks earlier. A female veterinary technician, aged 34 years, who sniffed the dog's vomitus on the paper towels to determine whether it smelled like food, immediately developed abdominal pain and nausea. The gastrointestinal symptoms persisted for only 20 minutes, and she did not seek medical care.

Veterinary staff members need to be aware of this occupational hazard and the phosphine product precautions posted on the American Veterinary Medical Association website. Moreover, pet owners and clinicians also are at risk for PH_3 poisoning through interaction with animal or human patients who have ingested Zn_3P_2. Using alternative methods of gopher and mole control, such as snap traps, could reduce unintentional rodenticide poisoning.

Reproduced from Centers for Disease Control and Prevention, *MMWR*, Occupational Phosphine Gas Poisoning at Veterinary Hospitals from Dogs that Ingested Zinc Phosphide—Michigan, Iowa, and Washington, 2006–2011, 2012;61(16): 286-288.

- Tetrachloroethylene (perchloroethylene)
- 2-Butanone (methyl ethyl ketone)

In the past, solvents were often used by workers without the benefit of goggles and a breathing mask (FIGURE 4.9). Nowadays, persons who work with solvents wear personal protective equipment combined with environmental controls such as hoods to reduce their risk of exposure to solvents. Depending on the solvent, the health effects of both acute and long-term exposures can range from negligible, with few observable health outcomes, to severe. Examples of the latter effects include neurologic injuries, potential for carcinogenicity, hearing loss, and adverse reproductive outcomes.

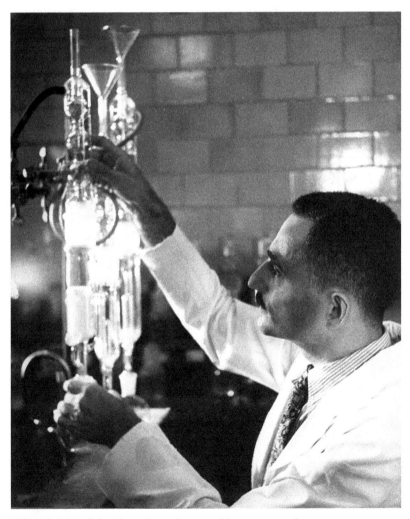

FIGURE 4.9   Scientist using solvents without protection

Perry, 1942. Courtesy of Centers for Disease Control and Prevention, Public Health Image Library/Barbara Jenkins, NIOSH.

Notably, exposures to organic solvents have been associated with persistent and severe neurologic injuries, including organic solvent syndrome. Organic solvent syndrome refers to a cluster of neurologic symptoms—for example, impaired memory, confusion, restlessness, and insomnia—associated with inhalation of solvents.[38] Organic solvent encephalopathy refers to long-term neurologic damage from solvent exposure as indicated by headache, memory impairment, and confusion.[39] An example of a highly neurotoxic compound is carbon disulfide, one of the first organic solvents used by industry. Historically, carbon disulfide was used to work latex gum into rubber sheets.[38]

Use of solvents in an inadequately ventilated workspace increases exposure levels. Adverse neurologic effects from such exposures are highly preventable. Houck et al., for example, linked a case involving solvent-related neurologic injuries with the poorly ventilated basement of a factory.[39] Use of ventilation and respirators could have reduced or prevented these injuries.

Some workers are imperiled by more than one solvent simultaneously during the course of their work. Combinations of solvents are called mixed solvents; they include, for example, the combination of toluene, methyl ethyl ketone, and mineral spirits. One setting in which mixed solvents are used is the screen printing industry. White et al. studied screen printing workers who had been exposed to mixed solvents.[40] High acute and chronic exposures to solvents were associated with impaired performance on neuropsychological tests. The researchers concluded that exposures to mixed solvents can affect central nervous system functioning even though clinical disease may not be readily observable.[40] In another example of neurologic effects of exposure to mixed solvents, a 57-year-old painter developed symptoms consistent with chronic toxic encephalopathy after many years of exposure to solvents in poorly ventilated areas.[41]

Benzene

"Benzene is a colorless liquid with a sweet odor. It evaporates into the air very quickly and dissolves slightly in water."[42] As a result of its use in gasoline and as an industrial solvent, widespread human exposure to benzene occurs quite frequently. This chemical is found naturally in gasoline and crude oil, and as a component of cigarette smoke. High levels of benzene exposure are related to leukemia and other blood disorders.

In the past, benzene was used in Turkey as a solvent in the manufacture of leather goods. Muzaffer Aksoy, a Turkish hematologist, discovered through clinical observations that many patients afflicted with leukemia were leather workers.[43]

In 1974, Aksoy reported a positive association between benzene exposure and leukemia on the basis of epidemiologic research. His work led to the restriction in many countries of occupational benzene exposures, which must be kept to negligible levels in the United States. However, the effects of low levels of exposure have not been delineated fully.[44]

Formaldehyde

Formaldehyde is a colorless, flammable gas that has a distinct, pungent smell.[45] Uses of formaldehyde include the production of plywood, resins (urea-formaldehyde resins), fertilizer, paper, food preservatives, as well as antiseptics and other household products. Classified as a volatile organic compound, formaldehyde also is a known human carcinogen. Volatile organic compounds (VOCs) are "organic chemical compounds whose composition makes it possible for them to evaporate under normal indoor atmospheric conditions of temperature and pressure."[46]

Toluene

"Toluene is a clear, colorless liquid with a distinctive smell."[47] Toluene is an excellent solvent that is added to many products including paints, thinners, adhesives, and gasoline. Exposure to toluene at high levels can affect the brain and neurologic system. However, in one study among workers exposed to low levels of toluene (less than 100 parts per million [ppm]), only weak associations were found between long-term exposures and tests of psychomotor performance (e.g., steadiness, aiming, and peg board tests).[48] The authors suggested that further research is needed. Also, toluene exposure has been reported to exacerbate the hearing loss that can occur in noisy work environments.[49]

Tetrachloroethylene (Perchloroethylene)

Tetrachloroethylene (also called perc or perchloroethylene) is a solvent that is widely used in the dry cleaning industry. "It is a clear, colorless liquid that has a sharp, sweet odor and evaporates quickly."[50] The EPA classifies perc as a "likely human carcinogen." Noncarcinogenic outcomes of long-term exposures to perc may include human nervous system effects, reproductive and development hazards, and health risks to the kidney, liver, and immune and hematologic systems.[50]

2-Butanone (Methyl Ethyl Ketone)

The chemical 2-butanone (methyl ethyl ketone [MEK]) is "a colorless liquid with a sharp, sweet odor."[51] As a result of its ability to evaporate rapidly and dissolve many substances, 2-butanone is used frequently in coatings and paints; it is also used in cleaners and glues. The primary health effects of exposure to 2-butanone are mild irritation of the nose, throat, skin, and eyes. No known deaths have been reported from breathing 2-butanone. Exposed workers often include painters and employees who use 2-butanone as a cleaning agent. Workers who use this solvent should prevent skin and eye contact; they should wash off the chemical from their bare skin should contact occur. An eyewash kit should be available at the worksite in case the chemical is unintentionally splashed into a worker's eyes.[52]

Chemicals Used in the Manufacture of Plastics

Two examples of chemicals used in the manufacture of plastics are styrene and vinyl chloride, both of which are possible human carcinogens. Vinyl chloride is associated with a rare form of liver cancer known as angiosarcoma of the liver.

Styrene

"Styrene is a colorless liquid that evaporates easily. In its pure form, styrene has a sweet smell."[53] Styrene is a constituent of many consumer products that contain plastics and rubber. It is used for the manufacture of plastics, rubber, and resins. Examples of such products include drinking cups, carpets, electrical and home insulation, and packaging materials.

Approximately 90,000 U.S. employees are potentially exposed to styrene each year. High-risk exposure groups include those in jobs in the reinforced-plastics industry, in rubber production, and in settings where styrene-polyester resins are produced. Affected workers may include those who build boats, tubs, and showers.[54]

Styrene can affect the central nervous system, causing loss of balance, a feeling of intoxication, headaches, fatigue, and dizziness.[54] In addition, this chemical is considered a possible carcinogen, although not all research supports its carcinogenic effects. For example, Ruder et al. found no excesses in mortality from leukemia or lymphoma among a cohort of 5204 boat-building workers exposed to styrene between 1959 and 1978.[55] Highly exposed workers had excess mortality from urinary tract cancer, but this result could have been due to chance, given the small number of cases found.

Vinyl Chloride

Vinyl chloride (vinyl chloride monomer) is a colorless gas that burns easily, is unstable at high temperatures, and has a mild, sweet odor.[56] Vinyl chloride

is used mainly for the manufacture of polyvinyl chloride (PVC), an ingredi-
ent in many plastics. Workers exposed to vinyl chloride are those involved
with the chemical's manufacture.

According to the Agency for Toxic Substances and Disease Registry
(ATSDR), "Studies of workers who have breathed vinyl chloride over many
years showed an increased risk for cancer of the liver."[56] The EPA classifies vinyl chloride as a human carcinogen.[56] Epidemiologic studies as well
as case reports have indicated that long-term, chronic occupational exposure to vinyl chloride is associated with liver cancer—specifically, a very
uncommon tumor called angiosarcoma of the liver.[57]

In 1974, the first three deaths from angiosarcoma of the liver among
workers at a plant involved with the manufacture of PVC were reported
to the National Institute for Occupational Safety and Health (NIOSH).[58]
This event evoked intense public and medical interest.[59] One year later in
1975, a total of 29 cases had been reported worldwide among vinyl chloride polymerization workers.[60]

In 1977, Fox and Collier reported evidence suggesting that angiosarcoma of the liver was the only form of cancer associated with exposure to
vinyl chloride monomer.[61] However, later information from the ATSDR
indicates that vinyl chloride exposure may be related to other types of cancer. For example, investigators conducted a follow-up study of the incidence
of cancer mortality in a cohort of 454 male workers exposed to vinyl chloride and polyvinyl chloride. Their study suggested that vinyl chloride was
associated with the development of malignant melanomas.[62]

Metals

Many venues exist for workers' exposures to metals. Consequently, the
adverse health effects of these exposures make a substantial contribution to the burden of occupational illnesses. One such route of exposure
is via inhalation of metal fumes from welding or other forms of working metals. The term metal fume fever (MFF) refers to "a self-limiting
inhalation fever attributed to a number of metal oxide fumes. The [etio-
logic] history is characterized by fever, headache, myalgia, fatigue, and
dyspnoea."[63(p. 269)] Metal fume fever also is known as brass founder's
ague, zinc shakes, and Monday morning fever. One of the most common forms of metal fume fever is associated with zinc oxide fumes
from welding. Kaye et al., for example, described the case of a former
plumber who developed metal fume fever following exposure to metal
fumes after using a torch to remove a steel tank.[63]

One potential effect of occupational exposure to metals is increased
cancer risk. In a case-control study of lung cancer risk among welders,

TABLE 4.5   Examples of Heavy Metals

• Beryllium	• Lead
• Cadmium	• Mercury
• Chromium/hexavalent chromium	• Nickel

more than 2000 individuals with lung cancer and a similar number of controls were examined with respect to welding as a risk factor for lung cancer. Analysis of data collected from Eastern European countries, Russia, and the United Kingdom supported a positive association between welding and the occurrence of lung cancer. This finding was plausible, as welders can be exposed to mixtures of fumes and gases from the welding process itself as well as other carcinogens that may be present in the workplace.[64]

Heavy Metals

A heavy metal is a metal that has a high atomic weight with a specific gravity that exceeds the specific gravity of water by five or more times. Examples of heavy metals are shown in **TABLE 4.5**.

Heavy metals including lead, mercury, and cadmium are significant occupational and environmental health hazards. Continuing occupational lead exposure is associated with hypertension, reduced kidney function, and impaired cognition. Mercury is a neurotoxin associated with the psychiatric condition known as "mad hatter's disease." Cadmium exposure is thought to be a risk factor for osteoporosis.[65] Occupational health policies regarding exposure of workers to toxic heavy metals have not kept pace with new knowledge regarding their health effects.

Beryllium

Beryllium is a metal used in the nuclear weapons industry because of its high melting point and other desirable properties. The EPA classifies beryllium as a probable human carcinogen. Other health effects from beryllium exposure include beryllium sensitization (an allergic reaction) and chronic beryllium disease (lung tissue scarring that affects breathing). Beryllium sensitization was reported among workers at the Nevada test site for nuclear weapons. These workers had been involved with beryllium cleanup or worked in a building where beryllium parts were machined.[66]

Cadmium

Elemental cadmium exists as a soft, silver-white metal.[67] It is found in nature in ores in combination with zinc, lead, and copper.[68] Uses of cadmium include electroplating and manufacturing products that contain polyvinyl chloride, paint pigments, alloys of cadmium, and in rechargeable nickel-cadmium batteries.[69] The health effects of cadmium exposure have been identified as "osteomalacia [softening of the bones], osteoporosis, painful bone fractures, and kidney dysfunction."[69(p. 2)]

Significant occupational exposures to cadmium come from nonferrous metal smelting operations.[69] In particular, one of the occupational environments in which exposure to cadmium can take place is the construction field. According to the Occupational Safety and Health Administration (OSHA), approximately 70,000 workers in the U.S. construction industry have potential exposure to cadmium. Among the high-risk construction activities for exposure to this heavy metal are welding metals that contain cadmium, working on existing structures where cadmium-containing materials are present, having contact with surfaces that are coated with cadmium-containing paints, and disposing of cadmium-contaminated materials.[70]

Another important occupational setting for cadmium exposure is the jewelry industry. Wittman and Hu presented a case study of a young female worker who had three years of employment in a jewelry-making metal shop where she mixed precious metals with cadmium.[71] The worker developed left flank pain and increased frequency of urination. Medical examinations revealed a substantial body burden of cadmium and cadmium-related nephropathy.

In the workplace, inhalation is one of the most important mechanisms for entry of cadmium into the body.[67] For example, workers may be exposed to cadmium by breathing dusts and fumes that contain cadmium during the smelting of cadmium metal and electroplating activities.[67] Inhalation of cadmium fumes can be deadly.[68] When high concentrations of cadmium are inhaled, severe lung damage or even death may result. The metal is able to migrate to the kidneys and liver; the primary target organs for cadmium are the kidneys, where this heavy metal accumulates; such accumulation can produce irreversible renal tubular dysfunction.[69] Chronic inhalation of lower levels of cadmium causes the metal to accumulate in the kidneys. The result may be kidney disease, which may progress to severe kidney damage.[68] In addition, workers exposed to cadmium have an increased risk of kidney stones. Cadmium exposure over long time periods is associated with skeletal damage—for example, osteomalacia and osteoporosis. The condition called itai-itai (ouch-ouch) disease was first noted in Japan among persons exposed to cadmium-contaminated water; it causes excruciating pain over the entire body and, in severe cases, broken bones when victims attempt to move on their own.

The EPA classifies cadmium as a probable human carcinogen.[67] Swedish workers in a battery factory who were exposed to both cadmium and nickel had significantly increased risks of nose and nasal sinus cancers.[72]

Chromium/Hexavalent Chromium

The two primary forms of chromium that occur in the environment are trivalent chromium (Cr III) and hexavalent chromium (Cr VI).[73] "Hexavalent chromium is a toxic form of the element chromium. Hexavalent chromium compounds are man-made and widely used in many different industries."[74(p. 1)] Exposure to hexavalent chromium can occur among workers involved with chrome plating, production of stainless steel and chromates (salts of chromic acid; used as anti-corrosive agents), and leather tanning. EXHIBIT 4.3 presents information on the health effects of hexavalent chromium.

Hexavalent chromium is much more toxic than trivalent chromium. Acute effects of inhalation of trivalent chromium include respiratory effects (e.g., shortness of breath, coughing, and wheezing). Chronic exposure to Cr VI is associated with nasal ulcerations, bronchitis, and pneumonia. A human carcinogen, hexavalent chromium when inhaled increases the risk of human lung cancer. This heavy metal is also suspected of causing complications during pregnancy and childbirth.[73]

Another potential consequence of chromium exposure is genetic damage. Sialkot, Pakistan, is the site where many of the world's surgical instruments are manufactured. This industry employs large numbers of children who have high levels of exposure to metals including chromium and nickel, which are carcinogens. Sughis et al. found evidence of DNA damage among a sample of boys aged 10 to 14 years.[75] Zhang examined electroplating workers in Hangzhou, China, who had low levels of exposure to hexavalent chromium (Cr VI); occupational exposure to hexavalent chromium was found to induce DNA damage.[76]

Lead

Many types of occupational exposures to lead exist in the United States. For example, manufacturing and recycling of automobile batteries may expose workers to lead. Two hazardous components of batteries are lead and sulfuric acid. The use of protective gear such as gloves and eyewear is essential for workers in battery manufacture (FIGURE 4.10).

The adverse health consequences of lead have been known since antiquity, although their significance seems to have been forgotten until the end of the Middle Ages. Early in the 18th century, Ramazzini commented on the adverse effects of occupational exposure to lead. He provided the example of lead poisoning (plumbism) among potters who worked with lead. During the 19th century, awareness of lead poisoning among plumbers and manufacturers of white lead (a paint pigment) increased. In the early 20th century, researchers observed that persons involved with the manufacture of lead experienced adverse renal effects and renal failure. During the 19th

---

EXHIBIT 4.3   Health Effects of Hexavalent Chromium

Sources of Hexavalent Chromium

Major industrial sources of hexavalent chromium include the following:

* Chromate pigments in dyes, paints, inks, and plastics
* Chromates added as anticorrosive agents to paints, primers and other surface coatings
* Chrome plating by depositing chromium metal onto an item's surface using a solution of chromic acid
* Particles released during smelting of ferrochromium ore
* Fumes from welding stainless steel or nonferrous chromium alloys
* Impurities present in Portland cement

How Hexavalent Chromium Can Harm Employees

Workplace exposure to hexavalent chromium may cause the following health effects:

* Lung cancer in workers who breathe airborne hexavalent chromium
* Irritation or damage to the nose, throat, and lung (respiratory tract) if hexavalent chromium is breathed at high levels
* Irritation or damage to the eyes and skin if hexavalent chromium contacts these organs in high concentrations

How Employees Can Be Exposed to Hexavalent Chromium

Employees can inhale airborne hexavalent chromium as a dust, fumes, or mist during the course of the following activities:

* Producing chromate pigments and powders; chromic acid; and chromium catalysts, dyes, and coatings
* Working near chrome electroplating
* Welding and hotworking stainless steel, high-chrome alloys and chrome-coated metal
* Applying and removing chromate-containing paints and other surface coatings

Skin exposure can occur during direct handling of hexavalent chromium-containing solutions, coatings, and cements.

Reproduced from U.S. Department of Labor. Occupational Safety and Health Administration (OSHA). OSHA FactSheet. Health Effects of Hexavalent Chromium. U.S. DOL, OSHA. DSG 7/2006.

---

and 20th centuries, abortions were known to occur among women who were working in industries that used lead; also, lead poisoning events happened among miners in lead mines.[77]

At present, occupational exposure to lead occurs in a number of venues, particularly construction. Plumbers, welders, and painters are among those

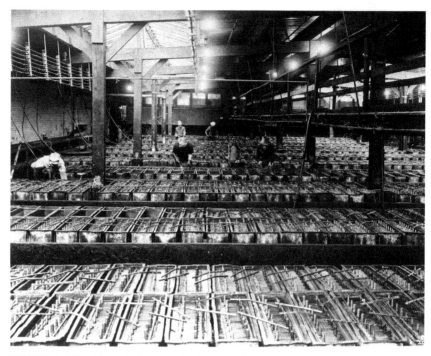

FIGURE 4.10   Historic image of a battery factory.
Courtesy of Centers for Disease Control and Prevention, Public Health Image Library/Barbara Jenkins, NIOSH, 1938.

workers with the highest exposure levels. "In construction, lead is used frequently for roofs, cornices, tank linings, and electrical conduits. In plumbing, soft solder, used chiefly for soldering tinplate and copper pipe joints, is an alloy of lead and tin. Soft solder has been banned for many uses in the United States."[78(p. 5)]

Also potentially exposed are workers involved with lead paint abatement. Lead-based paint remediation workers remove lead-based paint from older houses built before 1978. Not only can the workers themselves be exposed, but they can transfer the lead to their family members. For example, these workers may contaminate the floorboards of their automobiles with lead, which can be brought into their homes.[79]

The International Agency for Research on Cancer has classified lead (inorganic lead) as a probable carcinogen. However, a study of occupational use of lead did not support a relationship between lead exposure and lung cancer risk. When researchers conducted a case-control study of 1593 men with incident lung cancer and 1426 controls, they reported no increase in risk of lung cancer among persons exposed to lead.[80]

With respect to lead exposures and cardiovascular disease risk factors, investigators conducted a cross-sectional study of 497 male workers in a battery recycling plant. They found an association between high blood lead levels and diastolic blood pressure, but not with other risk factors for ischemic heart disease such as increased levels of triglycerides, cholesterol, and low-density lipoproteins.[81]

Lead remains an important occupational hazard for many workers. The use of lead is increasing worldwide, particularly as a result of its incorporation in batteries. Occupational exposures to lead are a major cause of elevated blood lead levels. Occupational protections of adults who work with metals such as lead need to be increased.[82]

Mercury

Mercury is present in several chemical forms, including elemental mercury (a metal), inorganic forms, and methylmercury compounds (one of the organic forms of mercury). Mercury is a highly poisonous substance, which causes mercurialism (poisoning by mercury). The three classical symptoms of mercurialism are gingivitis, tremors, and erethism (also known as mad hatter's disease or simply the hatter's shakes). Occupational exposures to mercury have resulted from mining cinnabar ore (the source of metallic mercury), refining gold, producing felt hats, manufacturing sodium hydroxide, and filling dental cavities with silver–mercury amalgams.[83]

Mad hatter's disease causes behavioral and personality changes, which are marked by shyness, excitability, memory loss, and insomnia.[83] In the United States, this condition was linked to the manufacture of felt hats before World War II (FIGURE 4.11). At that time, the hatter's shakes were common among immigrant millinery workers in New Jersey. With the advent of the war, mercury that had previously been used in hat manufacturing was redirected to weapons manufacturing, which resulted in the decline of this occupational disease.[84] EXHIBIT 4.4 describes a 38-year-old man who demonstrated symptoms of erethism from exposure to toxic levels of inorganic mercury.

Nickel

Nickel is widely dispersed in the environment from both natural and human-made sources.[86] Industrial processes make widespread use of nickel and its compounds in such applications as the manufacture of alloys, batteries and coins, nickel-containing jewelry, stainless steel cooking ware, and eating implements.[87] High levels of nickel pollution and exposure occur primarily in settings involved with the production of goods that contain nickel as well as nickel refining, electroplating, and welding.[86–88] Workers also can be exposed to nickel from tobacco smoke and from fossil fuels.

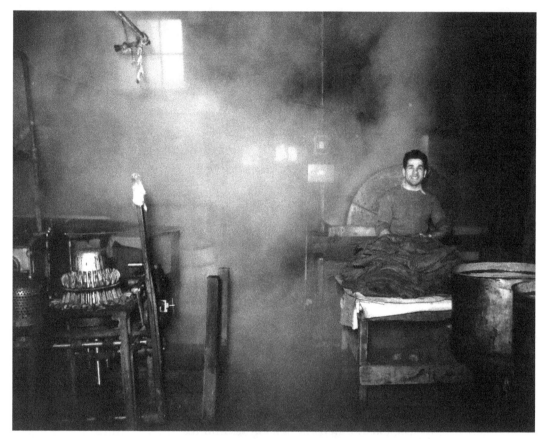

FIGURE 4.11   Mercury exposure in the hat-making industry

Courtesy of Centers for Disease Control and Prevention, Public Health Image Library/Barbara Jenkins, NIOSH, USPHS, 1938.

EXHIBIT 4.4   A 38-Year-Old Man Exposed to Toxic Levels of Inorganic Mercury

In this case study, the worker presented with numerous physical and psychiatric health issues, including muscle spasm, tremor, skin rash, and erethism—the psychiatric syndrome more commonly known as mad hatter's disease. "The main features of mad hatter's disease or 'erethism' are as follows: the sufferer becomes nervous, timid, and shy, blushes readily and gets embarrassed in social situations, objects to being watched and seeks to avoid people, becomes irritable and quarrelsome, with marked mood lability."[85(p. 95)] Over a five-day period, the employee was involved in cleaning a tank for holding phenylmercury ammonium acetate. The worker wore protective clothing and a respirator, but nevertheless developed erethism. Initial symptoms of this worker's condition were panic, headaches, and twitching and shakiness. During the subsequent four-year interval, the employee was unable to resume work due to disability. In addition to having continuing twitching and shakiness, the patient developed muscle spasms that caused falling with injuries and reported lightheadedness and difficulty in thinking clearly.

Data from O'Carroll RE, Masterton G, Dougall N, et al. The neuropsychiatric sequelae of mercury poisoning. The Mad Hatter's disease revisited. *Br J Psychiatry*. 1995;167(1):95–98.

The main bodily sites where exposure to nickel from work-related activities can occur are the lungs and skin, with inhalation being the main avenue for toxic exposure.[88] The principal adverse health effects from nickel exposure are lung cancer, fibrosis of the lungs, and skin allergies.[86,88] Nickel dermatitis is skin irritation from chronic skin contact with the metal.[87] Human exposure to nickel dust and nickel subsulfide (a nickel compound) may produce respiratory effects and increase the risk of lung and nasal cancers.[87] The EPA classifies nickel refinery dust and nickel subsulfide as group A human carcinogens.[87] According to the EPA, a group A carcinogen is one that has adequate evidence from human studies that it causes cancer.

Rubber, Petroleum, and Fossil Fuel–Based Products

Occupational exposures to natural rubber and synthetic rubber, petroleum-based products (tars and mineral oils, asphalt), and fossil fuels (diesel exhaust) have elicited concerns about these materials' potential carcinogenic effects. The suspected outcomes of exposure to them include scrotal cancer and lung cancer. Exposure to asphalt has been investigated as a risk factor for lung cancer mortality. For example, Hooiveld et al. analyzed data from a cohort of asphalt workers in the Netherlands.[89] The investigators concluded that the association of occupational exposure to asphalt with lung cancer was confounded by smoking and was reduced when smoking levels were controlled in the data analysis.

Soot, Tars, and Mineral Oils

Soot, tars, and mineral oils may contain polycyclic aromatic hydrocarbons. Polycyclic aromatic hydrocarbons (PAHs) "are a group of chemicals that are formed during the incomplete burning of coal, oil, gas, wood, garbage, or other organic substances, such as tobacco and charbroiled meat. There are more than 100 different PAHs. PAHs generally occur as complex mixtures (for example, as part of combustion products such as soot), not as single compounds."[90 (p. 1)] Inhalation, skin contact, and ingestion are the primary modes of entry of PAHs into the human body. Some PAHs are animal or human carcinogens.

Occupational exposures to PAHs occur in a variety of occupations. Metal machinists often have exposures to cutting oils and consequently have increased risk of scrotal cancer from carcinogens in these oils.[91] In addition to metal machinists, laborers such as chimney sweeps, coal distillers, shale oil workers, cotton mule spinners, and wax pressmen may have exposures to carcinogenic PAHs.

Research has examined the association of PAHs with injurious outcomes other than cancer—for example, cardiovascular and respiratory effects. One group of investigators analyzed data from a cohort of 7026 workers who had acute and chronic exposures to polycyclic aromatic hydrocarbons in a Canadian aluminum smelter. Ischemic heart disease was associated with chronic occupational exposures to PAHs among workers who had high levels of such exposures.[92]

Workers can be exposed to PAHs from engine exhaust and from working in industries involved with chemical production, mining, metal working, and oil refining, The introduction of protective measures such as splash guards, protective clothing, and showering facilities as well as switching to newer, more refined cutting oils has contributed to decreases in mortality from scrotal cancer, one of the forms of cancer linked to use of cutting oils.[91]

Diesel Exhaust

Diesel exhaust from diesel-powered equipment is a hazard in many occupations, especially when the emissions can reach concentrated levels in poorly ventilated areas such as mines (FIGURE 4.12). Exhaust from diesel

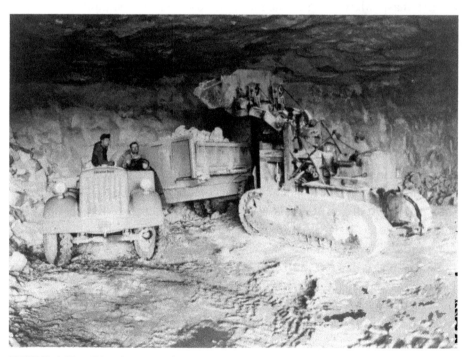

FIGURE 4.12   Diesel-powered equipment used in underground mines
Courtesy of the US Department of Labor MSHA Image Library.

and other petroleum fuels has been the subject of extensive research, particularly in regard to occupational carcinogenesis. For example, Silverman et al. studied the relationship between exposures to diesel exhaust and lung cancer mortality while controlling for the effects of confounding factors such as smoking.[93] They performed a case-control study of more than 12,000 workers who were believed to have been exposed to respirable elemental carbon (REC), which is a component of diesel exhaust. The researchers determined that cumulative exposure to REC was associated with lung cancer risk; they concluded that their finding provided additional support for a causal association between exposure to diesel exhaust and lung cancer in humans.

The association of risk of lung cancer with exposure to diesel motor exhaust was evaluated among 6000 German potash miners.[94] The exposure of concern was respirable elemental carbon. No evidence was found for an association between the REC exposure and lung cancer risk.

Lindquist et al. conducted a case-control interview study of 125 patients with acute leukemia.[95] Patients and controls were interviewed regarding their exposure to gasoline, diesel, and motor exhausts. The results suggested that exposure to petroleum products such as fuels and exhaust was related to the development of acute leukemia.

Other Chemicals and Substances

Additional chemically associated occupational hazards include arsenic, flavorings used in the food industry, and antineoplastic (cancer treatment) drugs and pharmaceuticals. Arsenic is a dangerous substance because of its carcinogenic properties; occupational exposures to arsenic may occur, for example, in the cutting of wood that has been treated with arsenic wood preservatives and the smelting of metals. Food industry workers exposed to flavorings used in foods are thought to be at increased risk of pulmonary diseases. Occupational exposures to pharmaceuticals have been linked to a plethora of health hazards, including cancer, allergic reactions, hormone disruption, and genetic damage.

Arsenic

"Arsenic is a naturally occurring element that is widely distributed in the Earth's crust"[96(p. 1)] and is toxic to humans. Frequently called a metal, arsenic is more correctly referred to as a metalloid, because it has the properties of both a metal and a nonmetal. The most common form of arsenic, called inorganic arsenic, is found in combination with other elements such as oxygen, chlorine, and sulfur. Organic arsenic is arsenic joined with carbon and hydrogen.

Ingestion of low levels of inorganic arsenic over long time periods is associated with melanosis, a condition in which the skin darkens and lesions appear on the soles of the feet and palms of the hands. Inorganic arsenic is classified as a known human carcinogen associated with increased risk of liver, bladder, and lung cancer. Occupational exposure to arsenic may potentially occur during smelting of copper or lead, while treating woods, or during use of arsenic-containing pesticides.

Although inhaled arsenic in occupational settings is a risk factor for lung cancer, less is known about the relationship between arsenic exposure and skin cancer. A case-control study of 618 incident cases of non-melanoma skin cancer (NMSC) found that exposure to sunlight in combination with arsenic exposure may increase the risk of NMSC.[97]

Diacetyl Flavorings Used in the Food Industry

Diacetyl, a flavoring used by the food industry, is a natural by-product of fermentation and is also synthesized by chemical manufacturers. This substance imparts a distinctive buttery flavor to a variety of food products, including microwave popcorn, snack foods, candies, baked goods, and pet foods.[98]

Employees exposed to diacetyl have an increased risk of developing obliterative bronchiolitis (OB), also called bronchiolitis obliterans (BO) or popcorn lung. OB is "a rare, irreversible form of fixed obstructive lung disease, [which] has been identified in workers exposed to flavoring chemicals while working in the microwave-popcorn and flavoring-manufacturing industries."[99] [(p. 305)] Workers who develop OB can become disabled by this condition. In addition, OB can become life threatening, such that severely affected patients require lung transplants. Because of this condition's rarity, some workers who have OB may have been misdiagnosed with other conditions such as asthma, bronchitis, or emphysema.[98]

In 2000, eight former employees of a microwave popcorn facility with OB became known to the CDC. These and subsequent additional cases apparently were exposed to microwave popcorn flavorings and diacetyl.[100] In California, two cases of bronchiolitis obliterans occurred among flavorings workers exposed to diacetyl during the period of 2004 through 2007.[101] From 2008 through 2012, the CDC recorded two cases of OB among workers exposed to flavorings in a small coffee-processing facility in Texas.[99] EXHIBIT 4.5 describes one of these cases in more detail.

> **EXHIBIT 4.5   Obliterative Bronchiolitis in a Coffee-Processing Facility—Texas, 2008–2012**
>
> In October 2007, a nonsmoking, previously healthy Hispanic woman aged 34 years began work at the coffee-processing facility. Initially hired to work in the quality control laboratory, after 3 months she moved briefly to housekeeping, and then to the flavoring room. There, whole roasted coffee beans were mixed with liquid flavorings in an open process, ground, and packaged. Her primary tasks included operating the grinding and packing machines for these flavored coffee beans. After 1 year in this room, in January 2009, she transferred to a similar job in the unflavored coffee area, and in October 2011, she was dismissed. The woman first sought care in November 2008, approximately 1 year after beginning work at the facility. She reported cough, shortness of breath on exertion, and occasional wheezing, which did not improve when away from work. Additional concerns included fatigue, throat dryness, constant thirst, and vertigo. Initial lung function testing showed severe obstruction responsive to bronchodilators.... . She was hospitalized, and upon discharge was placed on antihistamines, inhaled steroids, and bronchodilators for possible asthma.
>
> Despite initial improvement, 1 year later the woman visited a pulmonologist, describing worsening symptoms. Workup included repeat lung function testing, which demonstrated a worsening obstructive defect. Inspiratory and expiratory high-resolution computed tomography (HRCT) of the chest showed diffuse bronchial wall thickening, a prominent mosaic pattern, mild cylindrical bronchiectasis, and a small amount of fibrotic upper lobe scarring. Although inhaled steroids and mucus clearance therapy improved her cough, her dyspnea continued to worsen; an open lung biopsy was performed, which revealed constrictive bronchiolitis (the histopathologic correlate of obliterative bronchiolitis) with both narrowed and obliterated airways with surrounding fibrous tissue and a variable mixed chronic inflammatory cell infiltrate. Based on this result, she received a diagnosis of obliterative bronchiolitis.
>
> At the patient's most recent evaluation in April 2012, she continued to describe symptoms of severe shortness of breath with even light exertion, paroxysmal cough, and an inability to tolerate smells. Lung function testing at that time showed continued air trapping and severe obstruction marginally responsive to bronchodilators, and HRCT demonstrated disease progression. The patient currently is awaiting a lung transplant.
>
> Reproduced from Centers for Disease Control and Prevention (CDC). Obliterative bronchiolitis in workers in a coffee-processing facility–Texas, 2008-2012. *MMWR.* 2013;62(16):305.

Antineoplastic Drugs/Pharmaceuticals

In a classic 1947 paper, Watrous wrote, "In recent years the pharmaceutical industry has come to occupy a unique position in regard to problems of industrial hygiene and toxicology; practically no other single commercial enterprise presents such a wide variety of potentially toxic exposures or such a rapidly-changing advent of new chemical substances."[102(p. 111)]

Pharmaceutical compounding is the preparation of customized medications requested by healthcare providers. Compounding pharmacists can be exposed to the following types of hazardous medications: antineoplastic agents (anticancer drugs), hormone medications, and antibiotics. Antineoplastic drugs have been associated with congenital malformations, nausea, and allergic reactions. Exposure to hormones can be associated with abnormal menstruation, testicular dysfunction, and masculinization or feminization of exposed workers.[103] Exposure to antibiotics may cause serious allergic reactions.

An antineoplastic drug is used in cancer chemotherapy. Stücker et al. studied the effects of exposure to antineoplastic drugs among female nurses who worked with these compounds.[104] These authors reported an association of spontaneous abortions with antineoplastic drugs among exposed female nurses.

According to OSHA, "Worker exposure to hazardous drugs has been identified by OSHA as a problem of increasing health concern. Preparation, administration, manufacturing, and disposal of hazardous medications may expose hundreds of thousands of workers, principally in healthcare facilities and the pharmaceutical industry, to potentially significant workplace levels of these chemicals."[105] The potential health effects of exposure to hazardous medications include birth defects, cancer, damage to organs, disruption of fertility, and genetic harm.

SUMMARY

Workers in many fields are exposed to potentially hazardous chemicals during the course of their employment. Also, employees who come into contact with such chemicals may unknowingly transport them home and expose family members. Classes of dangerous chemicals include persistent organic pollutants (POPs), polycyclic aromatic hydrocarbons (PAHs), and volatile organic compounds (VOCs). Among their various forms, chemical hazards may be present as liquids, aerosols, and gases. Chemicals may act as asphyxiants and have other adverse physiologic properties. Dioxin, an extremely toxic material, is a POP, as are polychlorinated biphenyls. Formaldehyde, classified as a VOC, is considered to be a human carcinogen. Perchloroethylene, a solvent used in the dry cleaning industry, produces neurologic effects and unconsciousness when present in high concentrations. Toxic gases encountered at work include carbon monoxide, hydrogen sulfide, and phosphine.

Another group of hazardous materials found in the work environment are toxic metals (e.g., lead and mercury) and elements (e.g., arsenic). Some heavy metals are directly toxic, others are carcinogenic, and still others are associated with adverse health outcomes such as metal fume fever. Examples of miscellaneous occupational exposures to hazardous substances include contact with flavorings used in foods (e.g., popcorn flavoring, the cause of popcorn lung) and contact with pharmaceuticals (e.g., antineoplastic drugs), as in the case of healthcare workers.

STUDY QUESTIONS AND EXERCISES

1. Define the following terms:
   A. Pesticide
   B. Solvent
   C. Heavy metal
   D. Volatile organic compound
   E. Polychlorinated biphenyls
2. What is the significance for occupational health of notorious releases of chemicals (for example, in Seveso, Italy, and Bhopal, India) into the community?
3. Give five examples of categories of chemicals used in the workplace. Describe three possible modes of occupational exposure to these chemicals.
4. Give the names of two pesticides used in agriculture and describe how workers might be exposed to these pesticides. What are possible health effects of pesticide exposure?
5. State and define five physiologic properties of chemicals.
6. What is meant by the term *carcinogen*? Give an example of a chemical carcinogen.
7. Name two or more occupations that might involve exposures to toxic heavy metals. Under which circumstances might workers unintentionally transport toxic heavy metals into their homes?
8. What are two examples of toxic gases used in occupational settings?
9. Toxic chemicals can present hazards to employees in the food and pharmaceutical industries. Provide an example of an exposure associated with obliterative bronchiolitis (OB) and describe potential long-term sequelae of this condition. Name three possible adverse health outcomes that have been associated with workers' exposures to pharmaceuticals and antineoplastic drugs.
10. Give two examples of how workers can be exposed to diesel exhaust. Describe two potential health effects of such exposure.

REFERENCES

1. Collins JJ. Workplace hazards in the chemical industry. In: Friis RH, ed. *The Praeger handbook of environmental health*. Vol. 4. Santa Barbara, CA: Praeger; 2012:1–20.
2. American Chemistry Council. Jobs in chemistry. n.d. http://www.americanchemistry.com/jobs. Accessed October 13, 2013.
3. International Labour Organization. New chemicals, old risks: why careful monitoring must be maintained. n.d. http://www.ilo.org/global/about-the-ilo/newsroom/news/WCMS_075502/lang--en/index.htm. Accessed October 15, 2013.
4. Greenberg RS, Mandel JS, Pastides H, et al. A meta-analysis of cohort studies describing mortality and cancer incidence among chemical workers in the United States and Western Europe. *Epidemiology*. 2001;12(6):727–740.
5. Schecter A, Colacino JA, Harris TR, et al. A newly recognized occupational hazard for US electronic recycling facility workers: polybrominated diphenyl ethers. *J Occup Environ Med*. 2009;51:435–440.

6. U.S. Department of Labor, Occupational Safety and Health Administration (OSHA). *Stay healthy and safe while giving manicures and pedicures: a guide for nail salon workers.* OSHA 3542-05-2012. n.d.

7. Centers for Disease Control and Prevention, National Institute for Occupational Safety and Health (NIOSH). *Protect your family: reduce contamination at home.* DHHS (NIOSH) Publication No. 97-125. n.d.

8. Agency for Toxic Substances and Disease Registry (ATSDR). *How to reduce your exposure to chemicals at home, work, and play.* Atlanta, GA: ATSDR; n.d.

9. Centers for Disease Control and Prevention. Take-home lead exposure among children with relatives employed at a battery recycling facility—Puerto Rico, 2011. *MMWR.* 2012;61(47):967–970.

10. Centers for Disease Control and Prevention, National Institute for Occupational Safety and Health. Chemical safety. http://www.cdc.gov/niosh/topics/chemical-safety/. Accessed October 15, 2013.

11. U.S. National Library of Medicine. Haz-map glossary. n.d. http://hazmap.nlm.nih.gov /glossary. Accessed January 10, 2014.

12. U.S. Environmental Protection Agency. Persistent organic pollutants: a global issue, a global response. n.d. http://www.epa.gov/international/toxics/pop.html. Accessed October 24, 2013.

13. U.S. Environmental Protection Agency. Dioxins and furans. n.d. http://www.epa. gov/osw/hazard/wastemin/minimize/factshts/dioxfura.pdf. Accessed September 24, 2013.

14. Davy CW. Legislation with respect to dioxins in the workplace. *Environ Int.* 2004;30:219–233.

15. Schecter A, Birnbaum L, Ryan JJ, Constable JD. Dioxins: an overview. *Environ Res.* 2006;101:419–428.

16. Menzel HM, Bolm-Audorff U, Turcer E, et al. Occupational exposure to dioxins by thermal oxygen cutting, welding, and soldering of metals. *Environ Health Perspect.* 1998;106(suppl 2):715–722.

17. Manuwald U, Garrido MV, Berger J, et al. Mortality study of chemical workers exposed to dioxins: follow-up 23 years after chemical plant closure. *Occup Environ Med.* 2012;69:636–642.

18. Collins JJ, Bodner K, Aylward LL, et al. Mortality rates among trichlorophenol workers with exposure to 2,3,7,8-tetrachlorodibenzo-*p*-dioxin. *Am J Epidemiol.* 2009;170:501–506.

19. U.S. Environmental Protection Agency. Polychlorinated biphenyl (PCB). n.d. http:// www.epa.gov/osw/hazard/tsd/pcbs/about.htm. Accessed January 10, 2014.

20. Mallin K, McCann K, D'Aloisio A, et al. Cohort mortality study of capacitor manufacturing workers, 1944–2000. *J Occup Environ Med.* 2004;46(6):565–576.

21. Prince MM, Hein MJ, Ruder AM, et al. Update: cohort mortality study of workers highly exposed to polychlorinated biphenyls (PCBs) during the manufacture of electrical capacitors, 1940–1998. *Environ Health.* 2006;5:13.

22. U.S. Environmental Protection Agency. About pesticides. n.d. http://www.epa.gov /pesticides/about/index.htm. Accessed November 1, 2013.

23. Centers for Disease Control and Prevention, National Institute for Occupational Safety and Health. Pesticide illness and injury surveillance. n.d. http://www.cdc.gov /niosh/topics/pesticides/. Accessed January 9, 2014.

24. Das R, Steege A, Baron S, et al. Pesticide-related illness among migrant farm workers in the United States. *Int J Occup Environ Health.* 2001;7:303–312.

25. Goldner WS, Sandler DP, Yu F, et al. Pesticide use and thyroid disease among women in the Agricultural Health Study. *Am J Epidemiol.* 2010;171:450–464.

26. Engel LS, Checkoway H, Keifer MC, et al. Parkinsonism and occupational exposure to pesticides. *Occup Environ Med.* 2001;58:582–589.

27. Breast Cancer Fund. Triazine herbicides (atrazine). n.d. http://www.breastcancerfund.org/clear-science/radiation-chemicals-and-breast-cancer/pesticides.html. Accessed January 9, 2014.

28. Weisskopf MG, Moisan F, Tzourio C, et al. Pesticide exposure and depression among agricultural workers in France. *Am J Epidemiol.* 2013;178(7):1051–1058.

29. Centers for Disease Control and Prevention, National Institute for Occupational Safety and Health. Pesticide illness and injury surveillance: SENSOR-Pesticides program. n.d. http://www.cdc.gov/niosh/topics/pesticides/overview.html. Accessed August 12, 2013.

30. Ordin DL. Editorial: surveillance for pesticide-related illness—lessons from California. *Am J Public Health.* 1995;85(6):762–763.

31. U.S. Department of Labor. Occupational Safety and Health Administration. Glossary of terms. n.d. https://www.osha.gov/doc/outreachtraining/htmlfiles/hazglos.html. Accessed August 17, 2013.

32. Centers for Disease Control and Prevention, National Institute for Occupational Safety and Health. Carbon monoxide hazards from small gasoline powered engines. n.d. http://www.cdc.gov/niosh/topics/co/. Accessed September 2, 2013

33. Government of Alberta. *Carbon monoxide at the work site.* Alberta, Canada: Government of Alberta, Human Resources and Employment; 2009.

34. Thefreedictionary.com. Hydrogen sulfide. n.d. http://www.thefreedictionary.com/p/hydrogen%20sulfide. Accessed January 8, 2014.

35. Shivanthan MC, Perera H, Jayasinghe S, et al. Hydrogen sulfide inhalational toxicity at a petroleum refinery in Sri Lanka: a case series of seven survivors following an industrial accident and a brief review of medical literature. *J Occup Med Toxicol.* 2013;8:9.

36. Ng TP, Tsin TW, O'Kelly FJ. An outbreak of illness after occupational exposure to ozone and acid chlorides. *Br J Ind Med.* 1985;42:686–690.

37. Centers for Disease Control and Prevention. Chlorine gas exposure at a metal recycling facility—California, 2010. *MMWR.* 2011;60(28):951–954.

38. Spurgeon A. Watching paint dry: organic solvent syndrome in late-twentieth-century Britain. *Med Hist.* 2006;50:167–188.

39. Houck P, Nebel D, Milham S. Organic solvent encephalopathy: an old hazard revisited. *Am J Ind Med.* 1992;22:109–115.

40. White RF, Proctor SP, Echeverria D, et al. Neurobehavioral effects of acute and chronic mixed-solvent exposure in the screen printing industry. *Am J Ind Med.* 1995;28:221–231.

41. Feldman RG, Ratner MH, Ptak T. Chronic toxic encephalopathy in a painter exposed to mixed solvents. *Environ Health Perspect.* 1999;107(5):417–422.

42. Agency for Toxic Substances and Disease Registry. Benzene. n.d. http://www.atsdr.cdc.gov/substances/toxsubstance.asp?toxid=14. Accessed January 14, 2014.

43. Yaris F, Dikici M, Akbulat T. Story of benzene and leukemia: epidemiologic approach of Muzaffer Aksoy. *J Occup Health.* 2004;46:244–247.

44. Health Effects Institute. Validation of biomarkers in workers exposed to benzene: synopsis of research report 115. Boston, MA: Health Effects Institute; n.d.

45. Agency for Toxic Substances and Disease Registry. Formaldehyde. n.d. http:// www.atsdr.cdc.gov/substances/toxsubstance.asp?toxid=39. Accessed September 24, 2013.

46. U.S. Environmental Protection Agency. Volatile organic compounds (VOCs). n.d. http://www.epa.gov/iaq/voc2.html. Accessed January 10, 2014.

47. Agency for Toxic Substances and Disease Registry. Public health statement for toluene. n.d. http://www.atsdr.cdc.gov/ToxProfiles/tp56-c1-b.pdf. Accessed January 10, 2014.

48. Zupanic M, Demes P, Seeber A. Psychomotor performance and subjective symptoms at low level toluene exposure. *Occup Environ Med.* 2002;59:263–268.

49. Chang S-J, Chen C-J, Lien C-H, Sung F-C. Hearing loss in workers exposed to toluene and noise. *Environ Health Perspect.* 2006;114(8):1283–1286.

50. U.S. Environmental Protection Agency. Fact sheet on perchloroethylene, also known as tetrachloroethylene. n.d. http://www.epa.gov/oppt/existingchemicals/pubs /perchloroethylene_fact_sheet.html. Accessed September 24, 2013.

51. Agency for Toxic Substances and Disease Registry. *Tox FAQs: 2-butanone [MEK].* Atlanta, GA: U.S. Department of Health and Human Services, Public Health Service; 1995.

52. Centers for Disease Control and Prevention (CDC), National Institute for Occupational Safety and Health (NIOSH). 2-Butanone. In: *NIOSH pocket guide to chemical hazards.* DHHS (NIOSH) Publication No. 2005-149. U.S. Department of Health and Human Services, CDC, NIOSH; 2007.

53. Agency for Toxic Substances and Disease Registry (ATSDR). *Public health statement: styrene.* Atlanta, GA: U.S. Department of Health and Human Services, Public Health Service, ATSDR; 2012.

54. U.S. Department of Labor, Occupational Safety and Health Administration. Styrene. n.d. https://www.osha.gov/sltc/styrene. Accessed September 21, 2013.

55. Ruder AM, Ward EM, Dong M, et al. Mortality patterns among workers exposed to styrene in the reinforced plastic boatbuilding industry: an update. *Am J Ind Med.* 2004;45:165–176.

56. Agency for Toxic Substances and Disease Registry (ATSDR). *Public health statement: vinyl chloride.* Atlanta, GA: U.S. Department of Health and Human Services, Public Health Service, ATSDR; 2006.

57. Centers for Disease Control and Prevention. Epidemiologic notes and reports: angiosarcoma of the liver among polyvinyl chloride workers—Kentucky. *MMWR.* 1997;46(5):97–101.

58. Creech JL Jr, Johnson MN. Angiosarcoma of liver in the manufacture of polyvinyl chloride. *J Occup Med.* 1974;16(3):150–151.

59. Binns CHB. Vinyl chloride: a review. *J Soc Occup Med.* 1979;29:134–141.

60. Lloyd JW. Angiosarcoma of the liver in vinyl chloride/polyvinyl chloride workers. *J Occup Med.* 1975;17(5):333–334.

61. Fox AJ, Collier PF. Mortality experience of workers exposed to vinyl chloride monomer in the manufacture of polyvinyl chloride in Great Britain. *Br J Ind Med.* 1977;34:1–10.

62. Heldaas SS, Langård SL, Andersen A. Incidence of cancer among vinyl chloride and polyvinyl chloride workers. *Br J Ind Med.* 1984;41:25–30.

63. Kaye P, Young H, O'Sullivan I. Metal fume fever: a case report and review of the literature. *Emerg Med J.* 2002;19:268–269.

64. 't Mannetje A, Brennan P, Zaridze D, et al. Welding and lung cancer in Central and Eastern Europe and the United Kingdom. *Am J Epidemiol.* 2012;175(7):706–714.

65. Hu H. Exposure to metals. *Prim Care.* 2000;27(4):983–996.

66. Rodrigues EG, McClean MD, Weinberg J, Pepper LD. Beryllium sensitization and lung function among former workers at the Nevada test site. *Am J Ind Med.* 2008;51:512–523.

67. Agency for Toxic Substances and Disease Registry (ATSDR). *Public health statement: cadmium.* Atlanta, GA: U.S. Department of Health and Human Services, Public Health Service, ATSDR; 2012.

68. Järup L. Hazards of heavy metal contamination. *Br Med Bull.* 2003;68:167–182.

69. World Health Organization (WHO). *Exposure to cadmium: a major public health concern.* Geneva, Switzerland: WHO; 2010.

70. U.S. Department of Labor, Occupational Safety and Health Administration. Occupational exposure to cadmium in the construction industry. n.d. https:/www.osha.gov/doc/outreachtraining/htmlfiles/cadmium.html. Accessed October 29, 2013.

71. Wittman R, Hu H. Cadmium exposure and nephropathy in a 28-year-old female metals worker. *Environ Health Perspect.* 2002;110(12):1261–1266.

72. Järup L, Bellander T, Hogstedt C, Spång G. Mortality and cancer incidence in Swedish battery workers exposed to cadmium and nickel. *Occup Environ Med.* 1998;55:755–759.

73. U.S. Environmental Protection Agency. Chromium compounds. n.d. http://www.epa.gov/ttnatw01/hlthef/chromium.html. Accessed September 22, 2013.

74. U.S. Department of Labor, Occupational Safety and Health Administration (OSHA). *OSHA fact sheet: health effects of hexavalent chromium.* DSG 7/2006. U.S. Department of Labor, OSHA: n.d.

75. Sughis M, Nawrot TS, Haufroid V, Nemery B. Adverse health effects of child labor: high exposure to chromium and oxidative DNA damage in children manufacturing surgical instruments. *Environ Health Perspect.* 2012;120(10):1469–1472.

76. Zhang X-H, Zhang X, Wang X-C, et al. Chronic occupational exposure to hexavalent chromium causes DNA damage in electroplating workers. *BMC Public Health* 2011;11:224.

77. Hernberg S. Lead poisoning in a historical perspective. *Am J Ind Med.* 2000;38:244–254.

78. U.S. Department of Labor, Occupational Safety and Health Administration (OSHA). Lead in construction. OSHA 3142-09R. U.S. Department of Labor, OSHA; 2003.

79. Boraiko C, Wright EM, Ralston F. Lead contamination of paint remediation workers' vehicles. *J Environ Health.* 2012;75(7):22–27.

80. Wynant W, Siemiatycki J, Parent M-É, Rousseau M-C. Occupational exposure to lead and lung cancer: results from two case-control studies in Montreal, Canada. *Occup Environ Med.* 2013;70:164–170.

81. Ghiasvand M, Aghakhani K, Salimi A, Kumar R. Ischemic heart disease risk factors in lead exposed workers: research study. *J Occup Med Toxicol.* 2013;8:11.

82. Silbergeld EK, Weaver VM. Exposure to metals: are we protecting the workers? *Occup Environ Med.* 2007;64:141–142.

83. Satoh H. Occupational and environmental toxicology of mercury and its compounds. *Ind Health.* 2000;38:153–164.

84. Wedeen RP. Were the hatters of New Jersey "mad"? *Am J Ind Med.* 1989;16:225–233.

85. O'Carroll RE, Masterton G, Dougall N, et al. The neuropsychiatric sequelae of mercury poisoning: the mad hatter's disease revisited. *Br J Psychiatry.* 1995;167(1):95–98.

86. Kasprzak KS, Sunderman FW, Salnikow K. Nickel carcinogenesis. *Mutat Res.* 2003;533:67–97.

87. U.S. Environmental Protection Agency. Nickel compounds. n.d. http://www.epa.gov/ttnatw01/hlthef/nickel.html. Accessed September 22, 2013.

88. Zhao J, Shi X, Castranova V, Ding M. Occupational toxicology of nickel and nickel compounds. *J Environ Pathol Toxicol Oncol.* 2009;28(3):177–208.

89. Hooiveld M, Spee T, Burstyn I, et al. Lung cancer mortality in a Dutch cohort of asphalt workers: evaluation of possible confounding by smoking. *Am J Ind Med.* 2003;43:79–87.

90. Agency for Toxic Substances and Disease Registry (ATSDR). *Public health statement: polycyclic aromatic hydrocarbons (PAHs).* Atlanta, GA: U.S. Department of Health and Human Services, Public Health Service, ATSDR; 1995.

91. Coggon D, Inskip H, Winter P, Pannett B. Mortality from scrotal cancer in metal machinists in England and Wales, 1979–80 and 1982–90. *Occup Med.* 1996;46(1):69–70.

92. Friesen MC, Demers PA, Spinelli JJ, et al. Chronic and acute effects of coal tar pitch exposure and cardiopulmonary mortality among aluminum smelter workers. *Am J Epidemiol.* 2010;172:790–799.

93. Silverman DT, Samanic CM, Lubin JH, et al. The diesel exhaust in miners study: a nested case-control study of lung cancer and diesel exhaust. *J Natl Cancer Inst.* 2012;104:855–868.

94. Möhner M, Kersten N, Gellissen J. Diesel motor exhaust and lung cancer mortality: reanalysis of a cohort study in potash miners. *Eur J Epidemiol.* 2013;28:159–168.

95. Lindquist R, Nilsson B, Eklund G, Gahrton G. Acute leukemia in professional drivers exposed to gasoline and diesel. *Eur J Haematol.* 1991;47:98–103.

96. Agency for Toxic Substances and Disease Registry (ATSDR). *Public health statement: arsenic.* Atlanta, GA: U.S. Department of Health and Human Services, Public Health Service, ATSDR, 2007.

97. Surdu S, Fitzgerald EF, Bloom MS, et al. Occupational exposure to arsenic and risk of nonmelanoma skin cancer in a multinational European study. *Int J Cancer.* 2013;133:2182–2191.

98. U.S. Department of Labor, Occupational Safety and Health Administration. Hazard communication guidance for diacetyl and food flavorings containing diacetyl. n.d. https:/www.osha.gov/dsg/guidance/diacetyl-guidance.html. Accessed August 9, 2013.

99. Centers for Disease Control and Prevention. Obliterative bronchiolitis in workers in a coffee-processing facility—Texas, 2008–2012. *MMWR.* 2013;62(16):305–307.

100. Sahakian N, Kreiss K. Lung disease in flavoring and food production: learning from butter flavoring. *Adv Food Nutr Res.* 2009;55:163–192.

101. Centers for Disease Control and Prevention. Fixed obstructive lung disease among workers in the flavor-manufacturing industry—California, 2004–2007. *MMWR.* 2007;56(16):389–393.

102. Watrous RM. Health hazards of the pharmaceutical industry. *Br J Ind Med.* 1947;4:111–125.

103. U.S. Department of Labor, Occupational Safety and Health Administration. Potential health hazards associated with the process of compounding medications from pharmaceutical grade ingredients. n.d. https:/www.osha.gov/dts/tib/tib_data/tib20011221.html. Accessed October 29, 2013.

104. Stücker I, Caillard J-F, Collin R, et al. Risk of spontaneous abortion among nurses handling antineoplastic drugs. *Scand J Work Environ Health*. 1990;16:102–107.

105. U.S. Department of Labor, Occupational Safety and Health Administration. Hazardous drugs. n.d. https:/www.osha.gov/SLTC/hazardousdrugs/. Accessed October 29, 2013.

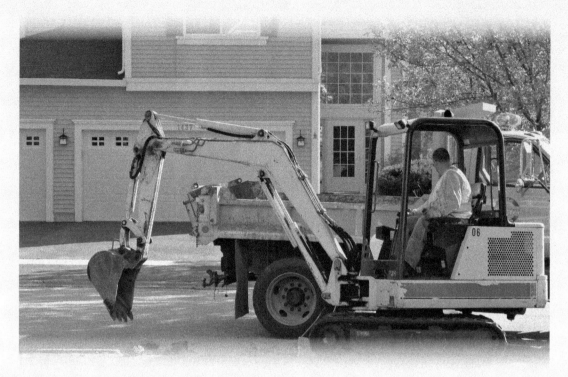

FIGURE 5.1 Occupational noise and vibration

© Flashon Studio/Shutterstock.

Every year, approximately 30 million people in the United States are occupationally exposed to hazardous noise. Noise-related hearing loss has been listed as one of the most prevalent occupational health concerns in the United States for more than 25 years. . . . Exposure to high levels of noise can cause permanent hearing loss. Neither surgery nor a hearing aid can help correct this type of hearing loss.

—U.S. Department of Labor, Occupational Safety and Health Administration[1]

CHAPTER 5

Physical Hazards in the Workplace

Learning Objectives

By the end of this chapter, you will be able to:

- Provide examples and categories of physical hazards encountered at work.
- Compare and contrast nonionizing and ionizing radiation.
- State the similarities and differences between work-related noise and vibration.
- Give examples of adverse health effects of work-associated extreme temperatures.
- Describe hazards associated with variations in atmospheric pressure.

Chapter Outline

- Introduction
- Noise in the Workplace
- Occupational Vibration
- Ionizing Radiation
- Non-ionizing Radiation
- Extreme Temperatures: High or Low
- Variations in Atmospheric Pressure
- Summary
- Study Questions and Exercises

Introduction

Workplace physical hazards include exposures to radiation, noise, and the related phenomenon of vibration, as well as exposures to extreme ambient temperatures and risks associated with atmospheric variations. Physical hazards occur in a wide variety of occupations and are an important cause of injuries. Workers impacted by physical hazards can endure permanent adverse health outcomes such as hearing and vision loss and, in some instances, mortality. This chapter considers the sources and impacts of physical hazards in the workplace in more detail.

One type of physical hazard covered in this chapter is oscillatory vibrations. The term oscillatory vibrations refers to noise from sources in the work environment as well as physical vibrations of the human body caused by machinery. These work-related physical hazards are associated with deleterious effects to hearing and the body. "Noise and vibration are both fluctuations in the pressure of the air (or other media), which affect the human body. Vibrations that are detected by the human ear are classified as sound. We use the term 'noise' to indicate unwanted sound."[1]

Noise and vibration are associated with fields such as construction, firearms testing, manufacturing, and entertainment (e.g., performing at rock concerts) as well as a plethora of other work settings. With respect to occupational exposure to noise, the Bureau of Labor Statistics estimates that as many as 125,000 U.S. workers have sustained permanent hearing loss since 2004; moreover, in a single year (2009), approximately 21,000 workers experienced hearing loss.[1] In addition to noise, two other forms of vibrations that affect the human body are called whole-body vibration and hand-transmitted vibration, both of which have been linked to musculoskeletal and other deleterious effects.

A second physical hazard is exposure to ionizing and non-ionizing radiation. "Radiation may be defined as energy traveling through space."[2] The various forms of radiation described in this chapter affect diverse groups of employees, ranging from electricians, electronics workers, and miners to employees in healthcare specialties, nuclear facilities, and science laboratories. Radiation is associated with a variety of adverse health outcomes, such as cancer, burns, and eye diseases.

A third physical hazard stems from atmospheric variations: heat, cold, and high and low air pressures. An example is extreme ambient temperatures—either high or low—that can cause heat stroke, heat exhaustion, frostbite, and death from hypothermia. Affected employees have a variety of occupations—for example, carpenters and laborers on construction projects whose assignment entails remaining outdoors on a blistering summer day or during the frigid winter. Similarly, farm workers

TABLE 5.1   Physical Hazards in the Work Environment

Physical Hazard	Example	Potential Occupational Exposures
Oscillatory vibrations	Noise and vibration	Construction, weapons firing ranges, manufacturing, truck driving
Atmospheric variations	Heat, cold, air pressure	Agriculture, construction, deep-sea diving, tunnel construction
Radiation: ionizing radiation	Alpha particles	Biologists, chemists, and physicists
	Beta particles	Dental assistants
	Protons	Physicians and veterinarians
	Neutrons	Radiologists/X-ray technicians
	Gamma rays and X-rays	Uranium miners
Radiation: non-ionizing radiation	Ultraviolet light	Many occupations, including laboratory workers, tanning booth operators, and welders
	Infrared radiation	Many occupations, including bakers, glass furnace workers, and kiln operators
	Microwaves Radio frequency radiation	Many occupations, including medical/diathermy personnel, plastic heat-sealing workers, and food product workers

often are required to harvest crops when the temperature has reached searing levels.

Variations in air pressures occur at high altitudes where air pressure is reduced and in pressurized environments in which atmospheric pressures are higher than at sea level. These pressure variations can impact workers at high altitudes or deep-sea divers and underground construction personnel. TABLE 5.1 summarizes the types of physical hazards in occupations that involve potential exposure to these physical hazards.

Noise in the Workplace

Noise-induced hearing loss is one of the leading forms of occupational illness.[3] Hearing loss is a significant concern for occupational health because the manufacturing sector in the United States employs approximately 16 million people, or around 13% of the workforce.[3] This section covers measurements of sounds, the physiology of hearing, hearing loss, and procedures for protecting workers against hearing loss. EXHIBIT 5.1 gives an overview of hearing loss among military veterans: Hearing impairment among veterans is the most frequent service-related disability.[4]

EXHIBIT 5.1   **Severe Hearing Impairment among Military Veterans**

Military service can entail harmful exposure to high-intensity noise from firearms, explosives, jet engines, machinery, and other sources during combat operations, [during] training, or in the course of general job duties. Such exposures can cause or contribute to hearing impairments, including hearing loss, if adequate hearing protection is not available and properly used. . . . Noise-induced hearing loss is a permanent disability, although the impairment sometimes can be rehabilitated with hearing aids.

Since 1978, the Department of Defense (DoD) policy has required each of the armed services to have in place HCPs [hearing conservation programs] incorporating noise hazard identification, safety signs and labels, noise mitigation, education and training, audiometric surveillance, and program evaluation. . . . However, a 2005 Institute of Medicine report identified certain shortcomings in military HCPs. . . . Between 10% and 18% of service members enrolled in military HCPs had standard threshold shifts* in hearing, . . . a prevalence two to five times higher than would be considered acceptable in a civilian, industrial HCPs [sic]. . . .

Noise-induced hearing loss is preventable. The observed association of SHI [severe hearing impairment] with military service, and particularly with service in the United States or overseas after September 2001, underscores the need for improved HCPs in the various service branches and the importance of hearing loss surveillance in military and VA health systems.

*A standard threshold shift is a change of 10 dB or more in the average hearing thresholds at 2000, 3000, and 4000 Hz in comparison with a baseline audiogram. (Refer to text for more information on these terms.)

Reproduced from Centers for Disease Control and Prevention (CDC). Severe hearing impairment among military veterans—U.S., 2010. *MMWR.* 2011;60(28):955–958.

Measures of Sound: Hertz and Decibels

Sound is classified according to its frequency and pressure. The term hertz (Hz) refers to the number of cycles per second (frequency) associated with the oscillation of a given sound wave, with high and low hertz numbers characterizing high and low tones, respectively. Human beings are able to perceive sounds in the range of approximately 20 Hz to 20,000 HZ.

The scale for measurement of sound pressure is called decibels (dBs). "Noise is measured in units of sound pressure levels called decibels, named after Alexander Graham Bell, using A-weighted sound levels (dBA). The A-weighted sound levels closely match the perception of loudness by the human ear. Decibels are measured on a logarithmic scale, which means that a small change in the number of decibels results in a huge change in the amount of noise and the potential damage to a person's hearing."[1] When a sound increases by 10 units on the decibel scale, its loudness becomes 10 times more powerful.[5] FIGURE 5.2 gives the levels of typical sounds in decibels.

Physiology of Hearing

The human ear translates the energy from sound waves into neurologic impulses that are heard as sound through the actions of the ear canal, eardrum, ossicles in the middle ear, cochlea, and the cochlear nerve (**FIGURE 5.3**). After sounds enter and pass through the ear canal, they cause the tympanic membrane (eardrum) to vibrate. These vibrations are transferred to the ossicles, a series of bones (hammer, anvil, and stirrup) in the middle ear. The ossicles amplify the sounds, which move the oval window of the cochlea. In turn, this movement causes fluid in the cochlea to move and stimulate hairs, which next activate cells that send neurologic impulses along the cochlear nerve to the brain. These impulses are perceived as sound. When workers are exposed to very intense sounds in an occupational setting, the delicate mechanisms in this sound pathway can be damaged.

Typical A-Weighted Sound Levels
(dB, re: 20 µPa)

– 140	Threshold of Pain
– 130	Jet Takeoff at 100 m
– 120	
– 110	Discotheque
– 100	
– 90	Jackhammer at 15 m
– 80	Heavy Truck at 15 m
– 70	Vacuum Cleaner at 3 m
– 60	Conversation at 1 m
– 50	Urban Residence
– 40	Soft Whisper at 2 m
– 30	North Rim of the Grand Canyon
– 20	
– 10	
– 0	Threshold of Hearing (1000 Hz)

FIGURE 5.2   Levels of typical sounds in decibels (dBs)

Reproduced from U.S. Department of Labor, Occupational Safety and Health Administration, Occupational noise exposure. https://www.osha.gov/SLTC/noisehearingconservation/index.html. Accessed August 23, 2013.

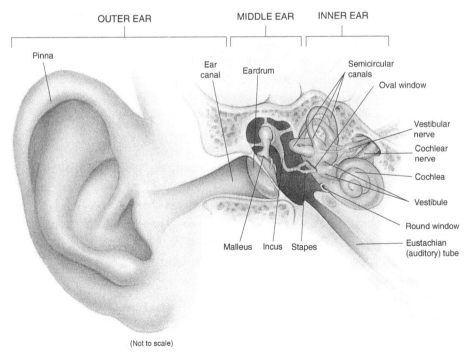

OUTER EAR   MIDDLE EAR   INNER EAR

Pinna

Ear canal

Eardrum

Semicircular canals

Oval window

Vestibular nerve

Cochlear nerve

Cochlea

Vestibule

Round window

Eustachian (auditory) tube

Malleus   Incus   Stapes

(Not to scale)

FIGURE 5.3   The sound pathway

Hearing Loss

Exposure to loud noises in the occupational environment may cause two types of changes in hearing sensitivity: a temporary threshold shift (TTS) in hearing sensitivity or a permanent threshold shift (PTS). A TTS is a short-term loss in hearing sensitivity that lasts for several hours—for example, 14 hours or longer in certain situations.[6] A PTS is "any change in hearing sensitivity, which is persistent."[6(p. 92)] A noise-induced permanent threshold shift (NIPTS) is "a permanent threshold shift [that] can be attributable to noise exposure."[6(p. 91)]

"Audiometry is the testing of a person's ability to hear various sound frequencies. The test is performed with the use of electronic equipment called an audiometer. This testing is usually administered by a trained technician called an audiologist."[7] Audiometry is essential to tracking hearing loss among employees who work in noisy occupations. The results of hearing tests for these employees can be compared periodically with baseline measurements of hearing taken when they began employment.

Protecting Workers Against Noise

To protect workers from high noise levels, a company may decide to monitor hearing hazards and, based on these assessments, introduce measures to reduce noise exposures. Several types of instruments and procedures for measurement of hazards are available. "The most common measurements are area surveys, dosimetry, and engineering surveys."[6(p. 13)] EXHIBIT 5.2 describes the purposes of hearing hazard exposure monitoring.

EXHIBIT 5.2 **Hearing Hazard Exposure Monitoring**

Hearing hazard exposure monitoring is conducted for various purposes:

- To determine whether hazards to hearing exist
- To determine whether noise presents a safety hazard by interfering with speech communication or the recognition of audible warning signals
- To identify employees for inclusion in the hearing loss prevention program
- To classify employees' noise exposures for prioritizing noise control efforts and defining and establishing hearing protection practices
- To evaluate specific noise sources for noise control purposes
- To evaluate the success of noise control efforts

Reproduced from Centers for Disease Control and Prevention, Franks JR, Stephenson MR, Merry CJ. eds. Preventing Occupational Hearing Loss: A Practical Guide. Cincinnati, OH: DHHS, CDC, NIOSH; 1996. Publication No. 96-110, p13.

Area Survey

In an area survey, "environmental noise levels are measured, using a sound level meter to identify work areas where employees' exposures are above or below hazardous levels, and where more thorough exposure monitoring may be needed. The result is often plotted in the form of a 'noise map,' showing noise level measurements for the different areas of the workplace."[6(p. 13)] "A sound level meter (SLM) is the basic instrument for investigating noise levels."[8] In the upper image in **FIGURE 5.4**, a woman is using a sound level meter to measure noise levels in a work area. "She will also measure exposure levels by placing the microphone in the hearing zone of the workers."[6(p. 15)]

Dosimetry

"Dosimetry involves the use of body-worn instruments (dosimeters) to monitor an employee's noise exposure over the work-shift. Monitoring results for one employee can also represent the exposures of other workers in the area whose noise exposures are similar. It may also be possible to use task-based exposure methods to represent the exposures of other workers in different areas whose exposures result from having performed the same task(s)."[6(p. 14)]

The lower image in Figure 5.4 shows a noise dosimeter. "A noise dosimeter measures and stores sound energy over time. It can be worn in the pocket, as shown [in Figure 5.4], or attached to the belt. The microphone is positioned on the shoulder in the hearing zone of the wearer. The wearer goes about a normal work shift while wearing the dosimeter."[6(p. 15)]

Engineering Surveys

"Engineering surveys typically employ more sophisticated acoustical equipment in addition to sound level meters. [This equipment furnishes] . . . information on the frequency/intensity composition of the noise being emitted by machinery or other sound sources in various modes of operation. These measurements are used to assess options for applying engineering controls."[6(p. 14)]

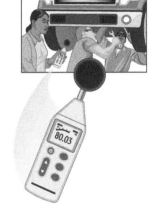

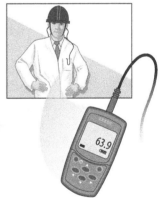

FIGURE 5.4 Sound level meter (upper image) and noise dosimeter (lower image)

Reproduced from Preventing Occupational Hearing Loss: A Practical Guide, Franks JR, Stephenson MR, Merry CJ, eds, Cincinnati, OH: DHHS, CDC, NIOSH. 1996. DHHS (NIOSH) Publication No. 96-110, p. 15

Hearing Loss and Occupational Noise

Hearing loss—the most commonly recorded occupational illness—can result from sustained exposure to occupational noise; exposure to sounds of 85 dB or higher may result in hearing loss.[5] According to the National Institute on Deafness and Other Communication Disorders (NIDCD), "when we are exposed to harmful noise—sounds that are too loud or loud sounds that last a long time—sensitive structures in our inner ear can be damaged, causing noise-induced hearing loss (NIHL). . . . NIHL can be caused by a one-time exposure to an intense 'impulse' sound, such as an explosion, or by continuous exposure to loud sounds over an extended period of time, such as noise generated in a woodworking shop."[5(p. 1)] Once hearing loss results from high noise levels, interventions such as surgery and hearing aids cannot reverse the loss.[1]

Occupational hearing loss accounts for nearly one out of nine cases of occupational illnesses in manufacturing and, therefore, is the most commonly recorded occupational illness. Moreover, occupational hearing loss tends to happen gradually over time. Because this disability usually develops gradually, many employees are unaware of their hearing loss.[3]

Occupational settings with high noise levels may include construction sites, airports, shooting ranges, steel foundries, boiler-making factories, and fishing vessels. FIGURE 5.5 shows a worker using a saw without hearing protection or other personal protective equipment. Commercial fishermen and other personnel working on fishing vessels are also exposed to high noise levels for long time periods. Often, these noise levels exceed recommended standards and pose risks for hearing loss.[9]

In addition to being implicated in diminished hearing, noise has been studied as a risk factor for conditions such as stress, annoyance, cardiovascular effects, and acoustic neuromas (intracranial tumors). For example, workers who had prolonged exposure to noise levels greater than 85 dBA were found to be at increased risk of hypertension in comparison with those who had noise exposures less than the 85 dBA level.[10] Another hypothesized consequence of occupational noise exposure is the development of acoustic neuromas. However, Edwards et al. did not observe an association between occupational noise exposure and acoustic neuroma.[11]

Occupational Vibration

Many occupations expose workers to vibration. For example, FIGURE 5.6 depicts a worker who is exposed to noise and vibration from a jackhammer.

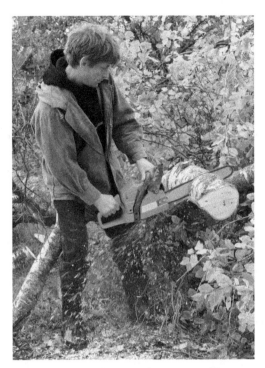

FIGURE 5.5   Worker using a saw without hearing protection or other personal protective equipment

© Gala_Kan/ShutterStock

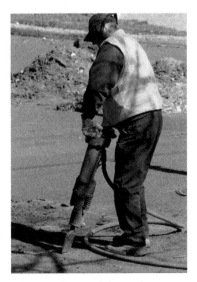

FIGURE 5.6   Worker exposed to noise and vibration from a jackhammer

Courtesy of U.S. Department of Labor, Occupational Safety and Health Administration.

Two important characteristics of vibration are its magnitude and its frequency. Magnitude of a vibration is defined by displacement velocity or acceleration; frequency is defined by cycles per second or hertz.[12] The health effects of exposure to vibration can include lower-extremity effects, low-back pain (LBP), sensorineural complaints, joint pain, vascular problems, and musculoskeletal impacts. The common types of vibration are whole-body vibration and hand–arm vibration (FIGURE 5.7).

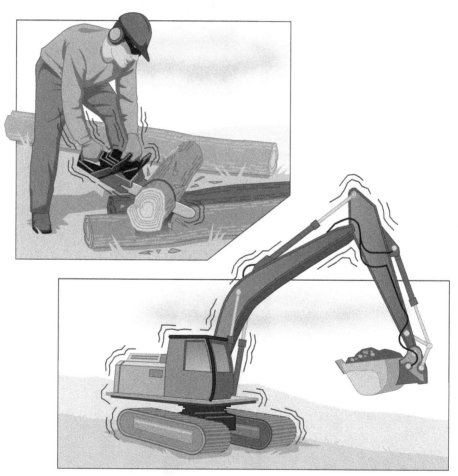

FIGURE 5.7   Occupational exposure to hand-arm vibration (HAV) [left panel] and whole body vibration (WBV) [right panel]

Courtesy of World Health Organization, Occupational Exposure to Vibration from Hand-held Tools, Teaching materials, http://www.who.int/occupational_health/pwh_guidance_no.10_teaching_materials.pdf?ua=1. Accessed February 14, 2014.

Whole-Body Vibration

Whole-body vibration (WBV) is defined as the form of vibration that "occurs when the human body is supported on a surface which is vibrating."[12(p. 58)] WPV occurs among heavy machinery operators—for example, bulldozer drivers, transport drivers, and operators of some other types of machinery.

Occupational exposures to whole-body vibration are common in many occupations. In a British study, workers whose exposures to WBV exceeded recommended standards included forklift truck drivers, agricultural owners and employees, and truck drivers. Among the sources of occupational exposures to WBV noted in this study were tractors, forklifts, trucks, and buses.[13]

Whole-body vibration is thought to contribute to low back pain. According to Bovenzi, "Long-term occupational exposure to intense WBV is associated with an increased risk for disorders of the lumbar spine and the connected nervous system."[12(p. 58)] The workers most likely to be affected by low back disorders from WBV include crane operators, bus drivers, tractor drivers, and fork-lift truck drivers.

The relationship between WBV and LBP was examined among a group of professional drivers. A dose–response pattern was reported between WBV and driving-related LBP. The findings suggested that exposure to WBV may contribute to LBP.[14] However, other research has suggested that occupational exposure to WBV is a less important contributor to LBP than lifting at work.[15] Nevertheless, although definitive evidence regarding a causal relationship is lacking, current information suggests that exposure to WBV should be kept at a minimum.[16]

A case-control study demonstrated that high levels of WBV were associated with increased odds of Parkinson's disease. An inverse relationship (protective effect) was found for low levels of WBV.[17] A hypothesized explanation for this finding is that higher-intensity WBV can cause micro-injuries to the head.

Hand-Transmitted Vibration/Hand–Arm Vibration Syndrome

Hand-transmitted vibration (HTV) is defined as vibration entering "the body through the hands."[12(p. 58)] This form of vibration occurs among people who use hand-held power tools. Prolonged exposure to HTV "from powered processes or tools is associated with an increased occurrence of symptoms and signs of disorders in the vascular, neurological, and osteoarticular systems of the upper limbs."[12(p. 60)] Examples of conditions associated with vibrating hand-held power tools are vibration-induced white finger (VWF) and Raynaud's phenomenon of occupational origin.[18]

Hand–arm vibration syndrome (HAVS) refers to the group of symptoms that result from hand-transmitted vibration.[19] "The syndrome includes vascular, neurological, and musculo-skeletal disorders that may become manifest individually or collectively."[20(p. 16)] For example, one musculoskeletal symptom of exposure to hand–arm vibration is neck pain.[21] The mechanisms underlying the development of HAVS are not understood fully.

One symptom of HAVS, vibration-induced white finger, is related to the influence of vibrations upon the circulatory and neurologic structures in the fingers. Another symptom of HAVS, Raynaud's phenomenon, consists of a combination of effects upon the vascular and neurologic systems that can be induced by vibration.[12] Raynaud's phenomenon is the most frequently observed symptom of occupational exposure to vibration.[22] In a French study of employees in poultry slaughterhouses and canning factories, investigators determined that Raynaud's phenomenon was associated with continuous repetition of tasks, exertion of the hands and arms, and taking breaks in a cold environment.[23]

Research with a sample of metalworkers reported a dose-response relationship between total lifetime dosage of hand–arm vibration and development of symptoms, which could include finger blanching, sensorineural complaints, and musculoskeletal issues.[24] Exposure over long time periods to hand-held vibrating tools usually is required to produce HAVS. However, Gerhardsson found that signs and symptoms of vibration exposure can appear after only short time periods among young workers.[25] HAVS is also reported to be associated with vascular symptoms that appear in the lower extremities of the body.[26]

Ionizing Radiation

The term radiation refers to "energy traveling through space."[2] Two forms of radiation are non-ionizing radiation and ionizing radiation, which are distinguished by their lower and higher energy levels, respectively. Together these two kinds of radiation make up the electromagnetic spectrum (FIGURE 5.8), an energy continuum that spans from the low-energy fields associated with electric power lines to the mid-level energy emitted by radio stations to the high levels of energy found in medical X-rays.

Ionizing radiation is an occupational hazard for workers in many settings, most notably health care, research laboratories, nuclear weapons

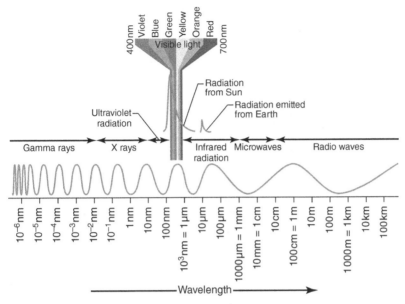

FIGURE 5.8   Electromagnetic spectrum

facilities, and nuclear power plants. Exposure to ionizing radiation should be minimized. Safeguards must be implemented to protect workers from excessive radiation that might have adverse health effects. In addition, employers must post warning signs to alert personnel to the presence of hazardous ionizing radiation sources (**FIGURE 5.9**).

Ionizing radiation is "[e]lectromagnetic (X ray and gamma) or particulate (alpha, beta) radiation capable of producing ions or charged particles."[27] It consists of either particulate energy (e.g., highly energetic protons, neutrons, and alpha [α] and beta [β] particles) or electromagnetic energy in the form of photons (e.g., gamma [γ] rays and X-rays). "All forms of ionizing radiation have sufficient energy to ionize atoms that may destabilize molecules within cells and lead to tissue damage."[2]

When ionization occurs, "An orbital electron is stripped from a neutral atom, producing an ion pair (a negatively charged electron and a positively charged atom)."[27] Ionizing radiation may damage any living tissue in the human body. "The body attempts to repair the damage, but sometimes the damage is of a nature that cannot be repaired or it is too severe or widespread to be repaired. Also mistakes made in the natural repair process can lead to cancerous cells."[28] The various types of radiation—alpha particles, beta particles, gamma rays, and X-rays (see the nearby box)—differ in their capacity to penetrate the human body (**FIGURE 5.10**).

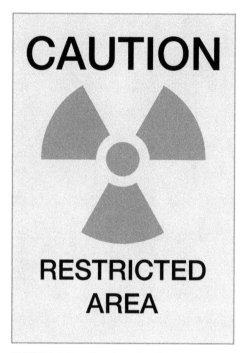

FIGURE 5.9   Caution sign for radiation-restricted area

Courtesy of U.S. Environmental Protection Agency.

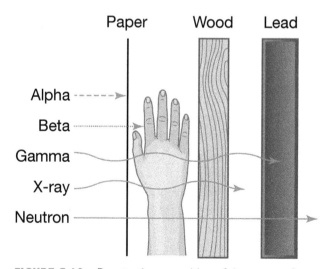

FIGURE 5.10   Penetrating capacities of the types of ionizing radiation

Reproduced from Canadian Nuclear Safety Commission. Working Safely with Nuclear Gauges. INFO-9999-4 (E) Revision 2. Ottawa, Canada: Canadian Nuclear Safety Commission; 2007, p. 7. http://nuclearsafety.gc.ca/pubs_catalogue/uploads/CC172-6 _e.pdf. Accessed February 14, 2014.

Definitions: Alpha Particles, Beta Particles, Gamma Rays, and X-Rays

- **Alpha particle**: A subatomic particle made up of the nucleus of a helium atom that is ejected from a radioactive atom. It has low penetrating power and a short travel range. Alpha particles can be stopped by a piece of paper and, therefore, generally fail to penetrate the skin. However, these particles cannot be considered harmless. When introduced into the body (e.g., through diet, skin wounds, or inhalation of uranium-bearing ores and radioactive dusts), alpha particles irradiate the body's cells and may act as carcinogens or initiate other adverse health effects.

- **Beta particle**: A particle that is emitted from the nucleus of a radioactive atom. It has moderate penetrating power and a travel range of up to a few meters in air. Beta particles will penetrate only a fraction of an inch (up to 2 cm) of skin tissue. Again, internal exposure is a factor in producing potentially adverse effects.

- **Gamma rays** (gamma radiation): High-energy rays that are part of the electromagnetic spectrum. Gamma rays, consisting of photons, are the most highly penetrating type of radiation; they are capable of passing through the body. When energy from photons interacts with bodily tissues, adverse effects such as cellular damage can result, even though the source of the photons is external to the body.

- **X-rays**: Penetrating electromagnetic radiation whose wavelengths are shorter than those of visible light. X-rays are used in medical diagnostic procedures because they are absorbed differentially by soft tissue and bone.

Sources: Adapted from Oak Ridge Associated Universities, Oak Ridge Institute for Science and Education, Radiation Emergency Assistance Center/Training Site. Guidance for Radiation accident management, basics of radiation: definitions. n.d. http://orise.orau.gov/reacts/guide/definitions.htm. Accessed February 7, 2014; and World Health Organization, International Agency for Research on Cancer. Ionizing radiation, Part 1: X- and gamma (γ)-radiation, and neutrons. *IARC Monographs*. 2000;75:36.

Radioactivity denotes "The spontaneous emission of radiation from the nucleus of an unstable atom. As a result of this emission, the radioactive atom is converted, or decays, into an atom of a different element that might or might not be radioactive."[27] Radioactive decay is associated with the spontaneous disintegration of radioactive materials. Types of radiation associated with radioactivity include alpha and beta particles and gamma and X-rays.[27] Radiation also includes neutrons, which are uncharged.

Related to the concept of radioactivity are the terms *isotope*, *nuclide*, *radioisotope*, and *radionuclide*. An isotope is "any of two or more species of atoms of a chemical element with the same atomic number (same number of protons) and nearly identical chemical behavior but with differing atomic mass or mass number (different numbers of neutrons) and different physical properties."[29] For example, carbon is an atom (atomic number 6), and two isotopes of carbon are carbon-12 and carbon-14. A nuclide is a nucleus with a specific number of protons and neutrons and a specific energy state; it includes radioactive and nonradioactive atoms. A radioisotope is a natural or artificially produced isotope that is radioactive. For this reason, a radioisotope also is called a radioactive isotope. An example is the radio-isotope of iodine, iodine-131 (^{131}I). There are more than one dozen radioiso-topes of uranium (atomic number 92) plus several nonradioactive isotopes. A radionuclide is an atom that has an unstable nucleus; when a radionuclide decays, it can emit X- or gamma rays and/or subatomic particles; ^{131}I is a radionuclide as well as a radioisotope. Often radionuclides are described in terms of their half-life, meaning the time that it takes their level of radioac-tivity to decrease by half; the half-life of a radionuclide can range from a very brief time to millions of years. For example, ^{131}I has an 8-day half-life; the half-life of ^{227}U is 1.3 minutes; and the half-life of ^{238}U is 4.47 billion years. Stable elements (nonradioactive) have an infinite to near-infinite half-life.

Measures of Ionizing Radiation

The unit of energy associated with emissions from a radioactive material (radionuclide) is the electron volt (eV). The units used for measurement of the amount of radioactivity, dosage, and exposure are shown in TABLE 5.2.

TABLE 5.2   Ionizing Radiation Measurements

	Radioactivity ("The spontaneous emission of radiation from the nucleus of an unstable atom.")	Absorbed Dose (The quantity of radiation absorbed.)	Dose Equivalent (Dose related to biological effect.)	Exposure ("A quantity used to indicate the amount of ionization in air produced by X- or gamma-ray radiation." Ions are electrically charged atoms or groups of atoms.")
Common units (Defined in Table 5.3)	Curie (Ci)	Rad	Rem	Roentgen (R)
SI units (Defined in Table 5.4)	Becquerel (Bq)	Gray (Gy)	Sievert (Sv)	Coulomb/kilogram (C/kg)

Data from Oak Ridge Associated Universities (ORAU). Guidance for Radiation Accident Management. Radiation Emergency Assistance Center/Training Site (REAC/TS). Measurement. http://orise.orau.gov/reacts/guide/measure.htm. Accessed February 12, 2014 and ORAU, Guidance for Radiation Accident Management: Basics of Radiation. Definitions. http://orise.orau.gov/reacts/guide/definitions.htm. Accessed February 7, 2014

The term common units, which refers to an earlier system of radiation measurement (**TABLE 5.3**), is often used in the United States. The abbreviation SI (System International) units, which denotes the International System of Units (**TABLE 5.4**), has been implemented more recently and has largely replaced the older system of common units.

Fractional units of radiation doses are expressed by using the following prefixes: *milli-* (m) and *micro-* (µ). In addition, the prefix *kilo-* (k) is used. For example, when these prefixes are applied to a rad, an mrad is 1/1000 of a rad; a µrad is 1/1,000,000 of a rad; a krad is 1000 times one rad, or 1000 rad. These prefixes may be applied to other measures of radiation (e.g., sievert and rem). Note that the amount of radioactivity (defined previously as curies or becquerels) present in a material does

TABLE 5.3   Common Units of Radiation

Curie (Ci)	A unit of measure used to describe the amount of radioactivity in a sample of material;[a] I Ci equals 3.7×10^{10} disintegrations per second.[b]
Rad	Radiation absorbed dose [common unit].[a] The former unit of absorbed dose of ionizing radiation.[c]
Rem	Roentgen equivalent in man. A measure of radiation dose related to biological effect (i.e., the equivalent dose or effective dose).[a] A rem is a measure of dose deposited in body tissue, averaged over the body. One rem is approximately the dose from any radiation corresponding to one roentgen of gamma radiation.[c]
Roentgen (R)	The unit of exposure from X- or gamma rays.[a]

Data from

[a] Oak Ridge Associated Universities, Radiation Emergency Assistance Center/Training Site. Guidance for radiation accident management: basics of radiation: definitions. http://orise.orau.gov/reacts/guide/definitions.htm. Accessed February 7, 2014.

[b] Oak Ridge Associated Universities, Radiation Emergency Assistance Center/Training Site. Guidance for radiation accident management: measurement. http://orise.orau.gov/reacts/guide/measure.htm. Accessed February 12, 2014.

[c] Lawrence Berkeley National Laboratory. Nuclear science glossary, Appendix A: glossary of nuclear terms. n.d. http://www.lbl.gov/abc/wallchart/glossary/glossary.html. Accessed February 12, 2014.

TABLE 5.4   International System of Units (SI Units) and Equivalent Common Units

Becquerel (Bq)	(Corresponds to radioactivity) The SI unit of activity, which is defined as one disintegration per second; 37 billion Bq = 1 curie; 1 Bq = 2.7 × 10^{-11} Ci.
Exposure	The SI unit of exposure is the coulomb per kilogram (C/kg). One R = 2.58 × 10^{-4} C/kg.
Gray (Gy)	(Corresponds to absorbed dose) The SI unit of absorbed dose; 1 gray = 100 rad; 1 rad = 0.01 Gy.
Sievert (Sv)	(Corresponds to dose equivalent) The SI unit of dose equivalent; 1 Sv = 100 rem; 1 rem = 0.01 Sv.

Data from Oak Ridge Associated Universities. Guidance for Radiation Accident Management. Radiation Emergency Assistance Center/Training Site (REAC/TS). Basics of Radiation: Definitions. http://orise.orau.gov/reacts/guide/definitions.htm. Accessed February 7, 2014; and Oak Ridge Associated Universities. Guidance for Radiation Accident Management, Radiation Emergency Assistance Center/Training Site (REAC/TS). Measurement. http://orise.orau.gov/reacts/guide/measure.htm. Accessed February 12, 2014.

not depend on its weight or size but rather on the particular radioactive element or isotope.

Modes by Which Radiation Enters the Body

Radiation can enter the human body by three means: external irradiation, contamination, and incorporation.

- External irradiation occurs when all or part of the body is exposed to penetrating radiation from an external source. During exposure this radiation can be absorbed by the body or it can pass completely through. A similar thing occurs during an ordinary chest x-ray.
- Contamination means that radioactive materials in the form of gases, liquids, or solids are released into the environment and contaminate people externally, internally, or both. An external surface of the body, such as the skin, can become contaminated, and if radioactive materials get inside the body through the lungs, gut, or wounds, the contaminant can become deposited internally.
- The third type of radiation injury that can occur is incorporation of radioactive material. Incorporation refers to the uptake of radioactive materials by body cells, tissues, and target organs such as bone, liver, thyroid, or kidney. In general, radioactive materials are distributed throughout the body based upon their chemical properties.[30]

Health Effects of Exposure to Ionizing Radiation

The dose of radiation is associated with the amount of bodily tissue damage that may occur. The following factors govern the amount of exposure to radiation that a person receives (dose delivered):

- Total amount of time of exposure to the radioactive source
- Distance from the radioactive source
- Degree of radioactivity (rate of energy emission) of a radioactive material

The amount of radiation dose that is absorbed—expressed as either grays or rads—may or may not be associated with acute health effects, depending on the individual's susceptibility and the amount of exposure as determined by the foregoing factors. The health effects of radiation exposure are described as either nonstochastic (acute) or stochastic (chronic) effects.[28]

Nonstochastic Effects

TABLE 5.5 shows the nonstochastic (acute) effects of varying levels of radiation exposure. Among the acute effects of radiation exposure are tissue

TABLE 5.5 Nonstochastic Health Effects of Whole-Body Exposure for an Average Person and Time to Onset Following Acute Exposure

Exposure (rem)	Health Effect	Time to Onset
5–10	Changes in blood chemistry	
50	Nausea	Hours
55	Fatigue	
70	Vomiting	
75	Hair loss	2–3 weeks
90	Diarrhea	
100	Hemorrhage	
400	Possible death	Within 2 months
1000	Destruction of intestinal lining	
	Internal bleeding and death	1–2 weeks
2000	Damage to central nervous system	
	Loss of consciousness and death	Minutes, hours, to days

Reproduced from U.S. Environmental Protection Agency. Radiation Protection: Understanding Radiation: Health Effects. http://www.epa.gov/radiation/understand/health _effects.html. Accessed February 7, 2014.

burns and radiation sickness (e.g., nausea, weakness, and loss of hair). At low levels, for example, an exposure of 5 rem, radiation usually does not produce immediately detectable harm. At high levels (e.g., an exposure of 350–400 rad or greater), ionizing radiation is capable of producing fatal injuries. The acute effects shown in Table 5.5 are cumulative, meaning that when a person experiences the health effect associated with an exposure at a higher level, the effects that occur at a lower level also will have been experienced. For example, subjects who experience hemorrhage at an exposure of 100 rem of radiation also will have developed changes in blood chemistry.[28]

Stochastic Effects

Stochastic effects are those associated with low levels of exposure to radiation over long time periods. The term *stochastic* means that there is an increased probability of the occurrence of an adverse health event. Among the effects linked potentially to low levels of exposure to radiation are carcinogenesis and genetic damage such as changes in DNA. These changes may be inherited by the progeny of exposed individuals who have experienced DNA damage. In some cases the damage to DNA is so severe that it is not transmitted (i.e., the germinal cells are incapable of viable cell division).

Sources of Ionizing Radiation

According to the National Committee on Radiation Protection and Measurements (NCRP), the total amount of radiation exposure experienced by the U.S. population can be broken down into 82% from natural sources and 18% from human-made sources (FIGURE 5.11). Natural background radiation is the source of natural radiation that impinges upon all of humanity. Of the 18% of total ionizing radiation exposure that comes from anthropogenic sources, medical X-rays and nuclear medicine are the most important sources. Approximately 2% of such exposure comes from occupational sources.[31]

Occupations Where Ionizing Radiation Is Encountered

According to the Occupational Safety and Health Administration (OSHA), "Ionizing radiation sources may be found in a wide range of occupational settings, including healthcare facilities, research institutions, nuclear reactors and their support facilities, nuclear weapon production facilities, and other various manufacturing settings, just to name a few. These radiation sources can pose a considerable health risk to affected workers if not

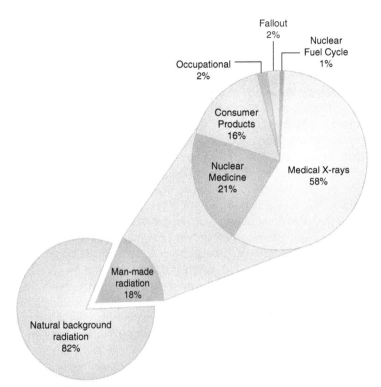

FIGURE 5.11 Pie chart showing radiation from natural and human sources

Reproduced from National Academy of Sciences Health Risks from Exposure to Low Levels of Ionizing Radiation: BEIR VII – Phase 2. Washington, DC: National Academies Press, 2006.

properly controlled."[32] Of historical note was radium poisoning among women who painted watch dials during the early 20th century (**EXHIBIT 5.3**).

Other personnel who might be exposed to ionizing radiation include physicians and health professionals as well as those situated in some manufacturing and service industries, defense installations, research institutions, universities, and the nuclear power industry. Industrial applications of ionizing radiation include the checking of welds and joints, security inspections, sterilization of foods and other materials, and analytic procedures. In the nuclear industry, approximately 800,000 employees worldwide are exposed to ionizing radiation; the corresponding number in medical facilities is more than 2 million. Less obvious exposures to ionizing radiation occur in underground mines (e.g., from radon), although levels of radiation can be lowered through adequate ventilation. Also less recognized are exposures of aircraft pilots and cabin personnel to cosmic rays. The total amount of exposure is correlated with the duration of a flight and is greater at higher altitudes than at lower altitudes. For example, on a long-distance flight between Paris and San Francisco, the estimated effective dose of cosmic radiation is 84.9 microsieverts (μSv).[33]

EXHIBIT 5.3   **Radium Poisoning among Watch Dial Painters**

The saga began shortly after the discovery of radium by Marie and Pierre Curie. The Curies had observed with "amazement and delight" that their newly found element (for which they shared the 1903 Nobel Prize in physics with Henri Becquerel, who had already discovered the radioactivity of elemental uranium) glowed in the dark! This property of radium was soon exploited. In 1902, the American electrical engineer William J. Hammer, using minute amounts of radium, invented a paint that could be used to treat watches and scientific instruments so they could be read in the dark. Because of the high cost of radium, $225,000 an ounce, Hammer did not pursue the commercial potential of his discovery in America. However, in Europe, particularly in Switzerland, radium-painted watch dials rapidly became popular. In 1914, the first major company to manufacture radium-painted dials in America was established in Newark, New Jersey.

Entry of the United States into the First World War in 1917 created a huge demand for a wide variety of radium-treated devices and the workers to manufacture them. Large numbers of young women were employed as dial painters, and they applied radium paint with a fine-tipped brush. Because workers were paid on a piecework basis, it was common to tip or point brushes with the tongue to facilitate application of the paint. Over time, this practice could result in substantial absorption of radium. It became apparent during the 1920s that many dial painters were dying prematurely and were suffering from a variety of acute and chronic diseases. Particularly frightening was the frequency of disfiguring cancers and osteomyelitis of the upper and lower jaw.

Reproduced from Winkelstein W. in Deadly glow: The radium dial worker tragedy by Ross Mullner. [Review] *Am J Epidemiol.* 2002;155(3):290–291.

Workers in Medical Fields

Medical fields that make use of ionizing radiation include medical imaging disciplines (e.g., diagnostic radiology, nuclear medicine, and fluoroscopy) and other medical specialties (e.g., orthopedic surgery, gastroenterology, and vascular surgery). The dangers of ionizing radiation can be lowered by minimizing the length of exposure, maintaining distance from radioactive sources, using shielding, and monitoring exposures to verify that they are occurring at safe levels. Especially important is safeguarding pregnant employees who use radiation in medical practice from exposure.[34]

Use of fluoroscopically guided medical interventional procedures has increased the total X-ray exposures of healthcare personnel. Medical interventions require exposure to greater amounts of radiation than diagnostic procedures. The interventional use of fluoroscopy also makes physical demands on healthcare personnel. Affected employees may include cardiologists, radiologists, surgeons, and pain management specialists. During such procedures, personnel must stand for long periods of time and wear heavy personal protective equipment. These factors, coupled with the need to maintain awkward positioning, may be associated with orthopedic injuries such as neck and back pain.[35]

Radiologists and medical specialists who implement procedures that expose them to ionizing radiation extensively in their practices may be at increased health risks from such exposures. However, these risks are believed to be low.[36] One possible effect of occupational exposure to ionizing radiation is the development of cataracts. Specifically, a 20-year prospective cohort study of 35,705 radiologic technologists suggested that low doses of ionizing radiation were associated with risk of cataracts.[37]

Among persons employed before 1950, epidemiologic research found that risk of leukemia, skin cancer, and female breast cancer was elevated among persons who used ionizing radiation for medical procedures. Since then, occupational doses of ionizing radiation among radiologists and radiologic technologists have demonstrated a declining trend over time. However, increases in exposure to ionizing radiation have arisen from greater use of fluoroscopically guided intervention and nuclear medicine procedures. This phenomenon necessitates additional research on the long-term health effects among medical workers who perform interventional procedures.[38]

Workers Involved with Processing Nuclear Materials

Mortality from cancer was examined among workers at a plutonium production factory in Hanford, Washington.[39] Researchers demonstrated that ionizing radiation exposure was related to cancer mortality primarily for radiation doses that occurred at older ages. Thus the occurrence of cancer depended on the age at which the exposure took place.

Starting in the mid-1950s, the Savannah River Site in South Carolina produced nuclear materials used by the U.S. nuclear weapons program. Researchers studied mortality among 18,883 workers at the installation; the workers had been hired between 1950 and 1986 and were followed through 2002.[40] Positive associations were found between external radiation doses and leukemia mortality.

The mortality and incidence of cancer among workers at the Port Hope, Ontario, Canada, radium and uranium refinery and processing plant was examined. These workers had not been employed in mining, but were exposed to radiation from radium, uranium, and gamma rays. "[N]o significant radiation-associated risks were observed for any cancer site or cause of death."[41(p. 1)]

Uranium Miners

Studies of uranium miners suggest that they are prone to dust-associated lung diseases, inhalation of toxic metals, and cancer from alpha radiation and radon. A large proportion of uranium miners in the former East Germany (1946–1990) developed lung diseases—for example, silicosis and bronchial carcinomas. These mines lacked safety procedures for control of dusts, which exposed miners to high levels of dust and alpha radiation.[42]

Lung cancer rates have been examined among miners exposed to radon, a radioactive gas associated with increased risk of lung cancer. Radon exposure is ranked only after smoking as a leading cause of lung cancer. According to the World Health Organization, "Studies of underground miners exposed occupationally to radon, usually at high concentrations, have consistently demonstrated an increased risk of lung cancer for both smokers and non-smokers."[43(p. 4)]

A historical cohort study examined lung cancer mortality among tin workers in Yunnan, China. Lung cancer mortality was associated with miners' exposures to arsenic, radon, and tobacco smoke.[44]

Workers at Nuclear Power Plants

Several disasters at nuclear power plants have exposed employees and first responders to high levels of ionizing radiation. An incident at the nuclear power plant in Chernobyl, Ukraine, on April 26, 1986, created a major public health disaster that necessitated high levels of radiation exposure among cleanup workers. More recently, the Fukushima Daiichi nuclear power plant disaster in March 2011 followed a major earthquake in northern Japan (FIGURE 5.12). While attempting to bring the runaway reactor under control, workers there also had high levels of radiation exposure. This episode demonstrated a need for greater involvement of occupational health professionals in managing health risks among recovery and emergency response workers.[45]

Monitoring Workers' Exposures to Ionizing Radiation

Monitoring ionizing radiation exposure involves conducting surveys of radiation in the occupational environment, measuring the presence of radiation on the bodies of workers, and assessing personal exposure to radiation. Several instruments are available for surveying radiation. The most commonly used device is the Geiger counter (FIGURE 5.13), which measures high-energy forms of ionizing radiation, but not alpha radiation or low-energy beta radiation. One of the uses of Geiger counters is for detecting the presence of radiation on the human body. Film badges measure personal exposure to radiation over a time period and should be worn by persons who use X-ray machines and radioactive materials (FIGURE 5.14).

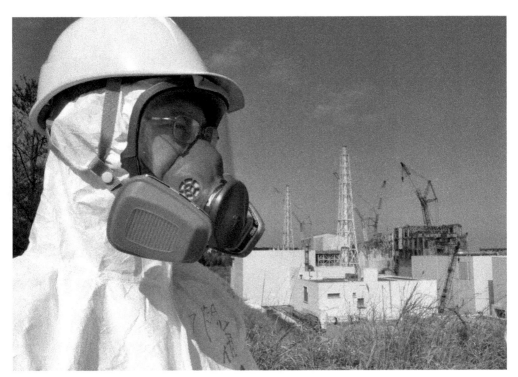

FIGURE 5.12   Fukushima Daiichi Power Plant

© Yoshikazu Tsuno/AFP/Getty Images

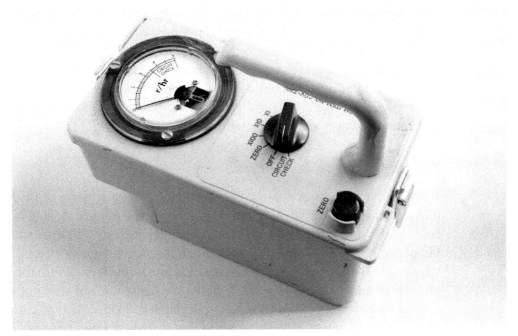

FIGURE 5.13   Geiger-Mueller tube (Geiger counter) used for detecting radiation

© albln/iStockphoto

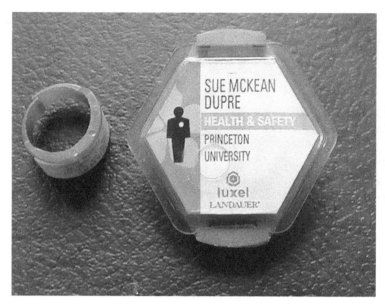

FIGURE 5.14 Radiation film badge

Courtesy of Princeton University Environmental Health and Safety.

Non-ionizing Radiation

"Non-ionizing radiation is described as a series of energy waves composed of oscillating electric and magnetic fields traveling at the speed of light. Non-ionizing radiation includes the spectrum of ultraviolet (UV), visible light, infrared (IR), microwave (MW), radio frequency (RF), and extremely low frequency (ELF). Lasers commonly operate in the UV, visible, and IR frequencies. Non-ionizing radiation is found in a wide range of occupational settings and can pose a considerable health risk to potentially exposed workers if not properly controlled."[46] TABLE 5.6 gives examples of types and sources of non-ionizing radiation.

Extremely Low-Frequency Magnetic Fields

Workers exposed to extremely low-frequency magnetic fields (ELF-MF) include electricians, welders, printers, telephonists, and some clerical workers.[47] The health effects of exposure to ELF-MF are not well understood, but one of the major concerns is the potential for carcinogenic effects. The International Agency for Cancer Research regards this type of radiation as possibly carcinogenic to humans.[48] Based on a case-control study of residential occupational exposures to 50-Hz magnetic fields (the type emitted by power lines), investigators concluded that there was a suggested association between such exposure and female breast cancer.[48] In contrast, childhood cancer was examined in relation to fathers' occupational exposure to

TABLE 5.6 Examples of Types and Sources of Nonionizing Radiation

Type of Non-ionizing Radiation	Description
Extremely low-frequency radiation (ELF)	ELF radiation at 60 Hz is produced by power lines, electrical wiring, and electrical equipment. Common sources of intense exposure include ELF induction furnaces and high-voltage power lines.
Radiofrequency (RF) and microwave (MW) radiation	MW radiation is absorbed near the skin, while RF radiation may be absorbed throughout the body. At high enough intensities, both will damage tissue through heating. Sources of RF and MW radiation include radio emitters and cell phones.
Infrared (IR) radiation	The skin and eyes absorb IR radiation as heat. Workers normally notice excessive exposure through heat sensation and pain. Sources of IR radiation include furnaces, heat lamps, and IR lasers.
Visible light radiation	The different visible frequencies of the electromagnetic (EM) spectrum are "seen" by our eyes as different colors. Good lighting is conducive to increased production, and may help prevent incidents related to poor lighting conditions. Excessive visible radiation can damage the eyes and skin.
Ultraviolet (UV) radiation	UV radiation has a high photon energy range and is particularly hazardous because there are usually no immediate symptoms of excessive exposure. Sources of UV radiation include the sun, black lights, welding arcs, and UV lasers.
Laser hazards	Lasers typically emit optical (UV, visible light, IR) radiation and are primarily an eye and skin hazard. Common lasers include the CO_2 IR laser; helium–neon, neodymium YAG, and ruby visible lasers; and the nitrogen UV laser.

Reproduced from U.S. Department of Labor. Occupational Safety and Health Administration. Non-ionizing radiation. https://www.osha.gov/SLTC/radiation_nonionizing/index.html. Accessed August 23, 2013.

ELF-MF. A case-control study of more than 2000 children with childhood cancers did not find a linkage between parental occupational exposure to ELF-MF and childhood cancer.[49]

Magnetic Resonance Imaging

Magnetic resonance imaging (MRI) is a medical imaging technique that uses intense magnetic fields instead of ionizing radiation to create images of the inside of the human body.[50] Advances in MRI procedures have increased the potential for work-associated exposures to magnetic fields.[51] Exposed workers can experience malfunctioning and heating up of implanted medical devices such as pacemakers and metal prostheses.

Ultraviolet Radiation

Ultraviolet (UV) radiation is a form of non-ionizing radiation that can affect many types of workers, especially those who work outdoors. Examples of such workers "include lifeguards, construction workers, agricultural workers, landscapers, gardeners, and other outdoor workers."[52] In addition to the sun, other sources of UV radiation include lights that emit UV rays (e.g., in laboratories), laser devices, and welding arcs. EXHIBIT 5.4 describes solar UV rays.

Radiation from Lasers

The acronym LASER (more commonly seen as the lowercase form, laser) is an acronym that stands for "light amplification by stimulated emission of radiation." "The laser produces an intense, highly directional beam of light. The most common cause of laser-induced tissue damage is thermal in nature."[53] Although the skin can be damaged by radiation from

---

EXHIBIT 5.4   Solar UV Rays

Ultraviolet rays are a part of sunlight that is an invisible form of radiation. UV rays can penetrate and change the structure of skin cells. There are three types of UV rays: ultraviolet A (UVA), ultraviolet B (UVB), and ultraviolet C (UVC). UVA is the most abundant source of solar radiation at the earth's surface and penetrates beyond the top layer of human skin. Scientists believe that UVA radiation can cause damage to connective tissue and increase a person's risk for developing skin cancer. UVB rays penetrate less deeply into skin, but can still cause some forms of skin cancer. Natural UVC rays do not pose a risk to workers because they are absorbed by the earth's atmosphere. Sunlight exposure is highest during the summer and between 10:00 a.m. and 4:00 p.m. Working outdoors during these times increases the chances of getting sunburned. Snow and light-colored sand reflect UV light and increase the risk of sunburn. At worksites with these conditions, UV rays may reach workers' exposed skin from both above and below. Workers are at risk of UV radiation even on cloudy days. Many drugs increase sensitivity to sunlight and the risk of getting sunburn. Some common ones include thiazides, diuretics, tetracycline, doxycycline, sulfa antibiotics, and nonsteroidal anti-inflammatory drugs, such as ibuprofen.

Reproduced from Centers for Disease Control and Prevention. National Institute for Occupational Safety and Health (NIOSH). UV radiation. http://www.cdc.gov/niosh/topics/uvradiation/. Accessed January 16, 2014.

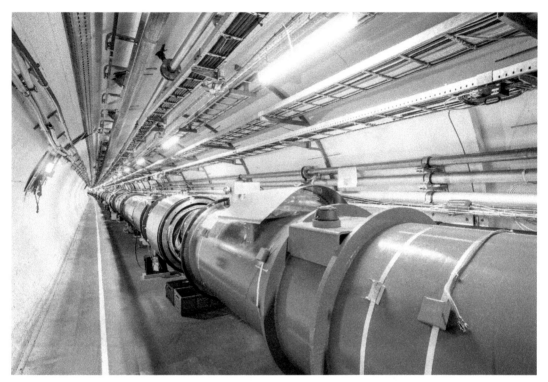

FIGURE 5.15   Stanford University-operated SLAC National Accelerator for producing X-ray laser pulses

© xenotar/iStockphoto

lasers, the human eye is usually more vulnerable to injury than the skin. Lasers pose hazards for serious injuries to the eye and skin from direct exposure and from secondary emissions.[54]

High-powered lasers for welding and cutting are used widely in industry. FIGURE 5.15 shows a laser used in research at Stanford University.

Microwave and Radiofrequency Radiation

Radiofrequency (RF) radiation (frequency range from 3 kilohertz [KHz] to 300 megahertz [MHz]) and microwave (MW) radiation (frequency range from 300 MHz to 300 gigahertz [GHz]) are both forms of electromagnetic radiation. Occupational exposure to MW radiation can occur in installations that involve the use of radar. Sources of exposure to both RF and MW radiation include "radios, cellular phones, the processing and cooking of foods, heat sealers, vinyl welders, high frequency welders, induction heaters, flow solder machines, communications transmitters, radar transmitters, ion implant equipment, microwave drying equipment, sputtering equipment and glue curing."[55] FIGURE 5.16 shows a mountain-top antenna farm with a collection of microwave and radiofrequency antennae.

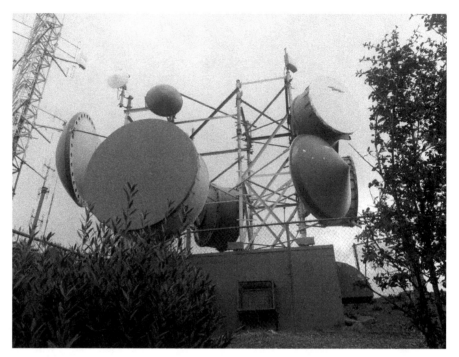

FIGURE 5.16   Microwave and radiofrequency antenna farm

Extreme Temperatures: High or Low

Very high and very low ambient temperatures can reduce the performance of workers.[56] Both extreme heat and cold are hazards for persons who must work outdoors or are involved with activities that bring them into contact with hot and cold environments. Workers exposed to such extreme temperatures can experience illnesses, injuries, and possibly mortality.

Heat Stress

In the context of the work environment, hyperthermia refers to "[o]verheating of the body, possibly due to extreme weather conditions. Unrelieved hyperthermia can lead to collapse and death, particularly in the elderly."[57] TABLE 5.7 gives reasons for preventing heat illness in the workplace.

Heat-related illnesses include heat rash, heat cramps, heat exhaustion, and heat stroke—a life-threatening condition that demands immediate medical attention.[58] Heat exhaustion is characterized by symptoms that include dizziness, headache, weakness, and nausea. Although heat exhaustion usually is not life threatening, persons with heat exhaustion need to receive appropriate interventions such as being moved to a cool area and provided with drinking water; they should not continue working.

TABLE 5.7   Why It Is Important to Prevent Heat Illness in the Workplace

- Heat illness can be a matter of life and death. Workers die from heat stroke every summer, and every one of these deaths is preventable.
- When heat stroke does not kill immediately, it can shut down major body organs, causing acute heart, liver, kidney, and muscle damage; nervous system problems; and blood disorders.
- Having a serious injury or death occur at work affects everyone at a worksite.
- Workers suffering from heat exhaustion are at greater risk for accidents, because they are less alert and can be confused.

Reproduced from U.S. Department of Labor. Occupational Safety and Health Administration (OSHA). Heat Illness Prevention Training Guide. OSHA 3437-04 N 2011.

In contrast, heat stroke is a serious and potentially fatal medical condition that requires immediate medical attention. Persons with heat stroke have symptoms that include high body temperature (104–106°F), convulsions, and skin surfaces that become red, hot, and dry. **FIGURE 5.17** gives additional information on heat exhaustion and heat stroke.

Two types of heat illness:

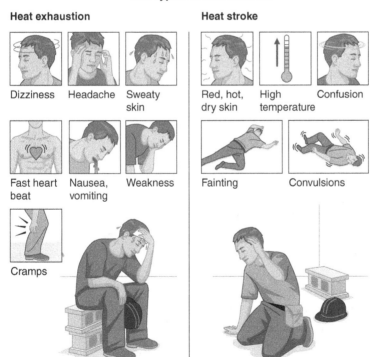

Heat kills — get help right away!

FIGURE 5.17   Two types of heat illness

Reproduced from U.S. Department of Labor, Occupational Safety and Health Administration, Water. Rest. Shade, https://www.osha.gov/SLTC/heatillness/3422_factsheet_en.pdf. Accessed February 13, 2014.

**NOAA's National Weather Service
Heat Index**

Temperature (°F)

Relative Humidity (%)	80	82	84	86	88	90	92	94	96	98	100	102	104	106	108	110
40	80	81	83	85	88	91	94	97	101	105	109	114	119	124	130	136
45	80	82	84	87	89	93	96	100	104	109	114	119	124	130	137	
50	81	83	85	88	91	95	99	103	108	113	118	124	131	137		
55	81	84	86	89	93	97	101	106	112	117	124	130	137			
60	82	84	88	91	95	100	105	110	116	123	129	137				
65	82	85	89	93	98	105	108	114	121	126	130					
70	83	86	90	95	100	108	112	119	126	134						
75	84	88	92	97	103	109	116	124	132							
80	84	89	94	100	106	113	121	129								
85	85	90	96	102	110	117	126	135								
90	86	91	98	105	113	122	131									
95	86	93	100	108	117	127										
100	87	95	103	112	121	132										

Likelihood of Heat Disorders with Prolonged
Exposure or Strenuous Activity

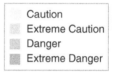

Caution
Extreme Caution
Danger
Extreme Danger

FIGURE 5.18   The National Weather Service Heat Index, U.S. National Oceanographic and Atmospheric Administration (NOAA)

Courtesy of U.S. Department of Labor, Occupational Safety and Health Administration. Using the heat index: A guide for employer, https://www.osha.gov/SLTC/heatillness/heat_index/pdfs/all_in_one.pdf. Accessed February 11, 2014.

FIGURE 5.18 depicts the danger levels for heat identified by the National Oceanographic and Atmospheric Administration (NOAA) in the National Weather Service Heat Index. The heat index levels that pose extreme dangers for heat-related disorders from strenuous activity are shown in color. Figure 5.18 also provides information about other hazard levels for various combinations of temperature and humidity levels.

TABLE 5.8 lists protective measures geared toward each risk level of the heat index. The heat index values shown have been changed to make them appropriate for the work environment; thus they differ from the NOAA heat index values, which are geared toward use by the public. Protective measures in excessive heat conditions range from making drinking water available on the worksite to rescheduling nonessential activities to days when the heat index is lower.

Occupational Settings with High Ambient Temperatures

Occupational settings with high ambient temperatures include both outdoor environments (especially when people work on a hot day unprotected from the sun) and indoor venues. According to OSHA, "Operations involving

TABLE 5.8   Using the Heat Index: A Guide for Employers

Heat Index	Risk Level	Protective Measures
91°F	Lower (caution)	• Provide drinking water. • Ensure that adequate medical services are available. • Plan ahead for times when the heat index is higher, including worker heat safety training. • Encourage workers to wear sunscreen.
91°F to 103°F	Moderate	In addition to the steps listed previously: • Remind workers to drink water often (about 4 cups/hour). • Review heat-related illness topics with workers: how to recognize heat-related illness, how to prevent it, and what to do if someone gets sick. • Schedule frequent breaks in a cool, shaded area • Acclimatize workers. • Set up a buddy system/instruct supervisors to watch workers for signs of heat-related illness.
103°F to 115°F	High	In addition to the steps listed previously: • Alert workers of high-risk conditions. • Actively encourage workers to drink plenty of water (about 4 cups/hour). • Limit physical exertion (e.g., use mechanical lifts). • Have a knowledgeable person at the worksite who is well informed about heat-related illness and able to determine appropriate work/rest schedules. • Establish and enforce work/rest schedules. • Adjust work activities (e.g., reschedule work, pace/rotate jobs). • Use cooling techniques. • Watch/communicate with workers at all times. When possible, reschedule activities to a time when the heat index is lower.
>115°F	Very high to extreme	Reschedule nonessential activity for days with a reduced heat index or to a time when the heat index is lower. Move essential work tasks to the coolest part of the work shift; consider earlier start times, split shifts, or evening and night shifts. Strenuous work tasks and those requiring the use of heavy or nonbreathable clothing or impermeable chemical-protective clothing should not be performed when the heat index is at or above 115°F. If essential work must be done, in addition to the steps listed previously: • Alert workers of extreme heat hazards. • Establish water drinking schedule (about 4 cups/hour). • Develop and enforce protective work/rest schedules. • Conduct physiological monitoring (e.g., pulse, temperature). • Stop work if essential control methods are inadequate or unavailable.

Reproduced from U.S. Department of Labor. Occupational Safety and Health Administation. Using the Heat Index: A Guide for Employers. https://www.osha.gov/SLTC/heatillness/heat_index/pdfs/all_in_one.pdf. Accessed February 11, 2014.

high air temperatures, radiant heat sources, high humidity, direct physical contact with hot objects, or strenuous physical activities have a high potential for causing heat-related illness. Workplaces with these conditions may include iron and steel foundries, nonferrous foundries, brick-firing and ceramic plants, glass products facilities, rubber products factories, electrical utilities (particularly boiler rooms), bakeries, confectioneries, commercial kitchens, laundries, food canneries, chemical plants, mining sites, smelters, and steam tunnels."[58] EXHIBIT 5.5 describes heat-related deaths among crop workers in the United States.

Cold Stress

FIGURE 5.20 shows an individual working outdoors in the snow. Such work is conducive to cold stress, which is associated with excessive loss of heat from the body. Cold stress can occur among persons who need to work outdoors on cold days as well as among individuals who work in unheated or poorly heated buildings. The adverse effects of work in very cold temperatures can be prevented—for example, by wearing appropriate clothing and shoes and moving periodically to heated areas.

EXHIBIT 5.5   Heat-Related Deaths among Crop Workers—United States, 1992–2006

Workers employed in outdoor occupations such as farming are exposed to hot and humid environments that put them at risk for heat-related illness or death. During 1992–2006, a total of 423 worker deaths from exposure to environmental heat were reported in the United States, resulting in an average annual fatality rate of 0.02 death per 100,000 workers. Of these 423 deaths, 102 (24%) occurred in workers employed in the agriculture, forestry, fishing, and hunting industries (rate: 0.16 death per 100,000 workers); 68 of the 102 deaths (67%) occurred in workers employed in the crop production or support activities for crop production sectors, resulting in an average annual fatality rate of 0.39 death per 100,000 crop workers. During 1992–2006, nearly all deceased crop workers were male, and 78% were aged 20–54 years. Analysis of fatality rates by 5-year periods suggests an increase in rates over time; however, those rates were based on small numbers of deaths, and the increase over time was not statistically significant (FIGURE 5.19).

Case Report

In mid-July 2005, a male Hispanic worker with an H-2A work visa (i.e., a temporary, non-immigrant foreign worker hired under contract to perform farm work), aged 56 years, was hand-harvesting ripe tobacco leaves on a North Carolina farm. He had arrived from Mexico 4 days earlier and was on his third day on the job. The man began work at approximately 6:00 a.m. and took a short mid-morning break and a 90-minute lunch break.

(Continues)

EXHIBIT 5.6   Heat-Related Deaths among Crop Workers—United States, 1992–2006 (*Continued*)

At approximately 2:45 p.m., the employer's son observed the man working slowly and reportedly instructed him to rest, but the man continued working. Shortly thereafter, the man's coworkers noticed that he appeared confused. Although the man was combative, his coworkers carried him to the shade and tried unsuccessfully to get him to drink water. At approximately 3:50 p.m., coworkers notified the employer of the man's condition. At 4:25 p.m., the man was taken by ambulance to an emergency department, where his core body temperature was recorded at 108°F (42°C) and, despite treatment, he died. The cause of death was heat stroke.

On the day of the incident, the local high temperature was approximately 93°F (34°C), with 44% relative humidity and clear skies. The heat index was in the range of 86–101°F (30–38°C) at mid-morning and 97–112°F (36–44°C) at mid-afternoon. Similar conditions had occurred during the preceding two days. The man had been given safety and health training on pesticides but nothing that addressed the hazards and prevention of heat-related stress. He reportedly spoke only Spanish. Fluids, such as water and soda, were always available to the workers in the field; however, whether the man drank any of these fluids is unknown.

Reproduced from Centers for Disease Control and Prevention, Heat-related deaths among crop workers-U.S., 1992–2006. *MMWR*. 2008;57(24): p. 649-651.

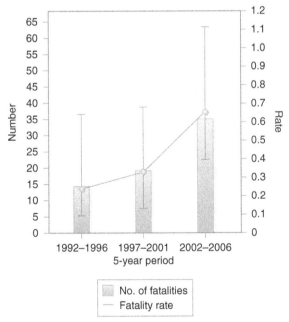

FIGURE 5.19   Number and rate (per 100,000 workers) of heat-related deaths among crop workers, by 5-year period—United States, 1992–2006.

Reproduced from Centers for Disease Control and Prevention, Heat-related deaths among crop workers—U.S., 1992–2006. *MMWR*. 2008;57(24):652.

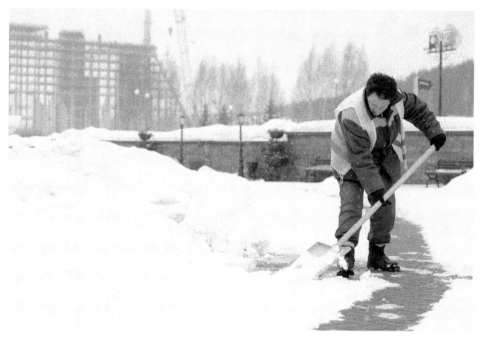

FIGURE 5.20 Cold stress
© Vadim Ratnikov/Shutterstock

Cold stress can result in several adverse health outcomes including hypothermia, frostbite, trench foot, and chilblains. Hypothermia refers to "[a] condition in which the body uses up its stored energy and can no longer produce heat. Often occurs after prolonged exposure to cold temperature."[59(p. 1)] **TABLE 5.9** lists the symptoms of hypothermia. The term frostbite denotes "[a]n injury to the body that is caused by freezing, which most often affects the nose, ears, cheeks, chin, fingers, or toes."[59(p. 1)] Trench foot is a painful and sometimes dangerous condition that occurs when the feet remain wet for long periods. Chilblains refer to swelling and itching of the skin that occurs when it is exposed to cold temperatures.

Variations in Atmospheric Pressure

Variations in atmospheric pressure in the job setting may include either high air pressure (hyperbaric) or low air pressure (hypobaric) environments. Such atmospheric pressure variations may lead to a variety of health risks.

Hyperbaric Environments

Hyperbaric environments are those with high ambient air pressures—that is, pressures greater than one atmosphere. Human beings are unable to adapt

TABLE 5.9 Symptoms of Hypothermia

Early Symptoms	Late Symptoms
Shivering	No shivering
Fatigue	Blue skin
Loss of coordination	Dilated pupils
Confusion	Slowed pulse and breathing
Disorientation	Loss of consciousness

Reproduced from Centers for Disease Control and Prevention, National Institute of Occupational Safety and Health (NIOSH). Protecting Yourself from Cold Stress. DHHS (NIOSH) Publication Number 2010-115.

biologically to high air pressures. At high air pressures, more gases than usual (e.g., nitrogen) become dissolved in the body's tissues and diffuse throughout the body. When air pressures are reduced suddenly, gas bubbles form as the gases become vaporized again, causing short-term muscle cramps, skin and joint pain, acute neurologic symptoms, and, in some instances, paralysis. This condition, which is known as the bends or decompression sickness (DCS), can occur when divers or other persons working at high atmospheric pressures return to conditions of normal atmospheric pressures. Permanent sequelae of DCS can include neurologic impairment and reduced health-related quality of life, as observed by researchers among former North Sea divers who had experienced DCS.[60]

Hyperbaric environments are encountered during underwater diving, while working in underground pressurized chambers, and in hyperbaric chambers used for medical treatments. Underwater operations connected with offshore drilling for oil are a source of exposure of workers to high-pressure environments. Caisson disease refers to an illness observed among workers who were subjected to high pressures while working underground during construction of the Brooklyn Bridge in the 1870s. This disease was actually decompression sickness caused by moving from an environment that had a high air pressure to one with normal atmospheric pressure.[61]

Another potential hazard of working under high atmospheric pressure is known as dysbaric osteonecrosis (DON). This occupational hazard is characterized by pain and changes in the joints such as joint deformity. At-risk workers include divers and caisson workers. Apparently the risk of DON can be reduced through training of exposed workers. For example, Bolte et al. reported that highly trained military divers did not appear to have an increased incidence of DON.[62]

Hyperbaric chambers use a high atmospheric pressure environment for the treatment of medical conditions such as carbon monoxide poisoning, nonhealing sores, and gangrene. Hyperbaric nurses are exposed to high gas pressures because they need to accompany patients undergoing treatment into the hyperbaric chamber in which the oxygen level is 100%. Although the nurses are exposed to high gas pressures, usually they breathe normal air and not pure oxygen. When the patients finish their treatments, the nurses are at risk of experiencing decompression sickness when air pressure returns to normal. Through the use of preventive measures (e.g., rotating nursing personnel and minimizing hyperbaric exposures), the risks of decompression sickness can be kept low among these workers. For example, none of the hyperbaric nurses in a Turkish study experienced decompression sickness.[63]

Hypobaric Environments

Hypobaric environments are characterized by reduced atmospheric pressures, such as those encountered at high altitudes and in outer space. Increased exposure of workers to high altitudes has occurred as a result of mining activities in Chile and Peru at elevations of about 4500 meters. Astronomers are another group of workers who must work at altitudes similar to those encountered by South American high-altitude miners. Although the human body sometimes is able to adapt to work at high elevations, some workers can develop high-altitude sickness, which includes acute mountain sickness (e.g., dizziness, light-headedness, fatigue, headache, and confusion), high-altitude pulmonary edema, and high-altitude cerebral edema.[64] Astronauts may develop muscle fiber atrophy after only a few days in outer space.

SUMMARY

Among the physical hazards encountered in the work environment are radiation (both ionizing and non-ionizing), noise and vibration, and atmospheric variations in temperatures and air pressure. Physical hazards are associated with a broad spectrum of work-associated morbidity and mortality. For example, workers' exposure to ionizing radiation may lead to an increased risk of some forms of cancer and adverse reproductive outcomes. Non-ionizing radiation from ultraviolet light, infrared radiation, radiofrequency sources, and microwaves can affect the eyes, injure the skin, and cause tissue burns.

Oscillatory vibrations include work-related noise and vibrations of the body. Excessive noise exposure is associated with temporary and permanent hearing loss and may have adverse psychological consequences. Vibration, both full-body and hand–arm, has been linked with adverse health effects ranging from musculoskeletal injuries to Raynaud's syndrome.

Atmospheric variations include hot and cold temperatures and hypobaric and hyperbaric conditions. Work-related high temperatures may cause heat stress, which can lead to fatal consequences. Low temperatures and resulting cold stress may produce frostbite and hypothermia. Among the effects of low atmospheric pressures (e.g., due to working at high altitudes) are pulmonary edema and loss of consciousness. The high atmospheric pressures encountered by deep-sea divers, some underground construction workers, and medical personnel who operate hyperbaric chambers may produce both acute effects, such as the bends and caisson disease, and longer-term effects, such as neurologic and bone and joint disease.

STUDY QUESTIONS AND EXERCISES

1. Define the following terms:
   A. Decibel (dB)
   B. Radioactivity
   C. Extremely low-frequency magnetic fields (ELF-MF)
   D. Raynaud's phenomenon
   E. Caisson disease
2. Provide three examples of physical hazards in the work environment. Describe occupational settings in which these physical hazards might be found.
3. What is meant by oscillatory vibrations? Describe the similarities and differences between noise and vibration.
4. Which health effects are associated with a noisy work environment? What are safe levels of exposure to excessive noise in the workplace? Describe some of the methods used to protect workers from occupationally associated noise.
5. What are some examples of occupations that expose workers to vibration? Describe health effects that have been attributed to whole-body and hand–arm vibration.
6. Distinguish between ionizing and non-ionizing radiation. Identify two sources of each kind of radiation.
7. Give some examples of occupations that may expose workers to ionizing radiation. Why should employees be concerned about ionizing radiation even at low levels?
8. Which types of occupational settings may expose employees to non-ionizing radiation? What are some of the possible health effects of exposure to non-ionizing radiation?
9. What are the possible health effects of occupational exposures to extreme—either high or low—temperatures? Which steps can employers and employees take to prevent adverse health effects of exposure to high temperatures?
10. Give examples of atmospheric variations that impact workers in various occupations. Describe some of the possible health effects that have been ascribed to work in low atmospheric pressure and high atmospheric pressure environments.

REFERENCES

1. U.S. Department of Labor, Occupational Safety and Health Administration. Occupational noise exposure. n.d. https://www.osha.gov/SLTC/noisehearingconservation/index.html. Accessed August 23, 2013.
2. U.S. Department of Labor, Occupational Safety and Health Administration. Radiation. n.d. https://www.osha.gov/SLTC/radiation/index.html. Accessed August 23, 2013.

3. Centers for Disease Control and Prevention, National Institute for Occupational Safety and Health (NIOSH), National Occupational Research Agenda. *Occupationally-induced hearing loss: employers and employees in manufacturing need your help.* DHHS (NIOSH) Publication No. 2010-136. Cincinnati, OH: DHHS (NIOSH); 2010.

4. Centers for Disease Control and Prevention. Severe hearing impairment among military veterans—United States, 2010. *MMWR.* 2011;60(28):955–958.

5. National Institute on Deafness and Other Communication Disorders (NIDCD). *Noise-induced hearing loss.* Publication No. 08-4233. Bethesda, MD: NIDCD; 2008.

6. Franks JR, Stephenson MR, Merry CJ, eds. *Preventing occupational hearing loss: a practical guide.* DHHS (NIOSH) Publication No. 96-110. Cincinnati, OH: DHHS, CDC, NIOSH; 1996.

7. Thefreedictionary.com. Audiometry. n.d. http://medical-dictionary.thefreedictionary.com/p/Audiometry. Accessed January 15, 2014.

8. U.S. Department of Labor, Occupational Safety and Health Administration. Instruments used to conduct a noise survey. n.d. https://www.osha.gov/dts/osta/otm/noise/exposure/instrumentation.html. Accessed January 14, 2014.

9. Neitzel RL. Noise exposures aboard catcher/processor fishing vessels. *Am J Ind Med.* 2006;49:624–633.

10. Chang T-Y, Hwang B-F, Liu C-S, et al. Occupational noise exposure and incident hypertension in men: a prospective cohort study. *Am J Epidemiol.* 2013;177(8):818–825.

11. Edwards CG, Schwartzbaum JA, Nise G, et al. Occupational noise exposure and risk of acoustic neuroma. *Am J Epidemiol.* 2007;166:1252–1258.

12. Bovenzi M. Health effects of mechanical vibration. *G Ital Med Lav Erg.* 2005;27(1):58–64.

13. Palmer KT, Griffin MJ, Bendall H, et al. Prevalence and pattern of occupational exposure to whole body vibration in Great Britain: findings from a national survey. *Occup Environ Med.* 2000;57:229–236.

14. Tiemessen IJH, Hulshof CTJ, Frings-Dresen MHW. Low back pain in drivers exposed to whole body vibration: analysis of a dose–response pattern. *Occup Environ Med.* 2008;65:667–675.

15. Palmer KT, Griffin MJ, Syddall HE, et al. The relative importance of whole body vibration and occupational lifting as risk factors for low-back pain. *Occup Environ Med.* 2003;60:715–721.

16. Lings S, Leboeuf-Yde C. Whole-body vibration and low back pain: a systematic, critical review of the epidemiological literature 1992–1999. *Int Arch Occup Environ Health.* 2000;73:290–297.

17. Harris MA, Marion SA, Spinelli JJ, et al. Occupational exposure to whole-body vibration and Parkinson's disease: results from a population-based case-control study. *Am J Epidemiol.* 2012;176(4):299–307.

18. Centers for Disease Control and Prevention, National Institute for Occupational Safety and Health. Vibration syndrome. n.d. http://www.cdc.gov/niosh/docs/83-110. Accessed September 24, 2013.

19. Centers for Disease Control and Prevention (CDC), National Institute for Occupational Safety and Health (NIOSH). *Occupational exposure to hand–arm vibration.* Cincinnati, OH: CDC (NIOSH); 1989.

20. Griffin MJ, Bovenzi M, Nelson CM. Dose–response patterns for vibration-induced white finger. *Occup Environ Med.* 2003;60:16–26.

21. Wahlström J, Burström L, Hagberg M, et al. Musculoskeletal symptoms among young male workers and associations with exposure to hand–arm vibration and ergonomic stressors. *Int Arch Occup Environ Health.* 2008;81:595–602.

22. Färkkilä M. Vibration induced injury. *Br J Ind Med.* 1986;43:361–362.

23. Kaminski M, Bourgine M, Zins M, et al. Risk factors for Raynaud's phenomenon among workers in poultry slaughterhouses and canning factories. *Int J Epidemiol.* 1997;26(2):371–380.

24. Sauni R, Pääkkönen R, Virtema P, et al. Dose–response relationship between exposure to hand–arm vibration and health effects among metalworkers. *Ann Occup Hyg.* 2009;53(1):55–62.

25. Gerhardsson L, Burstrom L, Hagberg M, et al. Quantitative neurosensory findings, symptoms and signs in young vibration exposed workers. *J Occup Med Toxicol.* 2013;8:8.

26. Schweigert M. The relationship between hand–arm vibration and lower extremity clinical manifestations: a review of the literature. *Int Arch Occup Environ Health.* 2002;75:179–185.

27. Oak Ridge Associated Universities. Basics of radiation. n.d. https://orise.orau.gov /reacts/guide/definitions.htm. Accessed February 7, 2014.

28. U.S. Environmental Protection Agency. Radiation protection: health effects: radiation and health. n.d. http://www.epa.gov/radiation/understand/health_effects.html. Accessed February 7, 2014.

29. *Merriam-Webster's collegiate dictionary.* 11th ed. Versailles, KY: Merriam-Webster; 2012.

30. Oak Ridge Associated Universities. Types of radiation exposure. n.d. http://orise. orau.gov/reacts/guide/injury.htm. Accessed February 7, 2014.

31. National Academy of Sciences. *Health risks from exposure to low levels of ionizing radiation: BEIR VII—Phase 2.* Washington, DC: National Academies Press; 2006.

32. U.S. Department of Labor, Occupational Safety and Health Administration. Ionizing radiation. n.d. http://www.osha.gov/SLTC/radiationionizing/. Accessed February 2, 2014.

33. International Atomic Energy Agency. Occupational exposure to radiation. n.d. http:// www.iaea.org/Publications/Booklets/RadPeopleEnv/pdf/chapter_9.pdf. Accessed October 18, 2013.

34. Dewar C. Occupational radiation safety. *Radiol Technol.* 2013;84(5):467–486.

35. Klein LW, Miller DL, Balter S, et al. Occupational health hazards in the interventional laboratory: time for a safer environment. *J Vasc Interv Radiol.* 2009;20:147–153.

36. Baker DG. How significant are the risks from occupational exposure to ionizing radiation? *Appl Radiol.* 1989;18(9):19–21, 24.

37. Chodick G, Bekiroglu N, Hauptmann M, et al. Risk of cataract after exposure to low doses of ionizing radiation: a 20-year prospective cohort study among US radiologic technologists. *Am J Epidemiol.* 2008;168:620–631.

38. Linet MS, Kim KP, Miller DL, et al. Historical review of occupational exposures and cancer risks in medical radiation workers. *Radiat Res.* 2010;174:793–808.

39. Wing S, Richardson DB. Age at exposure to ionising radiation and cancer mortality among Hanford workers: follow up through 1994. *Occup Environ Med.* 2005;62(7):465–472.

40. Richardson DB, Wing S. Leukemia mortality among workers at the Savannah River site. *Am J Epidemiol.* 2007;166:1015–1022.

41. Zablotska LB, Lane RSD, Frost SE. Mortality (1950–1999) and cancer incidence (1969–1999) of workers in the Port Hope cohort study exposed to a unique combination of radium, uranium and γ-ray doses. *BMJ Open.* 2013;3:e002159.

42. Schröder C, Friedrich K, Butz M, et al. Uranium mining in Germany: incidence of occupational diseases 1946–1999. *Int Arch Occup Environ Health.* 2002;75:235–242.

43. Zeeb H, Shannoun F, eds. *WHO handbook on indoor radon: a public health perspective.* Geneva, Switzerland: World Health Organization; 2009.

44. Hazelton WD, Luebeck EG, Heidenreich WF, Moolgavkar SH. Analysis of a historical cohort of Chinese tin miners with arsenic, radon, cigarette smoke, and pipe smoke exposures using the biologically based two-stage clonal expansion model. *Radiat Res.* 2001;156:78–94.

45. Mori K, Tateishi S, Hiraoka K, et al. How occupational health can contribute in a disaster and what we should prepare for the future: lessons learned through support activities of a medical school at the Fukushima Daiichi nuclear power plant in summer 2011. *J Occup Health.* 2013;55:6–10.

46. U.S. Department of Labor, Occupational Safety and Health Administration. Nonionizing radiation. n.d. https://www.osha.gov/SLTC/radiation_nonionizing/index.html. Accessed August 23, 2013.

47. Mee T, Whatmough P, Broad L, et al. Occupational exposure of UK adults to extremely low frequency magnetic fields. *Occup Environ Med.* 2009;66:619–627.

48. Kliukiene J, Tynes T, Andersen A. Residential and occupational exposures to 50-Hz magnetic fields and breast cancer in women: a population-based study. *Am J Epidemiol.* 2004:159:852–861.

49. Hug K, Grize L, Seidler A, et al. Parental occupational exposure to extremely low frequency magnetic fields and childhood cancer: a German case-control study. *Am J Epidemiol.* 2010;171:27–35.

50. U.S. Food and Drug Administration. Magnetic resonance imaging. n.d. http://www.fda.gov/Radiation-EmittingProducts/RadiationEmittingProductsandProcedures/MedicalImaging/ucm200086.htm. Accessed February 13, 2014.

51. Kännälä S, Toivo T, Alanko T, Jokela K. Occupational exposure measurements of static and pulsed gradient magnetic fields in the vicinity of MRI scanners. *Phys Med Biol.* 2009;54:2243–2257.

52. Centers for Disease Control and Prevention, National Institute for Occupational Safety and Health. UV radiation. n.d. http://www.cdc.gov/niosh/topics/uvradiation/. Accessed January 16, 2014.

53. U.S. Department of Labor, Occupational Safety and Health Administration. Laser hazards. n.d. https://www.osha.gov/SLTC/laserhazards/index.html. Accessed October 18, 2013.

54. Laser Institute of America. Hazards of laser welders, cutters, heat treaters and punch presses. Fact sheet. n.d. http://d12d0wzn4zozj6.cloudfront.net/pdf/OSHAIndustrial%20Fact%20Sheet.pdf. Accessed February 21, 2014.

55. U.S. Department of Labor, Occupational Safety and Health Administration. Radiofrequency and microwave radiation. n.d. https://www.osha.gov/SLTC/radiofrequencyradiation/index.html. Accessed January 16, 2014.

56. Rodahl K. Occupational health conditions in extreme environments. *Ann Occup Hyg.* 2003;47(3):241–252.

57. MedicineNet.com. Definition of hyperthermia. n.d. http://www.medterms.com/script/main/art.asp?articlekey=3848. Accessed January 14, 2014.

58. U.S. Department of Labor, Occupational Safety and Health Administration. Occupational heat exposure. n.d. https://www.osha.gov/SLTC/heatstress/index.html. Accessed August 23, 2013.

59. Centers for Disease Control and Prevention, National Institute for Occupational Safety and Health (NIOSH). *Protecting yourself from cold stress.* DHHS (NIOSH) Publication No. 2010–115. n.d.

60. Irgens Å, Grønning M, Troland K, et al. Reduced health-related quality of life in former North Sea divers is associated with decompression sickness. *Occup Med.* 2007;57:349–354.

61. Butler WP. Caisson disease during the construction of the Eads and Brooklyn Bridges: a review. *Undersea Hyperb Med.* 2004;31(4):445–459.

62. Bolte H, Koch A, Tetzlaff K, et al. Detection of dysbaric osteonecrosis in military divers using magnetic resonance imaging. *Eur Radiol.* 2005;15:368–375.

63. Uzun G, Mutluoğlu M, Ay H, Yildiz S. Decompression sickness in hyperbaric nurses: retrospective analysis of 4500 treatments. *J Clin Nurs.* 2011;20:1784–1787.

64. West JB. Health considerations for managing work at high altitudes. In: 37. Barometric pressure reduced. Dümmer W, ed. *Encyclopedia of occupational health and safety.* Stellman JM, ed. Geneva, Switzerland: International Labor Organization; 2011.

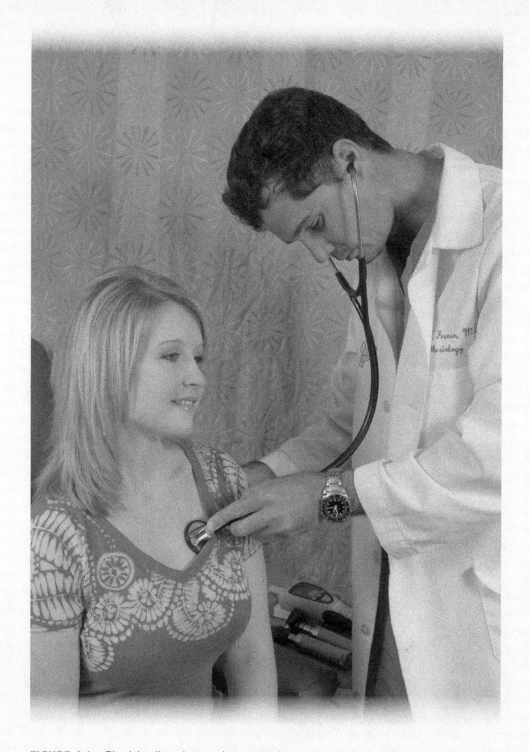

FIGURE 6.1 Physician listening to chest sounds

Courtesy of Centers for Disease Control and Prevention, Public Health Image Library.

Infectious disease agents are among the work-associated biological hazards of the healthcare setting. One of the modes of transmission of these agents is through contact with patients.

CHAPTER 6

Biological and Microbial Hazards in the Workplace

Learning Objectives

By the end of this chapter you will be able to:

- Describe three different categories of work-associated microbial agents.
- Discuss occupational hazards from blood and body fluids.
- Define the term *zoonotic diseases.*
- Give two examples of occupationally associated fungal diseases.
- Compare at least three occupations that pose a high risk for exposure to microbial agents.
- Describe methods of protecting at-risk employees against microbial agents.

Chapter Outline

- Introduction
- Categories of Work-Related Microbial Agents and Associated Diseases
- Occupational Exposures to Blood and Body Fluids
- Zoonotic Diseases
- Diseases Transmitted by Arthropod Vectors
- Fungal Diseases
- Other Agents
- Occupations in Which Workers Are at Risk of Exposure to Biohazards
- Methods for Protecting Employees Against Work-Related Biohazards
- Summary
- Study Questions and Exercises

Introduction

Hazardous biological agents (biohazards) pose significant occupational risks to workers in many fields and contribute substantially to the global burden of occupational morbidity worldwide. The term biohazard is composed of "[a] combination of the words biological hazard. [The term denotes organisms] or products of organisms that present a risk to humans."[1] Biohazards found in the workplace include agents of communicable (infectious) diseases. The term communicable disease means "[a]n illness due to a specific infectious agent or its toxic products that arises through transmission of that agent or its products from an infected person, animal, or reservoir to a susceptible host, either directly or indirectly through an intermediate plant or animal host, vector, or the inanimate environment."[2] If work related, such transmission occurs through direct or indirect contact with the agent in an occupational setting.

Of the estimated 2 million work-related deaths that occur globally each year, approximately 320,000 (16%) are caused by communicable diseases such as viral and bacterial infections.[3] As an example of the impact of job-related deaths from communicable diseases in the developed world, the European Union (EU) is estimated to experience 5000 deaths per year from infectious causes.[4] One of the major occupational hazards is the transmission of infectious diseases from exposure to blood and body fluids. However, many other types of work-related exposures to microbes are also possible.

In summary, work-related microbial agents pose significant hazards for illness and death of workers in some industries. This chapter covers the following topics with respect to occupational transmission of infectious agents:

- Agents transmitted by blood and body fluids
- Zoonoses
- Arthropod-borne infections
- Fungi
- Miscellaneous agents—for example, bacteria (e.g., foodborne bacteria, *Mycobacterium tuberculosis*, and *Helicobacter pylori*) and parasites

In addition to identifying categories of infectious agents, this chapter provides examples of infectious diseases, gives examples of occupations that pose risks of exposure to specific biohazards, and suggests methods for protecting workers against work-related biohazards.

Categories of Work-Related Microbial Agents and Associated Diseases

A diverse group of settings and materials represent potential hazards for exposure to microbial agents in the workplace. For example, such exposures can result from intentional commercial use of biological agents, contact with these agents in a clinical laboratory, or indirect contact as a result of occupational activities.[5] An example of the commercial use of biological agents includes addition of bacteria and molds to foods during production of cheese and bread. In clinical laboratories, technicians may come into contact with biohazards when culturing microorganisms collected from patients as part of a diagnostic procedure. Indirect contact with microbial agents can result from processing animal products such as hides or from disposal of waste materials that contain biohazards. EXHIBIT 6.1 lists other materials that can expose workers to biological agents.

TABLE 6.1 provides an overview of occupations that pose a risk of exposure to biohazards, the specific types of hazards and risks involved, and preventive measures for reducing exposures to them. Among these occupations are agriculture, forestry, metal and wood processing, textile manufacture, library and museum work, and construction. The types of microbial hazards associated with these work settings include bacteria, mites, viruses, and fungi (molds and yeasts).

Occupational Exposures to Blood and Body Fluids

Occupational exposures to blood and body fluids (BBF) are significant issues for physicians and nurses involved with direct patient care and operating

---

EXHIBIT 6.1   Materials that Can Expose Workers to Biological Agents

Hazardous biological agents occur in a wide range of materials used in the work environment. Some examples include the following:

* Natural or organic materials like soil, clay, and plant materials (e.g., hay, straw, cotton)
* Substances of animal origin (e.g., wool, hair)
* Food
* Organic dust (e.g. flour, paper dust, animal dander)
* Waste and wastewater
* Blood and other body fluids

Reproduced from European Agency for Safety and Health at Work (EU-OSHA). Biological agents. Bilbao, Spain: EU-OSHA; 2003.

TABLE 6.1   Biological Agents that Pose Occupational Hazards

Hazards/Risks	Occupations at Risk	Preventive Measures
Molds/yeasts, bacteria, and mites that cause allergies Organic dusts of grain, milk powder, or flour contaminated with biological agents Toxins such as botulinus toxins or aflatoxins	Food (cheese, yoghurt, salami) or food additive production, bakeries	Use closed processes [e.g., processes that prevent exposure of products to the work environment] Avoid aerosol formation Separate contaminated work areas Use appropriate hygiene measures
Several viral and bacterial infections such as HIV, hepatitis, or tuberculosis Needle stick injuries	Health care	Safe handling of infectious specimens, sharps waste, contaminated linen, and other material Safe handling and cleaning of blood spills and other body fluids Adequate protective equipment, gloves, clothing, and glasses Appropriate hygienic measures
Infections and allergies when handling microorganisms and cell cultures (e.g., of human tissues) Accidental spills and needle stick injuries	Laboratories	Microbiological safety cabinets Dust- and aerosol-reducing measures Safe handling and transport of samples Appropriate personal protection and hygiene measures Decontamination and emergency measures for spills Restricted access Biosafety label
Bacteria, fungi, mites and viruses transmitted from animals, parasites, and ticks Respiratory problems due to microorganisms and mites in organic dusts of grain, milk powder, flour, and spices Specific allergic diseases like farmer's lung and bird breeder's lung	Agriculture Forestry Horticulture Animal food and fodder production	Dust- and aerosol-reducing measures Avoiding contact with contaminated animals or equipment Protection against animal bites and stings Preservatives for fodder Cleaning and maintenance

(Continues)

TABLE 6.1   Biological Agents that Pose Occupational Hazards (*Continued*)

Hazards/Risks	Occupations at Risk	Preventive Measures
Skin problems due to bacteria and bronchial asthma due to molds/yeasts in circulating fluids in industrial processes such as grinding, pulp factories, and metal and stone cutting fluids	Metal processing industry Wood processing industry	Local exhaust ventilation Regular maintenance, filtering, and decontamination of fluids and machinery Skin protection Appropriate hygiene measures
Allergies and respiratory disorders due to molds/yeasts *Legionella*	Working areas with air-conditioning systems and high humidity (e.g., textile industry, print industry, and paper production)	Dust- and aerosol-reducing measures Regular maintenance of ventilation, machinery, and work areas Restrict number of workers Maintaining high hot (tap) water temperatures
Molds/yeasts and bacteria that cause allergies and respiratory disorders	Archives, museums, libraries	Dust and aerosol reduction Decontamination Adequate personal protective equipment
Molds and bacteria due to deterioration of building materials	Building and construction industry Processing of natural materials like clay, straw, and reed Redevelopment of buildings	Dust- and aerosol- reducing measures Appropriate personal protection and hygiene measures

Modified from European Agency for Safety and Health at Work (EU-OSHA). Biological agents. Bilbao, Spain: EU-OSHA; 2003.

room procedures, as well as for laboratory personnel and workers in a hospital's laundry room and waste disposal units. Also, such exposures are noteworthy hazards for correctional healthcare workers, because some prison populations have a higher prevalence of bloodborne diseases than other groups. In addition, prison violence can place healthcare personnel at risk of bites, stabbings, and other injuries. "Occupational exposure [to BBF] means reasonably anticipated skin, eye, mucous membrane, or parenteral contact with blood or other potentially infectious materials that

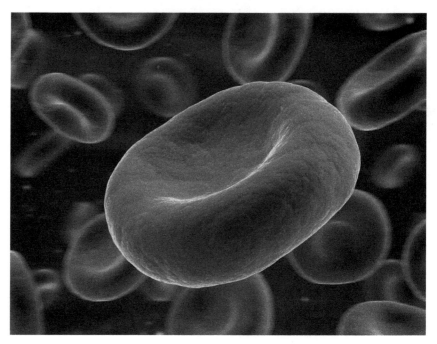

FIGURE 6.2   Red blood cells
© Sebastian Kaulitzki/ShutterStock, Inc.

may result from the performance of an employee's duties."[6] Human blood and blood components (e.g., red blood cells like those shown in **FIGURE 6.2**) should be regarded as a potential biohazards because they may contain infectious disease agents. Other potentially infectious materials from the human body include the following:[6]

- Human body fluids (e.g., semen, vaginal secretions, and saliva)
- Tissues or organs
- HIV-containing cells or tissue cultures

Contact with BBF increases the risk of employment-associated transmission of blood-borne microbes, including human immunodeficiency virus (HIV), hepatitis B virus (HBV), and hepatitis C virus (HCV). HIV is the infectious agent associated with acquired immunodeficiency syndrome (AIDS); HBV and HCV are both forms of viral hepatitis. All three viruses can be transmitted to healthcare workers through injuries with needles and cutting tools that are contaminated with infected blood.

Potential Types of Exposure to Blood and Body Fluids

Potential types of exposure to infections from blood and body fluids include unintentional needle sticks and cuts with surgical instruments (known as "sharps"), skin and other contact with microbes, and bites from patients. Doctors, nurses, other healthcare professionals, and custodians are among the workers who can have occupational exposures to blood and body fluids and are at increased risk of acquiring a blood-borne infection. EXHIBIT 6.2 defines some of the possible types of occupational exposures to human blood and tissues.

Relative Frequency of Types of Exposures to Blood and Body Fluids

Exposures to BBF are documented by the Centers for Disease Control and Prevention (CDC), which established the National Surveillance System for Health Care Workers (NaSH) for this purpose.[7] Operated as a voluntary program between 1995 and 2007, NaSH was implemented as a data source for the prevention of occupational exposures to biohazards that occurred among workers in the healthcare environment. FIGURE 6.3 provides data from NaSH concerning the routes of reported BBF exposures. As can be seen in the figure, percutaneous exposures were, by far, the most common route of exposure, accounting for more than 80% of all exposures.

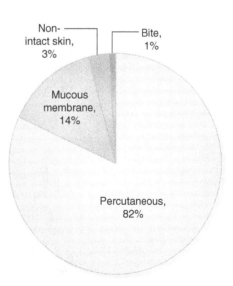

FIGURE 6.3   Routes of reported blood and body fluid exposures

Reproduced from Centers for Disease Control and Prevention, The National Surveillance System for Healthcare Workers, http://www.cdc.gov/nhsn/PDFs/NaSH/NaSH-Report-6-2011.pdf. Accessed September 27, 2013.

Occupational Transmission of Human Immunodeficiency Virus and Hepatitis B and C Virus

Prior to 2001, a total of 57 documented cases of HIV transmission from occupational exposures were recorded.[8] According to data from the National Occupational Mortality Surveillance (NOMS) system, employment in the healthcare field from 1984 to 2004 was related to increased mortality from blood-borne pathogens (HIV and HBV among males and HCV among both males and females).[9] Since early 2000, however, no confirmed cases of HIV transmitted to healthcare workers as a result of occupational exposure have been reported to the CDC. A vaccine for HBV is available that can be administered to protect healthcare workers against this virus. In contrast, no vaccines are available that afford protection against HIV and HCV.

Zoonotic Diseases

A zoonosis is "[a]n infection or infectious disease transmissible under natural conditions from vertebrate animals to humans. Examples include rabies and plague."[2] Skin contact with an infected animal, the bite or scratch of an animal, direct inhalation or ingestion (e.g., eating of contaminated food such as infected meats), or the bite of an arthropod vector are some of the methods for transmission of zoonotic pathogens. Employees who might come into contact with zoonotic disease agents include workers in facilities that house laboratory animals, farmers, abattoir workers, veterinarians, and persons who process hides from cattle. Three examples of diseases that can be transmitted occupationally from animals are anthrax, influenza, and Q fever. Some of the many zoonotic diseases and associated host animals (domestic and wild) are shown in **TABLE 6.2**.

Anthrax

Anthrax is "[a]n acute bacterial enzootic disease that can occur in three forms"[10(p. 22)] (*enzootic* means "present in certain species of animals"). The three types of anthrax are cutaneous (the most common form), pulmonary (called inhalational anthrax), and gastrointestinal. Untreated inhalational anthrax has a high case-fatality rate. Anthrax is caused by the bacterial agent *Bacillus anthracis*. One of the principal concerns regarding *B. anthracis* is the possibility that this agent might be used for bioterrorism. In 2001, for example, anthrax spores were mailed to members of the press and U.S. government officials for terrorist purposes.

According to the Food and Agriculture Organization (FAO) of the United Nations, "the most common form of anthrax in humans is a generally non-fatal

TABLE 6.2   Examples of Zoonotic Diseases (and Associated Animals)

Name/Type of Animal	Zoonotic Disease
Domestic Animals	
Cats	Rabies, parasites such as tapeworm, cat scratch fever, toxoplasmosis
Cattle	Anthrax, *Escherichia coli* O157:H7, Q fever, cryptosporidiosis, mad cow disease (bovine spongiform encephalopathy [BSE])
Dogs	Rabies, parasites such as tapeworm, leptospirosis, campylobacteriosis
Horses	Anthrax, salmonellosis, cryptosporidiosis, rabies (unusual)
Poultry (e.g., chickens and ducks)	Influenza, salmonellosis
Reptiles (e.g., pet turtles and snakes)	Salmonellosis
Sheep and goats	Anthrax, Q fever
Swine	Trichinosis, tapeworm, influenza, yersiniosis
Wild Animals	
Bats	Rabies (Bats are the major source of human rabies cases in the United States)
Birds	Psittacosis, cryptococcosis
Mammals (e.g., raccoons, skunks, foxes, deer)	Rabies, giardiasis, brucellosis
Rodents	Hantavirus, plague, tularemia

Data from Centers for Disease Control and Prevention, National Center for Infectious Diseases, Healthy pets healthy people, http://www.cdc.gov/healthypets/browse_by_animal .htm. Accessed January 30, 2014.

skin infection that strikes workers handling infected animals or animal products. (That anthrax is largely an 'occupational hazard' for humans is reflected in the common name given to its deadly pulmonary form: 'woolsorters' disease', contracted through the inhalation of spores in fleece.)"[11] The name woolsorters' disease referred to the 19th- and early 20th-century occupation of wool sorting in Yorkshire, England (as described in **EXHIBIT 6.3**); the disease was caused by *B. anthracis*.[12]

Eventually, when anthrax was recognized as the cause of woolsorters' disease and disinfection procedures were introduced, the condition became extremely rare.[12] However, during the early 1900s, when the disease was more common, explicit posters were used to warn workers of the dangers posed by anthrax.[13]

EXHIBIT 6.3   Woolsorters' Disease

Woolsorters' disease was a feared industrial disease associated primarily with Yorkshire's textile industry of the 19th and early 20th centuries… . Woolsorting was a common form of employment for British workers in the 19th and early 20th centuries. It involved separating the various qualities of wool of which a fleece is composed and then picking out the foreign substances such as locks, rag, and string that were so often found within a fleece.

Reproduced from Metcalfe N. The history of woolsorters' disease: a Yorkshire beginning with an international future? *Occup Med.* 2004;54:489

In more recent times, occupational exposures have been responsible for sporadic anthrax cases in the United States, typically as a result of contact with animal hides. **EXHIBIT 6.4** describes one such anthrax case.

Influenza

Influenza is an acute viral disease, often accompanied by symptoms that include fever, headache, and sore throat. Animal reservoirs for the influenza virus include aquatic birds (e.g., ducks), pigs, and several other species of animals. Farmers in close contact with poultry and swine can become infected with the influenza virus. **EXHIBIT 6.5** presents a case study of avian influenza among two poultry workers.

Q Fever

Q fever is caused by the infectious agent *Coxiella burnetii*, which is present in large amounts in the tissues of infected animals.[10] Q fever is "an occupational disease in persons whose work involves contact with animals, such as slaughterhouse workers, veterinarians, and farmers, although infection is not limited to these groups."[14] Cases of Q fever have been reported among military personnel deployed in Iraq. **FIGURE 6.5** shows a child playing with goats, a known reservoir of Q fever.

Tularemia

Also known as rabbit fever, tularemia is a bacterial disease caused by infection with *Francisella tularensis*. This disease is broadly distributed in the United States, occurring in all states except Hawaii. Typically found in rural areas, it is linked with wild animals such as rodents, rabbits, and hares. The bacterium may be transmitted in several ways, including the bite of an arthropod (e.g., tick or deer fly), coming into contact with infected

On August 29, 2007, the Connecticut Department of Public Health (CDPH) received a physician's report of a suspected cutaneous anthrax case [index case] involving a drum maker and one of his three children. On July 22, while sanding a newly assembled goat-hide drum in his backyard shed, the drum maker felt a sting on his right forearm. He then proceeded to an upstairs bathroom in his house to wash his arm. Two days later, a painless 2-cm papular [small conical] lesion with surrounding edema developed at the site. The man sought medical attention and was prescribed antibiotics for a presumptive infected spider bite.

On August 28, after the skin lesion progressed to an eschar [scab] with lymphangitic spread, the man consulted an infectious disease practitioner, who sent a biopsy specimen of the lesion to the Connecticut State Laboratory. A culture was negative, but *Bacillus anthracis* was detected by polymerase chain reaction (PCR). [PCR is a technique for making copies of DNA and can be used for detecting infectious disease agents.] The patient was administered ciprofloxacin for suspected cutaneous anthrax.

On August 31, the CDPH was notified of a second suspected case of cutaneous anthrax in the drum maker's child, aged 8 years, who developed a painless, 1-cm ulcer of 3 days' duration. Culture of the lesion was negative, but biopsy specimens tested positive for *B. anthracis* by PCR. The patient was treated with penicillin.

The index patient made traditional West African drums (known as djembe drums; FIGURE 6.4) by soaking animal hides in water, stretching them over the drum body, then scraping and sanding them. At the end of June, a contact in New York City told the index patient that he had some new goat hides from Guinea [in West Africa]. Shortly thereafter, the index patient purchased 10 of them, making the transaction on a street corner in New York City. Whether these goat hides were imported legally is unknown. The index patient used three of these hides to make drums during the time he developed anthrax.

All animal hides and drums in progress were stored in a backyard shed. Drum making usually occurred at the shed entrance. The affected child never participated in any drum making and had no known exposure to animal hides. He played indoors on carpeted floors and was prohibited from entering the shed.

On September 5 and 6, targeted environmental sampling was conducted collaboratively by the Federal Bureau of Investigation (FBI), the Environmental Protection Agency, and the Connecticut Department of Environmental Protection. The FBI chose to participate because anthrax is a select bioterrorism agent.

The following were culture positive for *B. anthracis*: six (24%) of 25 drum heads, including the recently sanded drum; 15 (42%) of 35 hides, some of which were exposed to ambient dust in the shed; all 16 shed samples, many indicating heavy growth; the car trunk; and 18 (26%) of 72 house specimens, including vacuum samples from the upstairs hallway and both affected patients' bedrooms and swab and wipe samples from the laundry room and upstairs bathroom.

Federal, state, and local officials completed a comprehensive remediation process that included fumigation of the house with chlorine dioxide [a type of pesticide used for *B. anthracis* decontamination]. The house and shed were cleared for occupancy on December 22, 2007, after all post-remediation samples had tested negative for anthrax. The findings underscore the potential hazard of working with untreated animal hides from areas with epizootic anthrax and the potential for secondary cases from environmental contamination, as in the case of the worker's child.

Modified from Centers for Disease Control and Prevention (CDC). Cutaneous anthrax associated with drum making using goat hides from West Africa—Connecticut, 2007 *MMWR*. 2008;57(23):628-629.

EXHIBIT 6.5 **Highly Pathogenic Avian Influenza A (H7N3) Virus Infection in Two Poultry Workers—Jalisco, Mexico, July 2012**

During June–August 2012, Mexico's National Service for Health, Safety, and Food Quality reported outbreaks of highly pathogenic avian influenza (HPAI) A (H7N3) virus in poultry on farms throughout the state of Jalisco.... This report describes two cases of conjunctivitis without fever or respiratory symptoms caused by HPAI A (H7N3) virus infection in humans associated with exposure to infected poultry.

- **Patient 1.** On July 7, a poultry worker, aged 32 years, complaining of pruritus in her left eye was examined at a clinic in Jalisco. Physical findings included redness, swelling, and tearing. Conjunctivitis was diagnosed; the patient was treated symptomatically and recovered fully.... [T]he patient had collected eggs in a farm where HPAI A (H7N3) virus was detected.

- **Patient 2.** A man, aged 52 years, who was a relative of patient 1 and worked on the same farm, developed symptoms consistent with conjunctivitis on July 10 and sought care at a local clinic on July 13. He was treated symptomatically and recovered without sequelae. When public health authorities became aware of this patient, they obtained eye swabs, which were [positive for] influenza A (H7).

Reproduced from Highly pathogenic avian influenza A (H7N3) virus infection in two poultry workers—Jalisco, Mexico, July 2012. *MMWR.* 2012;61(36):726.

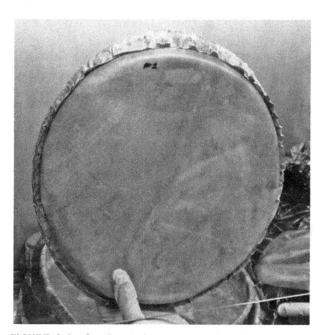

FIGURE 6.4 *Bacillus anthracis*-contaminated drum head made from goat hide from Guinea

Reproduced from Centers for Disease Control and Prevention (CDC). Cutaneous anthrax associated with drum making using goat hides from West Africa—Connecticut, 2007. MMWR. 2008;57(23):629

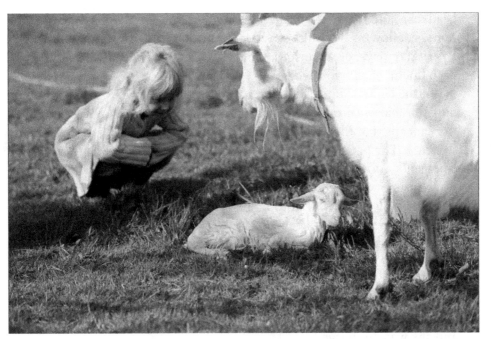

FIGURE 6.5   Child plays with goats, one of the primary reservoirs of Q fever

Courtesy of Centers for Disease Control and Prevention, Diagnosis and management of Q fever—U.S., 2013. *MMWR.* 2013;62:RR #3.

animal carcasses, consuming food or water that has been contaminated with the bacterium, or even breathing in the bacterium.[15] Occupationally exposed persons include those who might handle animals infected with *F. tularensis.*

Tularemia presents with a range of possible symptoms that are related to how the organism enters the body. Often, symptoms include skin ulcers, swollen lymph glands, painful eyes, and sore throat. Inhalation of the bacterium may cause sudden fever, chills, headaches, muscle aches, joint pain, dry cough, and progressive weakness; in some cases, pneumonia may occur.[10] Tularemia, which is treatable with antibiotics, may be a severe or fatal condition when untreated.

Rabies (Hydrophobia)

Rabies is an acute and highly fatal disease of the central nervous system caused by a virus transmitted most often through saliva from the bites of infected animals; globally, dog bites are the principal source of transmission of rabies to humans.[10] A disease that affects mammals, rabies causes encephalopathy and paralysis of the respiratory system. In the early stages of the disease, symptoms are nonspecific, consisting of apprehension, fever, headache, and malaise. The disease then progresses to paralysis, hallucinations, swallowing difficulties, and fear of water (called hydrophobia). After a period of days, death ensues. Only six cases of survival from rabies have been documented worldwide.

In the United States, human cases of rabies are rare. A case of abortive human rabies occurred in Texas beginning in early 2009. The term "abortive" means that the patient recovered without ever having received intensive care. The patient was a 17-year-old female who was seen in a hospital emergency room for symptoms that included severe headache, photophobia (sensitivity to light), neck pain, and fever. She was discharged after three days, when the symptoms resolved. Subsequently, after the headaches returned, she was rehospitalized and treated for suspected infectious encephalitis. During subsequent examinations, the patient revealed that while on a camping trip she had been bitten by flying bats. After serological tests were found to be positive for rabies, the patient was administered rabies immune globulin and rabies vaccine. Following these steps, the young woman was given supportive care until the symptoms resolved and she was discharged.

The hosts for rabies are wild animals—carnivores and bats. The CDC estimates that more than 90% of rabies cases occur in wild animals (e.g., skunks, raccoons, foxes, and coyotes) and the remainder in domestic animals. Before 1960, the majority of U.S. rabies cases occurred among domestic animals—dogs, cats, and cattle; today, however, most cases occur in the wild. In the United States, vaccination programs for domestic animals, measures to control animals, and public health laboratories for conducting rabies tests have changed the prevalence of rabies.

Environmental health programs have prevented human cases of rabies very successfully through post-exposure prophylaxis (PEP). In the United States, fatal human rabies cases have declined from approximately 100 cases annually in the early 1900s to one to two cases annually at the end of the 20th century. One reason for this decline has been the introduction of PEP, which is nearly 100% successful; the remaining fatal cases usually can be attributed to failure to seek medical attention. PEP consists of a series of vaccinations that should be given as soon as possible after the occurrence of an animal bite from a suspected rabid animal.

As mentioned earlier, outside the United States, rabid dogs are the most common source of rabies exposure and cause 99% of human rabies deaths. For this reason, an important component of rabies prevention is the control and vaccination of stray dogs. Within the United States, people are most likely to be exposed to rabies from bats.[10] Workers who could be exposed to the rabies virus are those who might touch a rabid bat or have other contact with rabid wild animals.

Plague

The bacterium *Yersinia pestis* is the infectious agent for plague, a condition that affects both animals and humans. Plague may be transmitted by the bite of a flea harbored by rodents. Historians believe that the plague epidemic during the Middle Ages (the "black death") was caused by fleas from infested rats. Although morbidity and case-fatality rates among persons infected with the disease remain high, prompt treatment with antibiotics is efficacious.[16] Nevertheless, human infections with *Y. pestis* remain a matter of great concern for authorities. Plague is distributed widely across the world, including the United States, South America, Asia, and parts of Africa.

One of the natural reservoirs for plague is wild rodents, such as the ground squirrels that make their homes in the western United States. Pets, such as house cats and dogs, may bring the wild rodents' fleas into homes or may even transmit plague on rare occasions from their bites or scratches. The condition known as bubonic plague begins with nonspecific symptoms such as fever, chills, and headache and then progresses into lymphadenitis (infected lymph nodes) at the site of the initial flea bite. Secondary involvement of the lungs, known as pneumonic plague, may also occur. The epidemiologic significance of this form of plague is that respiratory droplets from an infected person can transfer *Y. pestis* to other individuals. The case-fatality rate for untreated bubonic plague is high, in the range of 50% to 60%. Patients who are infected with the disease need to be placed in strict isolation and their clothing and other personal articles disinfected. Persons who have had contact with the patient should be placed under quarantine.

Environmental control of plague may be accomplished by encouraging the public to avoid enzootic areas, especially rodent burrows, and direct contact with rodents. Unfortunately, some people ignore posted warning signs in nature parks and risk contracting plague when they feed squirrels and chipmunks. Also, the number of rodents needs to be kept in check. Environmental health officials should inform the populace of the importance of preventing rats from entering buildings and should encourage the removal of food sources that could enable rats to multiply. Shipping areas and docks need to be patrolled because rats can be transferred to and from cargo containers and ships. Persons who handle wildlife as part of their work assignments should take care to wear gloves.[10] EXHIBIT 6.6 provides additional information regarding occupational risks to veterinary staff from plague.

Psittacosis

Psittacosis, a disease associated with the bacterial agent *Chlamydia psittaci*, is conveyed by dried bird droppings. Bird owners, pet shop employees, and veterinarians can be at risk of exposure from apparently healthy birds

> **EXHIBIT 6.6   Avoiding Occupational Risks from Plague**
>
> * Veterinary staff are at risk of developing plague if they have contact with infectious exudates, respiratory droplets, oral secretions, tissues, or fleas.
> * Any material used in examination of plague-suspected cats (cats are highly susceptible to this infection and a common source of plague infection in humans) should be disinfected, autoclaved, or incinerated.
> * Masks and gloves should be worn when examining and treating cats suspected of having plague.
> * Veterinarians should use appropriate personal protective equipment (PPE) before beginning a necropsy on a plague-suspected animal. PPE should include gloves, an N95 respirator or the equivalent, and protective eye equipment.
> * If any veterinary staff are exposed to infectious material, they should watch their health closely for 2 weeks following the exposure and discuss post-exposure prophylaxis or fever watch with a healthcare provider and public health officials.
>
> Reproduced from Centers for Disease Control and Prevention. Plague. Information for veterinarians. http://www.cdc.gov/plague/healthcare/veterinarians.html. Accessed February 17, 2014.

and asymptomatic birds that shed C. *psittaci*. Outbreaks of psittacosis in poultry processing plants have been reported.

Toxoplasmosis

Toxoplasma gondii is a type of protozoa transmitted most commonly to humans by felines. Animals may acquire this microorganism when they consume infected rodents and birds.[10,17] Cattle, sheep, goats, swine, and poultry also can become infected with *T. gondii*. Individuals who might be at risk are those who are in contact with infected meat, animals, soils, and cat feces. Workers who may be exposed to this pathogen include individuals who care for animals, those employed in meat processing, farmers, landscapers, laboratory employees, and healthcare personnel.

Leptospirosis

Leptospirosis, which is caused by a bacterium (a variety of spirochete), is an illness that shows great variations in severity, ranging from asymptomatic cases to fatal disease. The reservoirs for bacteria associated with leptospirosis are wild and domestic animals, which shed the bacteria in their urine, body fluids, and body tissues. The bacteria can then contaminate water—the most common source of human exposure.[18] At-risk employees include outdoor workers who are exposed to bodies of water contaminated with the bacteria. For example, farmers may acquire lepto-spirosis by wading in paddies that are flooded with contaminated water in rice- and sugar-producing areas. Other at-risk employees include those who have skin and body contact with infected waters in places where the bacteria may be present.

Yersiniosis

Most human cases of yersiniosis are caused by one species of bacteria, *Yersinia enterocolitica*. Pigs are one of the most important reservoirs for *Y. enterocolitica*. This infectious agent can cause acute diarrhea, fever, and abdominal pain, particularly in children, who account for most of the cases. Transmission of *Yersinia* might occur when persons who care for children handle contaminated pork products and do not wash their hands sufficiently before touching infants or their toys and baby bottles. Food handlers infected with *Yersinia* who do not maintain adequate personal hygiene—for example, proper hand washing—can transmit the disease to restaurant patrons or other consumers.

Hantavirus Pulmonary Syndrome

Hantavirus pulmonary syndrome (HPS) is a severe and sometimes fatal respiratory condition that is transmitted by rodent vectors.[19] This infection may be transmitted when aerosolized droppings from infected rodents are inhaled. For example, vacationers who return to a mountain cabin after an extended absence may stir up droppings when cleaning to make the cabin habitable. Occupational exposure to hantaviruses can occur among animal laboratory workers and individuals assigned to work in virus-infested buildings, especially if they stir up large amounts of dust.[20]

Diseases Transmitted by Arthropod Vectors

Arthropod vectors include ticks, mites, and mosquitoes, all of which can transmit bacterial, parasitic, or viral agents.[21] Persons employed in outdoor occupations such as farming, horticulture, construction, and landscaping are at risk of bites from arthropod vectors. Related potential hazards to outdoor workers are stinging and biting insects (fire ants, bees, and wasps) and venomous spiders and scorpions. One of the most dangerous consequences of a bite is a severe allergic reaction called anaphylactic shock; individuals who experience this reaction must receive prompt medical attention lest it prove fatal.[22] In the United States, as many as 100 persons die each year from allergic reactions to insect stings.

TABLE 6.3   Types of Work that Pose Risks of Tick-Borne Diseases

• Construction	• Farming
• Landscaping	• Railroad work
• Forestry	• Oil field work
• Brush clearing	• Utility line work
• Land surveying	• Park or wildlife management

Courtesy of Centers for Disease Control and Prevention, National Institute for Occupational Safety and Health, Tick-borne diseases. http://www.cdc.gov/niosh/topics /tick-borne/. Accessed September 28, 2013.

Tick-Borne Diseases

Tick-borne diseases include Lyme disease, Rocky Mountain spotted fever, tick-borne relapsing fever, and tularemia; these conditions are hazards for persons who work outside. TABLE 6.3 lists examples of outdoor occupations in which employees are at risk from the bite of infected ticks.

According to the CDC, Lyme disease is the most commonly reported tick-borne disease in the United States.[23] Its symptoms can include a characteristic skin rash, tiredness, fever, headache, and stiff neck. Untreated Lyme disease can progress to more severe neurologic, cardiovascular, and joint symptoms.[10]

Mosquito-Borne Agents

In the United States, mosquitoes carry viruses associated with several types of illness, including encephalitis, Dengue fever, and West Nile virus infection. According to the CDC, "the West Nile virus (WNV) is most often spread to people from the bite of an infected mosquito. The WNV normally cycles between mosquitoes and birds. However, people may be infected if they are bitten by a WNV-infected mosquito."[24] Persons who work outdoors can acquire WNV from the bites of infected mosquitoes. Laboratory workers who handle the tissues of WNV-infected birds also can contract WNV infection.

Fungal Diseases

"Fungal diseases may sound mysterious and dangerous, but they are often caused by fungi that are common in the environment. Fungi can be found in soil, on plants, trees, and other vegetation, and on our skin, mucous membranes, and intestinal tracts."[25] They produce the molds that appear after flooding and in damp environments (EXHIBIT 6.7). Fungi can be hazardous to outdoor workers who inhale dusts from soils and develop valley fever (coccidioidomycosis) in endemic regions of the United States. In addition, researchers have identified negative health effects from working in damp buildings, exposure to fungal enzymes used in food production, and employment in sawmills and libraries. On the positive side, fungi play a valuable role in food production as leavening agents and flavorings.

Coccidioidomycosis

Coccidioidomycosis (also known as valley fever) is an occupational hazard for workers exposed to dust from windblown soil in areas that range from southern and central California to southern Texas. Residing in the soil in endemic areas, spores from the fungus *Coccidioides immitis* can become airborne and lead to dangerous lung and other diseases following exposure.[10] In 2013, an outbreak of valley fever was reported among 28 employees at two solar electric generation facilities in San Luis Obispo County, California. Construction operations at those sites had involved scraping large acreages to permit installation of the solar panels.[26]

Histoplasmosis

Histoplasmosis is a fungal-associated disease that can occur among workers (e.g., those involved with demolition of old buildings) who come into contact with the infectious agent, *Histoplasma capsulatum*. *H. capsulatum*,

---

EXHIBIT 6.8   **Histoplasmosis Outbreak among Workers Who Renovated a House**

On May 19, 2013, a consulting physician contacted the Laurentian Regional Department of Public Health (Direction de santé publique des Laurentides [DSP]) in Quebec, Canada, to report that two masons employed by the same company to do demolition work were experiencing cough and dyspnea accompanied by fever. Other workers also were said to be ill. DSP initiated a joint infectious disease, environmental health, and occupational health investigation to determine the extent and cause of the outbreak. The investigation identified 14 persons with respiratory symptoms among 30 potentially exposed persons. A strong correlation was found between exposure to demolition dust containing bat or bird droppings and a diagnosis of histoplasmosis. Temporary suspension of construction work at the demolition site in Saint-Eustache, Quebec, northwest from Montreal, and transport of the old masonry elements to a secure site for burial were ordered, and information about the disease was provided to workers and residents. To prevent future outbreaks, recommendations included disinfection of any contaminated material, disposal of waste material with proper control of aerosolized dust, and mandatory use of personal protective equipment such as gloves, protective clothing, and adequate respirators.

Reprinted from Centers for Disease Control and Prevention (CDC). Histoplasmosis outbreak associated with the renovation of an old house—Quebec, Canada, 2013. *MMWR.* 2014;62(51):1041-1044.

---

a type of fungus that grows in the soil,[10] can be excreted in the droppings of birds, bats, and some other animals. Among infected individuals, the spectrum of illness can range from asymptomatic infections to acute respiratory symptoms and life-threatening illnesses. **EXHIBIT 6.8** presents a case study of a histoplasmosis outbreak among workers involved with a renovation project.

Workers in Damp Buildings

Leaks, high humidity, and flooding can create a damp environment in office buildings, schools, and other nonindustrial buildings. The result of excessive moisture can be the production of mold, other types of fungi, and bacteria. Damp environments in buildings increase the risk of respiratory symptoms and progression to more severe health problems among persons who have asthma or conditions (e.g., hypersensitivity pneumonitis) that make them hypersensitive to dampness and molds.[27] Hypersensitivity pneumonitis (HP) is "a disease in which the lungs become inflamed from breathing in foreign substances, such as molds, dusts, and chemicals. These substances also are known as antigens."[28] It is imperative to correct moisture problems in buildings to protect the health of employees and other occupants. The case report presented in **EXHIBIT 6.9** describes hypersensitivity pneumonitis in an office building.

Industrial Fungal Enzymes

The risk of occupational exposures to fungal enzymes has increased for some categories of workers as a result of the introduction of new fungal enzymes for commercial applications. Such fungal enzymes are used in many occupational settings—for example, agriculture, waste management, biotechnology, food processing, baking, and brewing in wine production. Examples of fungi used in food preparation include the cheese flavoring *Penicillium roqueforti* and yeasts used for fermentation and as leavening agents. Exposures to fungal enzymes can increase the risk of adverse health effects such as occupational asthma.[29]

Workers in Sawmills, Libraries, and Museums

Investigations have revealed the presence of molds in sawmills. Some library and museum environments afford a suitable domain for fungi and dust mites. A study of sawmills in Croatia found that workers could be exposed to airborne fungi from wood.[30] Researchers in Warsaw, Poland, demonstrated how fungi might be a potential allergen for museum workers.[31]

Other Agents

Other agents covered in this chapter are those responsible for foodborne illness, tuberculosis, and parasitic infections. Foodborne illness can affect persons who ingest pathogenic microorganisms present in food. An example of an occupationally associated communicable disease hazard is tuberculosis (TB), which can be transmitted to both patients and healthcare workers.[32] The bacterium *Helicobacter pylori*, a known cause of ulcers, is an occupational hazard for gastroenterologists.

Foodborne Illnesses

Foodborne illnesses (food poisoning) are unusual occupational diseases.[33] "These diseases may be occupationally related if they affect the food processors (e.g., poultry processing workers), food preparers and servers (e.g. cooks, waiters), or workers who are provided food at the worksite."[34] Outbreaks of foodborne illness can occur among large groups of persons who dine in company cafeterias or among military personnel fed in military canteens. Sometimes such illness is associated with contaminated food served at company potlucks. Yet another type of occupationally associated foodborne illness is transfer of foodborne agents from food workers to consumers. For example, an outbreak among patrons of a restaurant might be associated with restaurant employees who are infected with an agent of foodborne disease. Such an outbreak occurred during 2007 among individuals who purchased groceries from a grocery store delicatessen in Minnesota; stool samples from two food workers at the deli tested positive for *Salmonella* bacteria.[35]

Among the primary effects of foodborne illness are gastrointestinal (GI) symptoms of varying severity. Among the common bacterial agents that cause foodborne illness are *Salmonella*, *Staphylococcus aureus*, and *Clostridium perfringens*. The incubation period—that is, the time between ingestion of a contaminated food and development of illness symptoms—varies according to the agent involved.

Salmonellosis—a foodborne infection caused by *Salmonella* bacteria—accounts for more than 10% of all foodborne illness cases in the United States. Typically, the incubation period for salmonellosis is about 12–24 hours.

Staphylococcal food poisoning is an intoxication caused by a toxin (an enterotoxin) produced by the bacterium *Staphylococcus aureus*. The toxin develops when foods contaminated with *S. aureus* are not kept under refrigeration. An intoxication differs from a foodborne infection (e.g., a *Salmonella* infection) in that illness is caused by the effects of the bacterial toxin and not by the actions of an infectious agent. The incubation period for staphylococcal food poisoning is approximately 3 hours.

Food poisoning caused by *Clostridium perfringens* is an intoxication that has an incubation period of 10–12 hours. These bacteria live in the intestines of people and animals and, when transferred to foods, can produce a toxin associated with GI symptoms.

To prevent foodborne illness outbreaks, manufacturers of foodstuffs need to furlough workers who test positive for organisms such as *Salmonella* that are potentially transmissible in foods. The workers can return after subsequent testing has verified that the organisms have cleared from their bodies.

Tuberculosis

Globally, tuberculosis is a highly prevalent condition that can be transmitted from patients to healthcare workers. According to the CDC, in 2008 approximately one-third of the world's population was infected with TB.[36] The causative bacterial agent for TB is *Mycobacterium tuberculosis*.[10] A contagious and communicable disease, TB can become life threatening.

Persons infected with TB may not have any clinically observable symptoms. Nevertheless, these individuals may spread *M. tuberculosis* through the air when they expel air from their lungs by coughing or other means. Symptoms of active TB infection can include pulmonary symptoms such as cough and hemoptysis (coughing up blood). Other common TB symptoms include fever, tiredness, and weight loss.

In the United States, the prevalence of TB has shown a declining trend. Nevertheless, transmission of tuberculosis within the healthcare setting remains an occupational hazard. Rates of tuberculosis have increased among patients who are immunocompromised for various reasons—for example, as a result of HIV infection. Also of increasing concern are hazards from drug-resistant forms of tuberculosis (e.g., extensively drug-resistant [XDR] TB strains).[37] EXHIBIT 6.10 gives additional information about TB.

Helicobacter pylori

The bacterium *Helicobacter pylori*, which is recognized as a cause of gastritis and ulcers, is a potential occupational hazard for healthcare workers.

EXHIBIT 6.10   Tuberculosis in Healthcare Settings

Healthcare workers are at higher than average risk for TB. Sound TB infection control measures should be implemented in all healthcare facilities with patients suspected of having infectious TB. Transmission of TB in healthcare settings to both patients and healthcare workers has been reported from virtually every country of the world, regardless of local TB incidence. TB transmission occurs when droplet nuclei are aerosolized by patients with infectious pulmonary TB and inhaled by other persons. Transmission is most likely to occur from unrecognized or inappropriately treated TB. The risk for transmission varies by setting, occupational group, local prevalence of TB, patient population, and effectiveness of TB infection control measures.

Reprinted from Baussano P, Nunn P, Williams B, et al. Tuberculosis among health care workers. *Emerg Infect Dis.* 2011;17(3):488-494.

However, some groups of workers who have close contact with their patients are likely to be at greater risk than others. These employees may need to handle patients' fecal and oral materials. For example, the risk of transmission of *H. pylori* appears to be increased for gastroenterologists, endoscopy staff, and intensive care nurses.[38]

Parasitic Agents

A parasite is "an organism that lives on or in a host organism and gets its food from or at the expense of its host."[39] The three principal classes of disease-associated parasites for human beings are protozoa, helminths, and ectoparasites.

- Protozoa: Microscopic single-celled organisms. Protozoa that live in the human intestine can spread through the fecal–oral transmission route. Insect vectors transfer protozoa that live in human blood and tissues. Some of the diseases caused by protozoa are cryptosporidiosis, malaria, giardiasis, and amebiasis.
  - Cryptosporidiosis: The causative agent, *Cryptosporidium parvum,* produces gastrointestinal symptoms such as abdominal cramping and severe diarrhea. *C. parvum* has human and animal reservoirs and sometimes can be transmitted by polluted water.
  - Malaria: The organism that causes malaria (*Plasmodia*) is transmitted by mosquitoes in endemic countries.
  - Giardiasis: The organism responsible for giardiasis is *Giardia lamblia,* which can be acquired when water contaminated with the organism is ingested.

- Helminths: Large, multicellular organisms, which include intestinal parasites such as pinworms, hookworms, tapeworms, and roundworms. An example of an infection by helminths is ascariasis, an infection of the small intestine caused by worms.
- Ectoparasites: "[O]rganisms such as ticks, fleas, lice, and mites that attach or burrow into the skin and remain there for relatively long periods of time (e.g., weeks to months)."[39]

Occupational groups at risk for contracting parasitic diseases include veterinarians, who might come into contact with animal reservoirs and animal wastes. Another at-risk group consists of outdoor and agricultural workers who might contact contaminated water and soil or be bitten by insect vectors. Farmers who work barefoot in the soil, sewer maintenance personnel, and lifeguards who walk barefoot on the beach could be exposed to hookworm larvae.

Occupations in Which Workers Are at Risk of Exposure to Biohazards

Some occupations place workers at greater risk of exposure to biohazards than others. Especially important examples of the settings in which exposures to biohazards occur are health care, veterinary medicine, and waste management. TABLE 6.4 lists some of the employees who are at risk of exposures to these biological pathogens.

Healthcare Workers

Healthcare workers are at risk from infections transmitted by patients. An example noted previously was TB. Another example is infection with the Ebola virus. In late 2014, U.S. medical personnel who responded to the

TABLE 6.4 Examples of Employees Who Are at Risk of Exposure to Biohazards

Healthcare workers	Workers who have contact with animals
• Correctional healthcare workers	• Veterinarians
Public utility workers	• Agricultural workers
Workers exposed to sewage and wastewater	• Abattoir workers
• Sewage processing plant employees	Clinical laboratory workers
• Waste and refuse collectors	Morticians
• Landfill workers	Adult film entertainers

Ebola epidemic in West Africa became infected with the virus. At a Dallas hospital, nurses who attended to an Ebola patient from Liberia subsequently contracted the virus.

Also, personnel may develop infections from percutaneous injuries such as those caused by sharps. Percutaneous injuries are among the most significant hazards for healthcare workers. These injuries can occur across the healthcare field, including among prison healthcare workers.[40] Unfortunately, percutaneous injuries tend to be underreported; thus the extent of their frequency has not been ascertained fully. Some preventive measures are available, such as vaccination for the hepatitis B virus, to reduce the risk of HBV transmission from an unintentional sharps injury.

Clinical sites where exposures to BBF in the healthcare setting transpire include inpatient units of hospitals, operating rooms, rooms for clinical procedures, outpatient clinics, emergency treatment rooms, and clinical laboratories. The NaSH surveillance program reported that inpatient units and operating rooms were the most frequent locations for BBF exposures, accounting for 36% and 29% of exposures, respectively. FIGURE 6.6 provides more information about the work locations of BBF exposures.

The hospital environment can be an ideal environment for the development of nosocomial infections (outbreaks of infections in hospitals). "In the microbial setting, the hospital environment is a vast grass field for herds of bacteria."[41(p. 247)] The increasing resistance of some bacteria to antibiotics (e.g., methicillin-resistant *Staphylococcus aureus* [MRSA]) is a topic

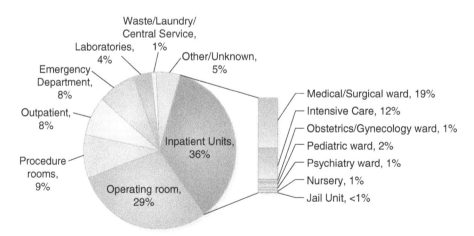

FIGURE 6.6   Work locations where reported blood and body fluid (BBF) exposures occurred

of growing concern for hospital epidemiologists.[42] One of the implications of bacterial resistance for occupational health is that healthcare workers need to maintain sanitary precautions such as hand washing to prevent the spread of microorganisms among patients.

Public Utility Workers

Public utilities render essential services to the community, including delivery of water and electrical power, sewage disposal, and waste and refuse collection. Employees of these companies are often exposed to hazardous microbes. For example, workers who maintain the sanitary sewer system can be exposed to sewage and wastewater. Such workers might come into contact with raw sewage and be exposed to pathogenic microorganisms and viruses (e.g., the hepatitis A virus [HAV]). However, no or a slightly increased risk of HAV was reported among participants in a study of 365 wastewater workers.[43] (Note that HAV is spread through the fecal-oral route.)

Collectors of household waste and refuse have potential exposure to toxic materials and biohazards. These materials could increase the risk of chronic respiratory symptoms such as cough, wheezing, and chronic bronchitis among waste collectors.[44] Finally, landfill workers who maintain disposal sites can be exposed to hazards from airborne dust and biologic hazards such as bacteria and fungi.[45]

Workers Who Have Contact with Animals

Occupational hazards in the field of veterinary medicine include exposures to X-rays, gases used in anesthesiology, chemicals, and to hazards from injuries caused by large animals.[46] Veterinarians and associated workers can acquire zoonotic diseases from infected animals under their treatment. Similarly, farmers and agricultural workers can become infected with zoonotic diseases such as Q fever and salmonellosis from cattle and other farm animals. Abattoir workers can develop infections (e.g., salmonellosis and *E. coli* infections) from animals that have been slaughtered for food production.

Clinical Laboratory Workers

The most important occupational danger in clinical microbiology laboratories is contamination from microbial agents. This danger directly affects laboratory personnel who work with the agents and indirectly impacts other persons who enter the laboratory. These other persons at risk of being exposed to microbial agents include janitors, clerical workers, maintenance

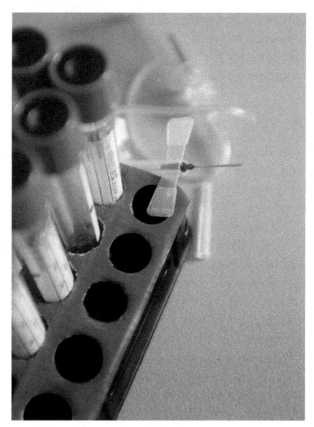

FIGURE 6.7   Blood-contaminated needle

Courtesy of Centers for Disease Control and Prevention, Public Health Image Library.

personnel, and visitors. For this reason, it is imperative for clinical laboratories to implement safe procedures throughout the facility for handling potentially infectious materials such as blood and body fluids.[47]

One of the microbial exposure risks to clinical laboratory workers is from percutaneous injuries. Surveillance data suggest "that the most serious exposure risk to clinical lab workers is from needles used to draw or transfer blood and from glass specimen and capillary tubes used to collect and store blood."[48(p. 72)] FIGURE 6.7 displays a blood-contaminated needle—one type of hazard encountered by clinical laboratory employees.

Mortuary Professionals

Personnel in the mortuary profession and workers involved with the exhumation of bodies can be exposed to biohazards. "Embalming is defined as the preservation of a body from decay, originally with spices, and now through the use of injection of a chemical embalming fluid. It involves replacing blood with a preservative solution (the embalming fluid) and treatment of the body cavity and organs with a similar preservative... . As the process involves direct contact with the body, exposure to blood and other body fluids, and the use of sharps (and hazardous chemicals), this process, of all of those carried out involving human remains, is likely to present the greatest risk of exposure to infectious micro-organisms."[49]

Adult Film Entertainers

Adult film entertainers are another group of workers at increased risk of exposure to blood-borne pathogens. The state of California reported that "[a] recent cluster of HIV infections in the adult film industry in Southern California has drawn attention to health hazards in these workplaces. Workers in this industry need to know there are laws written to protect them from injury and illness on the job, and to specify where to go for help if their employer doesn't follow those laws. Employers in the adult film industry must know how to protect their employees from health and safety hazards and understand the consequences of failing to comply with state regulations."[50] Persons employed in the adult film industry need to be informed about the hazards of HIV infection and blood-borne pathogens and ways to prevent infections with such agents.

Methods for Protecting Employees Against Work-Related Biohazards

A variety of procedures and methods are available to protect workers against biohazards. One group of measures involves the use of personal protective equipment such as gloves, face shields, and masks. Another relates to the design of facilities in which microbes are handled. The level of protection needs to be adjusted to the degree of hazard presented by a microbe. Some agents are not extremely hazardous (e.g., nonpathogenic *E. coli*), whereas others can cause life-threatening illnesses (e.g., Ebola virus) for which there are limited medical interventions and that have great potential for causing mass epidemics.

A vital issue for protecting workers against biohazards is to increase their awareness and knowledge of biological risks. Improved data are needed regarding this matter.[4] Although relatively little information is available on workers' awareness of biological hazards, some research has demonstrated differences among various occupations regarding workers' levels of knowledge about such hazards.[4]

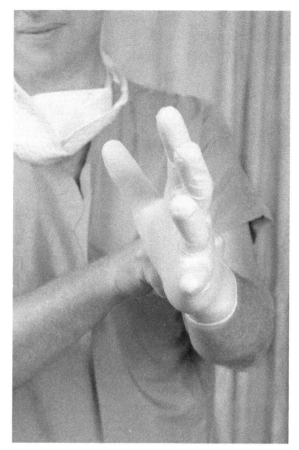

FIGURE 6.8   Latex gloves for protection against biohazards

Courtesy of Centers for Disease Control and Prevention, Public Health Image Library.

Precautions Related to Blood and Body Fluids

The CDC recommends that all patients' blood and body fluids should be regarded as potentially infectious and precautions should be taken for safe handling of these materials.[8] The transmission of infectious agents from blood and body fluids can be prevented through application of protective measures such as using barriers (e.g., wearing gloves and goggles), washing one's hands, and handling and disposing of sharps in a safe manner.

FIGURE 6.8 shows latex gloves used for protection against biohazards. Double gloving provides additional protection against transmission of blood-borne infections.[51] Another preventive procedure focuses on the safe use of sharps. "Blunt-tip suture needles ... which are not as sharp as standard (sharp-tip) suture needles, are designed to penetrate muscle and fascia and reduce the risk of needle sticks. Blunt tip suture needles are regulated

---

EXHIBIT 6.11   Precautions for Handling Body Fluids

Healthcare personnel are at risk for occupational exposure to blood-borne pathogens, including hepatitis B virus, hepatitis C virus, and human immunodeficiency virus. Exposures may occur through needle sticks or cuts from other sharp instruments contaminated with an infected patient's blood, or through contact of the eye, nose, mouth, or skin with a patient's blood. Important factors that influence the overall risk for occupational exposures to blood-borne pathogens include the number of infected individuals in the patient population and the type and number of blood contacts. Most exposures do not result in infection. Following a specific exposure, the risk of infection may vary with factors such as these:

* The pathogen involved
* The type of exposure
* The amount of blood involved in the exposure
* The amount of virus in the patient's blood at the time of exposure

Employers should have in place a system for reporting exposures so that they can quickly evaluate the risk of infection, inform employees about treatments available to help prevent infection, monitor employees for side effects of treatments, and determine if infection occurs. This may involve testing the blood of the exposed employee and that of the source patient and offering appropriate post exposure treatment.

Reprinted from Centers for Disease Control and Prevention (CDC). Exposure to blood: what healthcare personnel need to know. http://www.cdc.gov/HAI/pdfs/bbp/Exp_to_Blood.pdf, p. 1. Accessed August 27, 2013.

---

by the FDA and have been marketed in the [United States] for more than 25 years."[52] **EXHIBIT 6.11** describes precautions for handling body fluids.

Biosafety Levels

The biosafety levels (BSLs) of microbes relate to their virulence levels and the degree of hazard that they present. Different microbial agents differ in their degree of hazard. Four biosafety levels have been designated for microbes and other biological agents: BSL-1, BSL-2, BSL-3, and BSL-4 (**TABLE 6.5**).[53] These levels affect the design of clinical laboratories and other facilities in which microbes are handled. "Each level has specific controls for containment of microbes and biological agents. The primary risks that determine levels of containment are infectivity, severity of disease, transmissibility, and the nature of the work conducted. Origin of the microbe, or the agent in question, and the route of exposure are also important."[53] With extremely hazardous agents, personnel may need to conduct procedures involving the microorganisms under a safety hood and wear a biosafety suit (**FIGURE 6.9**).

TABLE 6.5   Biosafety Levels of Microbes

Biosafety Level (BSL)		Precautions
BSL-1	In a lab that is designated as BSL-1, the microbes are not known to consistently cause disease in healthy adults and present minimal potential hazard to laboratory workers and the environment. An example of a microbe that is typically worked with at a BSL-1 facility is a strain of *E. coli* that does not cause disease.	Laboratory practices • Standard microbiological practices are followed. • Work can be performed on an open lab bench or table. Safety equipment • Personal protective equipment, (lab coats, gloves, eye protection) are worn as needed. Facility construction • A sink must be available for hand washing. • The lab should have doors to separate the working space with the rest of the facility.
BSL-2	BSL-2 builds upon BSL-1. In a lab that is designated as BSL-2, the microbes pose moderate hazards to laboratory workers and the environment. The microbes are typically indigenous (found in the geographic area) and associated with diseases of varying severity. An example of a microbe that is typically worked with at a BSL-2 laboratory is *Staphylococcus aureus*.	Laboratory practices • Access to the laboratory is restricted when work is being conducted. Safety equipment • Appropriate personal protective equipment is worn, including lab coats and gloves. Eye protection and face shields can also be worn, as needed. • All procedures that can cause infection from aerosols or splashes are performed within a biological safety cabinet (BSC). • An autoclave or an alternative method of decontamination is available for proper disposals. Facility construction • The laboratory has self-closing doors. • A sink and eyewash are readily available.
BSL-3	BSL-3 builds upon the containment requirements of BSL-2. In a lab that is designated as BSL-3, the microbes can be either indigenous or exotic, and they can cause serious or potentially lethal disease through respiratory transmission. Respiratory transmission is the inhalation route of exposure. An example of a microbe that is typically worked with in a BSL-3 laboratory is *Mycobacterium tuberculosis*, the bacteria that causes tuberculosis.	Laboratory practices • Laboratory workers are under medical surveillance and might receive immunizations for microbes they work with. • Access to the laboratory is restricted and controlled at all times. Safety equipment • Appropriate personal protective equipment must be worn, and respirators might be required. • All work with microbes must be performed within an appropriate BSC. Facility construction • A hands-free sink and eyewash are available near the exit. • Exhaust air cannot be recirculated, and the laboratory must have sustained directional airflow by drawing air into the laboratory from clean areas toward potentially contaminated areas. Entrance to the lab is through two sets of self-closing and locking doors.

(Contnues)

TABLE 6.5   Biosafety Levels of Microbes (*Continued*)

Biosafety Level (BSL)	Precautions
BSL-4 BSL-4 builds upon the containment requirements of BSL-3 and is the highest level of biological safety. There are a small number of BSL-4 labs in the United States and around the world. The microbes in a BSL-4 lab are dangerous and exotic, posing a high risk of aerosol-transmitted infections. Infections caused by these microbes are frequently fatal and without treatment or vaccines. Two examples of microbes worked with in a BSL-4 laboratory include the Ebola and Marburg viruses.	In addition to BSL-3 considerations, BSL-4 laboratories have the following containment requirements: Laboratory practices • Change clothing before entering. • Shower upon exiting. • Decontaminate all materials before exiting. Safety equipment • All work with the microbe must be performed within an appropriate Class III BSC, or by wearing a full-body, air-supplied, positive-pressure suit. Facility construction • The laboratory is in a separate building or in an isolated and restricted zone of the building. • The laboratory has dedicated supply and exhaust air, as well as vacuum lines and decontamination systems.

Modified from Centers for Disease Control and Prevention (CDC). Recognizing the biosafety levels. http://www.cdc.gov/training/QuickLearns/biosafety/. Accessed January 20, 2014.

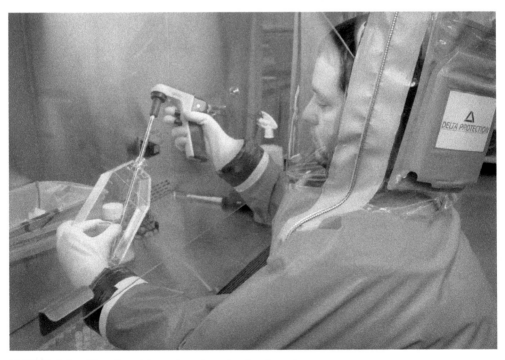

FIGURE 6.9   Biosafety suit and enclosed safety hood

Courtesy of Centers for Disease Control and Prevention, Public Health Image Library.

SUMMARY

Hazardous biological agents (biohazards) pose dangers to workers in a wide range of occupations and cause more than 300,000 work-related deaths across the globe each year. When transmission of a communicable disease occurs in a place of employment, it is considered a work-related illness. Work-associated biohazards include blood-borne viruses (HIV, HBV, and HCV) contained in blood and body fluids, vector-borne agents, zoonotic agents, and miscellaneous organisms such as bacteria, fungi, and parasites. Zoonotic diseases such as Q fever and anthrax can be transmitted through contact with animals and animal hides. Arthropod vectors are responsible for transmitting West Nile virus and Lyme disease. Infectious and communicable agents present in blood and body fluids present risks to healthcare personnel, public utility workers, veterinarians, and laboratory workers. Employees who are responsible for preparing foods for large producers and restaurants can transmit foodborne organisms to the public.

Occupational diseases caused by microbial and biological agents are highly preventable. The biohazard safety levels of organisms govern the types of precautions needed to minimize occupational exposures to these microorganisms. Transmission of biohazards can be prevented by taking measures such as hand washing, use of PPE, and avoiding percutaneous injuries and contact with mucous membranes.

STUDY QUESTIONS AND EXERCISES

1. Define the following terms:
   A. Biohazard
   B. Communicable disease
   C. Occupational exposure to blood and body fluids
   D. Zoonotic agent
   E. Biosafety levels (BSLs)
2. Medical advances such as the development of antibiotics and improved diagnostic procedures have improved the treatment of infectious diseases. In your own opinion, why are infectious diseases important (or not important) for the work environment, regardless of advances in medicine?
3. Describe how personnel in the following occupational settings might be exposed to biohazards:
   A. Medicine/health care
   B. Veterinary medicine
   C. Agriculture
   D. Clinical laboratories
   E. Waste collection, transport, and disposal
4. How are infections from contact with blood and body fluids most likely to be transmitted in the work environment? What are two examples of such infections? Which settings in the healthcare environment seem most likely to promote infections from contact with BBF?
5. How do the mechanisms for the spread of the hepatitis A virus in an occupational setting differ from those for the spread of hepatitis B and C?
6. Which kinds of biohazards can affect workers in institutions such as prisons? Conduct an online search on this topic and write a one-page essay on this topic.

7. Using your own ideas, describe why unrecognized cases of TB might endanger hospital personnel. What are some methods for protecting hospital patients and personnel from the spread of tuberculosis?

8. Which steps can be taken to prevent nosocomial infections? Why is MRSA a concern for hospitals?

9. Which occupational health measures can be taken to protect workers from infectious diseases that originate from agricultural and farming practices?

10. Give examples of parasitic agents of disease. Which occupational groups might be exposed to these agents?

REFERENCES

1. U.S. Department of Labor, Occupational Safety and Health Administration. Glossary of terms. n.d. https://www.osha.gov/doc/outreachtraining/htmlfiles/hazglos.html. Accessed August 17, 2013.

2. Porta M, ed. *A dictionary of epidemiology.* 5th ed. New York, NY: Oxford University Press; 2008.

3. Driscoll T, Takala J, Steenland K, et al. Review of estimates of the global burden of injury and illness due to occupational exposures. *Am J Ind Med.* 2005;48:491–502.

4. De Guisti M, Corrao CRN, Mannocci A, et al. Occupational biological risk knowledge and perception: results from a large survey in Rome, Italy. *Ann Ist Super Sanita.* 2012;48(2):138–145.

5. European Agency for Safety and Health at Work (EU-OSHA). *Biological agents.* Bilbao, Spain: EU-OSHA; 2003.

6. U.S. Department of Labor, Occupational Safety and Health Administration. Bloodborne pathogens. n.d. https://www.osha.gov/pls/oshaweb/owadisp.show_document?p_id=10051&p_table=STANDARDS. Accessed November 22, 2013.

7. Centers for Disease Control and Prevention. The National Surveillance System for Healthcare Workers (NaSH). n.d. http://www.cdc.gov/nhsn/PDFs/NaSH/NaSH-Report-6-2011.pdf. Accessed September 27, 2013.

8. Centers for Disease Control and Prevention. Occupational HIV transmission and prevention among health care workers. n.d. http://www.cdc.gov/hiv/resources/factsheets/PDF/hcw.pdf. Accessed September 27, 2013.

9. Luckhaupt SE, Calvert GM. Deaths due to bloodborne infections and their sequelae among health-care workers. *Am J Ind Med.* 2008;51:812–824.

10. Heymann DL, ed. *Control of communicable diseases manual.* 19th ed. Washington, DC: American Public Health Association; 2008.

11. United Nations, Food and Agriculture Organization. Anthrax in animals: spotlight, 2001. 2001. http://www.fao.org/ag/magazine/0112sp.htm. Accessed August 27, 2013.

12. Metcalfe N. The history of woolsorters' disease: a Yorkshire beginning with an international future? *Occup Med.* 2004;54:489–493.

13. Stark JF. A poster of pustules: representations of early twentieth century industrial anthrax in Britain. *Endeavour.* 2011;35(1):23–30.

14. Centers for Disease Control and Prevention. Diagnosis and management of Q fever—United States, 2013. *MMWR.* 2013;62(RR #3):1–30

15. Centers for Disease Control and Prevention. Frequently asked questions (FAQ) about tularemia. n.d. http://www.bt.cdc.gov/agent/tularemia/faq.asp. Accessed February 17, 2014.

16. Centers for Disease Control and Prevention. Plague. n.d. http://www.cdc.gov/plague/. Accessed February 17, 2014.

17. Canadian Centre for Occupational Health and Safety. Toxoplasmosis. n.d. http://www.ccohs.ca/oshanswers/diseases/toxoplasmosis.html. Accessed February 3, 2014.

18. World Health Organization. Leptospirosis. n.d. http://www.who.int/zoonoses/diseases/leptospirosis/en/#. Accessed February 3, 2014.

19. Centers for Disease Control and Prevention. Hantavirus pulmonary syndrome (HPS). n.d. http://www.cdc.gov/hantavirus/hps/index.html. Accessed February 3, 2014.

20. U.S. Department of Labor, Occupational Safety and Health Administration. Hantavirus. n.d. https://www.osha.gov/SLTC/hantavirus/. Accessed February 3, 2014.

21. Centers for Disease Control and Prevention, National Institute for Occupational Safety and Health (NIOSH). Protecting yourself from ticks and mosquitoes. n.d. http://www.cdc.gov/niosh/docs/2010-119/pdfs/2010-119.pdf. Accessed September 28, 2013.

22. Centers for Disease Control and Prevention, National Institute for Occupational Safety and Health. Insects and scorpions. n.d. http://www.cdc.gov/niosh/topics/insects/. Accessed September 28, 2013.

23. Centers for Disease Control and Prevention, National Institute for Occupational Safety and Health. Tick-borne diseases. n.d. http://www.cdc.gov/niosh/topics/tick-borne/. Accessed September 28, 2013.

24. Centers for Disease Control and Prevention, National Institute for Occupational Safety and Health. West Nile virus. n.d. http://www.cdc.gov/niosh/topics/westnile/. Accessed September 28, 2013.

25. Centers for Disease Control and Prevention. Fungal diseases. n.d. http://www.cdc.gov/fungal/. Accessed February 6, 2014.

26. Cart J. 28 workers get valley fever at solar construction plant construction sites. *Los Angeles Times.* May 1, 2013. AA1, AA2.

27. Centers for Disease Control and Prevention, National Institute for Occupational Safety and Health (NIOSH). *NIOSH alert: preventing occupational respiratory disease from exposures caused by dampness in office buildings, schools, and other nonindustrial buildings.* DHHS (NIOSH) Publication No. 2013-102. 2012.

28. National Heart, Lung, and Blood Institute, National Institutes of Health. What is hypersensitivity pneumonitis? n.d. http://www.nhlbi.nih.gov/health/health-topics/topics/hp/. Accessed January 23, 2014.

29. Green BJ, Beezhold DH. Industrial fungal enzymes: an occupational allergen perspective. *J Allergy.* 2011;682574. doi: 10.1155/2011/682574.

30. Klarić MŠ, Varnai VM, Calušić AL, Macan J. Occupational exposure to airborne fungi in two Croatian sawmills and atopy in exposed workers. *Ann Agric Environ Med.* 2012;19(2):213–219.

31. Wiszniewska M, Walusiak-Skorupa J, Pannenko I, et al. Occupational exposure and sensitization to fungi among museum workers. *Occup Med.* 2009;59(4):237–242.

32. Centers for Disease Control and Prevention, National Institute for Occupational Safety and Health. Tuberculosis. n.d. http://www.cdc.gov/niosh/topics/tb/. Accessed January 23, 2014.

33. Key MM, Henschel AF, Butler J, et al. *Occupational diseases: a guide to their recognition.* Washington, DC: U.S. Department of Health, Education, and Welfare (NIOSH); 1977.

34. U.S. Department of Labor, Occupational Safety and Health Administration. Foodborne disease. n.d. https://www.osha.gov/SLTC/foodbornedisease/. Accessed January 22, 2014.

35. Hedican E, Miller B, Ziemer B, et al. Salmonellosis outbreak due to chicken contact leading to a foodborne outbreak associated with infected delicatessen workers. *Foodborne Pathog Dis.* 2010;7(8):995–997.

36. U.S. Department of Labor, Occupational Safety and Health Administration. Tuberculosis. n.d. https://www.osha.gov/SLTC/tuberculosis/. Accessed January 23, 2014.

37. Baussano I, Nunn P, Williams B, et al. Tuberculosis among health care workers. *Emerg Infect Dis.* 2011;17(3):488–494.

38. De Schryver AA, Van Winckel MA. *Helicobacter pylori* infection: epidemiology and occupational risk for health care workers. *Ann Acad Med Singapore.* 2001;30:457–463.

39. Centers for Disease Control and Prevention. Parasites: about parasites. n.d. http://www.cdc.gov/parasites/about.html. Accessed February 17, 2014.

40. Gershon RRM, Sherman M, Mitchell C, et al. Prevalence and risk factors for blood-borne exposure and infection in correctional healthcare workers. *Infect Control Hosp Epidemiol.* 2007;28:24–30.

41. Cua A, Lutwick LI. The environment as a significant cofactor for multiply resistant nosocomial infections. *Semin Respir Infect.* 2002;17(3):246–249.

42. Lipsitch M, Bergstrom CT, Levin BR. The epidemiology of antibiotic resistance in hospitals: paradoxes and prescriptions. *Proc Natl Acad Sci USA.* 2000;97(4):1938–1943.

43. Venczel L, Brown S, Frumkin H, et al. Prevalence of hepatitis A virus infection among sewage workers in Georgia. *Am J Ind Med.* 2003;43:172–178.

44. Yang C-Y, Chang W-T, Chuang H-Y, et al. Adverse health effects among household waste collectors in Taiwan. *Environ Res.* 2001;85(3):195–199.

45. Kitsantas P, Kitsantas A, Travis HR. Occupational exposures and associated health effects among sanitation landfill employees. *Environ Health.* December 2000; 17–24.

46. Epp T, Waldner C. Occupational health hazards in veterinary medicine: physical, psychological, and chemical hazards. *Can Vet J.* 2012;53:151–157.

47. Baron S, ed. *Medical microbiology.* 4th ed. Galveston, TX: University of Texas Medical Branch at Galveston; 1996.

48. Jagger J, Perry J, Parker G. Lab workers: small group, big risk. *Nursing.* 2003;33(1):72.

49. Health and Safety Executive, United Kingdom. Controlling the risks of infection at work from human remains. n.d. http://www.hse.gov.uk/pubns/web01.pdf. Accessed August 27, 2013.

50. State of California, Department of Industrial Relations. Vital information for workers and employers in the adult film industry. n.d. http://www.dir.ca.gov/dosh/AdultFilmIndustry.html. Accessed August 27, 2013.

51. Korniewicz D, El-Masri M. Exploring the benefits of double gloving during surgery. *AORN J.* 2012;95(3):328–336.

52. U.S. Food and Drug Administration (FDA), National Institute for Occupational Safety and Health (NIOSH), and Occupational Safety and Health Administration (OSHA). FDA, NIOSH & OSHA joint safety communication: blunt-tip surgical suture needles reduce needlestick injuries and the risk of subsequent bloodborne pathogen transmission to surgical personnel. 2012. http://www.cdc.gov/niosh/topics/bbp/pdfs/Blunt-tip_Suture_Needles_Safety.pdf. Accessed February 22, 2014.

53. Centers for Disease Control and Prevention. Recognizing the biosafety levels. n.d. http://www.cdc.gov/training/QuickLearns/biosafety/. Accessed January 20, 2014.

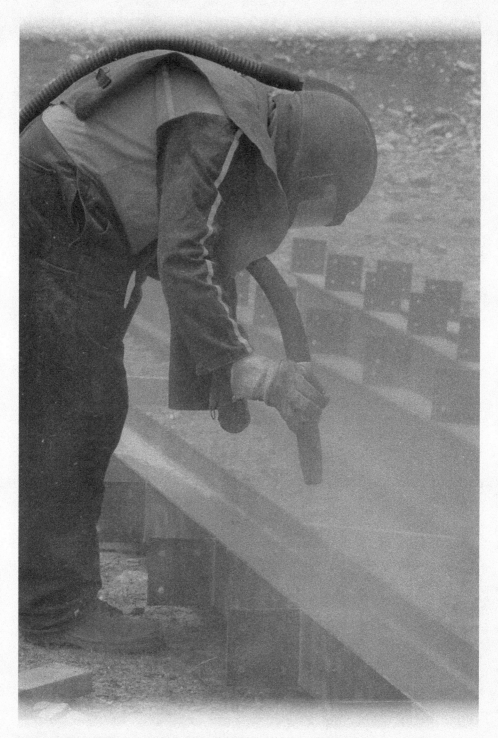

FIGURE 7.1   Worker sandblasting a wall

© Lakeview Images/Shutterstock

The National Institute for Occupational Safety and Health (NIOSH) admonishes that abrasive blasting with sands containing crystalline silica can cause serious or fatal respiratory diseases.

CHAPTER 7

Examples of Major Occupational Diseases

Learning Objectives

By the end of this chapter, you will be able to:

- Describe the significance of occupational diseases for the United States.
- State possible effects of the work environment on respiratory health, including asthma.
- Describe how occupational exposures may be related to cancer.
- Describe two possible linkages between occupations and adverse reproductive outcomes.
- State possible associations between occupational exposures and skin conditions.

Chapter Outline

- Introduction
- Occupational Lung Diseases
- Occupationally Associated Cancers
- Occupational Skin Diseases (Occupational Dermatoses)
- Occupations and Reproductive Hazards
- Summary
- Study Questions and Exercises

Introduction

The International Labour Organization has declared occupational diseases to be a "hidden epidemic" that causes untold suffering and loss.[1] Work-related diseases also are significant for American society with respect to their prevalence, contributions to the burden of mortality and morbidity, and economic costs. Estimates suggest that more than 53,000 deaths from fatal occupational illnesses occurred in the United States in 2007, with a cost of $46 billion; the corresponding estimates for nonfatal illnesses were 427,000 cases and $12 billion in costs.[2] These numbers may underestimate the actual costs substantially: Occupational disease tends to be an under-recognized phenomenon.[3] In addition, many conditions not considered to be occupationally associated diseases actually may have an occupational component.

Occupational illnesses are adverse health outcomes—for example, disease and disability—linked with exposures that occur in the work environment. As one occupational health authority has stated, "Disease and disability have been endemic to the American workplace. Unguarded machinery and unregulated conditions produced so many accidents that the muckrakers compared the hazards at work with the risks of war. By the early 20th century, the intensification of work and the introduction of new technologies produced extraordinary health hazards. Higher concentrations of toxic dust and new chemical poisons created serious chronic diseases for much of the industrial workforce despite an improvement in health statistics for the American population as a whole."[4(p. 525)] Today, more and more potentially hazardous substances are being used in the workplace. The health impacts of these substances may not be confined to a specific occupational setting, as they have potential to impact the larger community environment.[5]

Health Disparities and the Occurrence of Occupational Diseases

Occupational health disparities are differences among populations in the occurrence of adverse health outcomes and other health-related conditions.[6] For example, some populations and subgroups of populations in the United States are disproportionately affected by adverse health outcomes such as unintentional injuries and chronic illnesses. One of the goals of *Healthy People 2020* is the elimination of health disparities.

Factors associated with occupational health disparities include socio-economic status, the organization of work, race and ethnicity, nativity (e.g., being foreign-born), gender, and age.[7] These variables have been reviewed in other chapters. However, an example related to racial and ethnic differences is morbidity and mortality from occupational lung diseases. African Americans have higher mortality rates from silicosis than whites, but lower mortality rates for malignant mesothelioma. In comparison with other groups, Native Americans have higher rates of lung cancer from radon exposure because of their frequent employment in uranium mines. Hispanics tend to be employed more frequently than other ethnic and racial groups in high-risk jobs such as cleaning buildings, stonemasonry, and cement work; these occupations place them at risk for respiratory diseases such as silicosis.[8]

Types of Work-Associated Illnesses

Illnesses linked with occupations run the gamut from relatively benign and self-limiting conditions to serious, life-threatening health outcomes. Some occupational diseases are short-lived, others build up gradually over time, and still others result in workplace chronic diseases. Workplace chronic diseases are longstanding illnesses and adverse health effects that arise from occupational exposures. This chapter covers prevalent illnesses and diseases linked with workplace exposures; examples are respiratory diseases, skin diseases, occupationally associated cancers, and adverse reproductive effects (TABLE 7.1).

Occupational Lung Diseases

Occupational lung diseases are the most common work-related illness; also, they are noteworthy for their potential severity as well as their preventability.[8] **Occupational lung diseases** are defined as "a group of illnesses caused by either repeated or extended exposures or a single, severe exposure to irritating or toxic substances that lead to acute or chronic respiratory ailments."[8(p. 63)]

Occupational lung diseases have been known for millennia. For example, early writers expounded on such diseases during the periods of classical history in Greece and Rome. Debilitating occupational lung diseases have shown worrisome increases in the modern era and continue to be problematic for contemporary society.[11] Particularly concerning is the observation that the frequency of occupational lung diseases is increasing in the developing world, possibly as a result of the transfer of manufacturing operations from developed market economies to less developed countries, where protection of workers' safety tends to be more lax.[12]

Occupational lung diseases can be classified according to two broad pathophysiological types: pulmonary fibrosis and obstructive airway disease.[12] Pulmonary fibrosis is marked by restricted lung volume and increased

TABLE 7.1   Selected Occupationally Associated Diseases and Adverse Health Outcomes

Disease or Adverse Health Outcome	Examples
Allergies: Occupational allergies contribute greatly to morbidity among the working population.[9]	Allergies to molds and mites (e.g., farm workers can be exposed to microscopic mites, which can cause allergic diseases)[10]
Cancer	Bladder cancer
	Female breast cancer
	Leukemia
	Lung cancer
	Mesothelioma
	Skin cancer
Occupational lung diseases	Asbestosis
	Asthma
	Byssinosis
	Coal workers' pneumoconiosis
	Mesothelioma
	Silicosis
Reproductive hazards	Female (spontaneous abortions; preterm birth)
	Male (infertility)
Skin diseases (dermatologic conditions)	Latex skin allergies
	Skin cancer

interstitial pulmonary markings shown in chest X-rays. (*Interstitial* refers to the interstitium, a part of the lungs' structure.) Obstructive occupational lung diseases comprise lung conditions that prevent affected individuals from exhaling air completely, causing air to remain in the lungs. This effect can be due to narrowing of the airways or lung damage. Illnesses in this category include asthma and chronic obstructive pulmonary disease (COPD).[13]

Risk Factors for Occupational Lung Diseases

Risk factors for occupational lung diseases include exposures to biological agents, contact with ionizing radiation, inhalation of toxic chemicals and allergens, and inhalation of dusts—especially chronic breathing of dusts. Usually occupational lung diseases are linked with long-term exposures to agents such as "mineral and/or organic dusts, smoke, fumes, gases, mists, sprays and vapors. It is possible, however, to develop occupational lung diseases from several or single exposures, the latter usually due to industrial accidents such as chlorine spills."[14(p. 4)] Lung disease severity is correlated with the nature of the material that has been inhaled, the intensity of the exposure, and the time period over which exposure occurs.[11]

One category of occupational lung diseases (not occupation specific) results from the aggravation of preexisting lung conditions such as asthma.[8] Another type of work-related lung diseases (occupation specific) arises from specific occupational exposures to hazardous materials associated with a particular occupation or a specific kind of exposure. These conditions include asbestosis (from breathing asbestos), byssinosis (brown lung disease from inhaling cotton fibers), and coal workers' pneumoconiosis (from exposure to coal dust). In addition, indirect exposures of both individuals who do not work directly with hazardous substances and family members (via take-home exposures) can result in lung diseases. Other chapters in this text review the effects of biologic agents, physical hazards (e.g., ionizing radiation), and toxic chemicals on lung diseases; this chapter focuses on lung diseases associated with dusts.

The Role of Dusts in the Etiology of Lung Diseases

In the context of the occupational environment, dusts are solid particles that become suspended in the air as a result of activities such as construction, mining, agriculture, and manufacturing. Dusts encountered in the work environment include those from mineral sources (inorganic dusts) and organic sources (organic dusts). Activities that produce inorganic dusts (which include particles of silica, coal, and mineral fibers such as asbestos and fiberglass) include mining, construction, agriculture, and manufacturing processes. The construction industry, for example, can expose workers to large amounts of inorganic dust.

Examples of occupations associated with organic dusts, which include wood particles, cotton fibers, and particles from plastics (e.g., Styrofoam), are employment in the production of rubber and related products, textile weaving, and shoe repair. Workers in the shoe manufacturing and repair industries come into contact with solvents, glues, cleaning agents, and airborne particles that contain leather dust. Exposure to leather dust is thought to increase the risk of nasal cancer.[15] EXHIBIT 7.I describes two case studies of dust exposure: one that involved a grain elevator and the other grinding animal bones and horns.

Prolonged and even short-term exposure to dusts can be the cause of significant lung disease with many adverse consequences and can even result in death. Dusts can act synergistically with other exposures—for example, smoking—to exacerbate adverse health effects. Dusts can overwhelm

---

EXHIBIT 7.1   Case Studies of Exposures to Organic Dusts

Kansas Grain Elevator Explosion

When dust from grain stored in grain elevators becomes suspended in air, it may form a highly explosive mixture whose ignition can result in catastrophic injuries and deaths. A spark from machinery or a cigarette can set off a lethal explosion. In October 2011, a massive grain elevator explosion at the Bartlett Grain Company in Atchison, Kansas, killed six employees and injured two others.[16] The Occupational Safety and Health Organization (OSHA) cited the company for willful and serious violations related to operation of the grain elevator, including allowing dust to accumulate and then failing to shut off ignition sources that might cause an explosion while removing dust from the facility.[17]

Dust from Grinding Animal Bones and Horns

For many generations, craftsmen in India have hand-carved animal bones and horns into a variety of items, such as jewelry and eating utensils.[18] One of the health-related consequences of working in this industry is dust-associated pulmonary effects. Workers may spend many decades in this occupation, which pays the equivalent of a few dollars per day. The work requires that the laborers sit for as long as 10 hours daily. Snow-like clouds of airborne dust are inhaled and descend on the workers' hair and skin. The airborne dusts make breathing difficult and, when inhaled, are associated with high levels of tuberculosis. Workers, many of whom are children, also may suffer from injuries caused by power tools.

---

the body's defense mechanisms and damage vital organs, as shown in **FIGURE 7.2** and described in **EXHIBIT 7.2**. Potential adverse health outcomes associated with dust exposure include silicosis (from exposure to dusts from sand), pulmonary emphysema, lung cancer, and COPD. Notably, silicosis increases susceptibility to tuberculosis.

Types of Occupational Lung Diseases

Common occupation-specific lung diseases include work-related asthma, pneumoconioses, hypersensitivity pneumonitis, and sick building syndrome. The most common form of occupational lung disease is occupational asthma.[8] **TABLE 7.2** lists the occupational lung diseases discussed in this chapter.

Work-Related Asthma

"Work-related asthma (WRA) includes work-exacerbated asthma (preexisting or concurrent asthma worsened by factors related to the workplace environment) and occupational asthma (new onset asthma attributed to the workplace environment)."[21] Estimates of the prevalence of adult asthma cases from occupational exposures vary widely.[22,23] The Centers for Disease

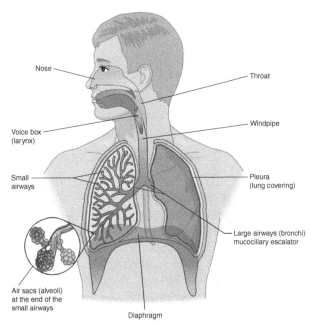

FIGURE 7.2   What dust can do to you

Reproduced from U.S. Department of Labor, Mine Safety and Health Administration,
National Mine Health and Safety Academy, Dust—What You Can't See CAN Hurt You!

EXHIBIT 7.2   Description of what Happens when a Worker Inhales Dust

[Figure 7.2 provides an overview of the respiratory system. As the worker breathes, air containing dust particles passes through the nose. At this stage, some of the large dust particles can be swallowed or expelled—for example, by sneezing.]

Air then passes through the windpipe (*trachea*) into the bronchial tubes (*bronchi*). In these tubes, a mucus blanket moistens the air, preventing the walls from drying out. It also traps particles that get past the nose and mouth. Special cells with whip-like projections (*cilia*) move the trapped particles up the larger air tubes to the mouth, where they will be swallowed or spit out. The cilia and mucus blanket are called the *mucociliary escalator.*

Particles that get past the mucociliary escalator are called *respirable*, and are generally less than 10 micrometers (μ) in diameter. A micrometers is about 1/25,000 of an inch. (Note: A human hair is about 40 micrometers in diameter.) These particles, which are invisible to the naked eye, move through smaller and smaller tubes called *bronchioles*, finally ending in *alveolar sacs* and *alveoli* (air sacs). *Remember—when you see dust in the air, there's a lot more that's invisible and respirable!*

Exchange of oxygen and carbon dioxide takes place in our more than 300 million alveoli, which have walls so thin that gases can easily pass through. The entire blood volume of the body (approximately 5 liters) passes through the lungs each minute when we are resting. Special cells called *macrophages*, which are part of the lungs' defenses, engulf some of the particles that make it to the alveoli. When there is too much dust, the number of macrophages builds up to the point that they cannot pass out of the bronchioles to be cleared. Particles begin to build up in the air sacs, interfering with the oxygen–carbon dioxide exchange. Eventually these respirable particles cause scarring (*fibrosis*) in the air sacs, making it very hard to breathe. Diseases that cause this scarring are called *pneumoconioses.*

Reprinted from the U.S. Department of Labor. Mine Safety and Health Administration. Dust—What You Can't See CAN Hurt You. http://www.msha.gov/S&HINFO/blacklung/DUST99.PDF. Accessed September 5, 2013.

TABLE 7.2 Examples of Occupational Lung Diseases

- Occupational lung cancer
- Work-related asthma
- Occupational pneumoconioses
  - Asbestosis
  - Asbestosis-associated mesothelioma
  - Byssinosis (brown lung disease)
  - Coal workers' pneumoconiosis (black lung disease)
  - Silicosis
- Hypersensitivity pneumonitis: "[I]nflammation of the lungs due to breathing in a foreign substance, usually certain types of dust, fungus, or molds.... Hypersensitivity pneumonitis usually occurs in people who work in places where there are high levels of organic dusts, fungi, or molds."[19]
- Sick building syndrome: "An illness affecting workers in office buildings, characterized by skin irritations, headache, and respiratory symptoms, and thought to be caused by indoor pollutants, microorganisms, or inadequate ventilation."[20]

Data from Centers for Disease Control and Prevention. National Institute for Occupational Safety and Healt, Pneumoconioses, http://www.cdc.gov/niosh/topics/pneumoconioses/. Accessed February 26, 2014; American Lung Association (ALA). What are occupational lung diseases? http://www.lung.org/assets/documents/publications/lung-disease-data/ldd08 -chapters/ldd-08-old.pdf. Accessed February 9, 2014.

Control and Prevention (CDC) reported that between 2006 and 2009, 9% of all employed persons had work-related asthma (**FIGURE 7.3**).[21]

Occupational and work-aggravated asthma are defined as follows:

- "Work-aggravated asthma [WAA] is defined as concurrent asthma worsened by nontoxic irritants or physical stimuli in the workplace."[24(p. 1084)]
- "Occupational asthma is defined as a disease characterized by variable airflow limitation and/or bronchial hyperresponsiveness due to causes and conditions attributable to a particular working environment and not to stimuli encountered outside the workplace."[24(p. 1084)] Sometimes this type of asthma is also called work-related new-onset asthma (NOA) and results from occupational exposure to sensitizing or irritating materials.[23]

Occupational asthma is an important topic for occupational health given that it is the most frequently occurring type of work-related lung disease in developed countries.[25,26] When persistent, this condition can be highly debilitating and can negatively impact an affected person's quality of life and income potential. The main types of occupational asthma include immunologic asthma and nonimmunologic asthma.[22] Immunologic asthma

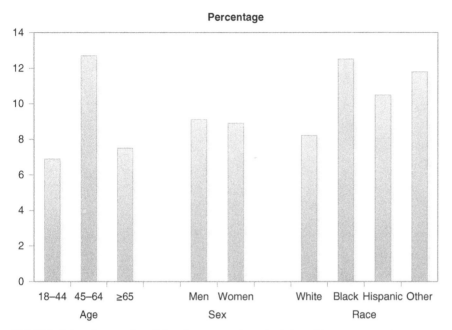

FIGURE 7.3   Proportion (%) of ever-employed adults with current asthma who have work-related asthma

Data from Centers for Disease Control and Prevention, Work-related asthma—38 states and District of Columbia, 2006–2009. *MMWR.* 2012;61(20).

occurs after a latency period of exposure to an etiologic agent; during the latency period, sensitization to the agent occurs. Nonimmunologic asthma, which does not involve a latency period, occurs soon after exposure to an irritant in the workplace.

Among the employees at risk of occupational asthma are animal handlers, food producers, construction workers, painters, and healthcare personnel. Healthcare workers, for example, may potentially be exposed to respiratory hazards such as airborne latex, cleaning products, disinfectants, pharmaceuticals, solvents, and medications that have become aerosolized. Some of these exposures may be asthmagenic as well.[27] TABLE 7.3 identifies selected major causes of occupational asthma and workers at risk of occupational asthma.

In summary, programs for prevention of occupational asthma are crucial for reducing the prevalence of this common work-related lung disease. In fact, "[p]revention of new cases is the best approach to reducing the burden of asthma attributable to occupational exposures."[25(p. 697)]

Occupational Pneumoconioses

Pneumoconiosis is defined as "the accumulation of dust in the lungs and the tissue reactions to its presence. For the purpose of this definition,

TABLE 7.3 Selected Major Causes of Occupational Asthma and Workers at Risk

Agents	Workers at Risk
Animals	
Animal proteins	Animal handlers, laboratory research workers
Prawns, crabs	Processors of these foods
Egg protein	Egg producers
Plants	
Grain dust	Grain storage workers
Wheat, rye, soy flours	Bakers, millers
Latex	Healthcare workers
Green coffee bean	Coffee roasters
Enzymes	
Proteases from *Bacillus subtilis*	Detergent industry workers
Pancreatin, papain, pepsin	Pharmaceutical industry workers
Fungal amylase	Bakers
Wood Dusts	
Western red cedar, redwood	Sawmill workers, joiners, carpenters
Chemicals	
Diisocyanates	Polyurethane, plastics, varnish workers
Acid anhydrides	Epoxy resins, alkyd resins, plastics workers
Complex amines	Photographers, shellac workers, painters
Azodicarbonamide	Plastics, rubber workers
Reactive dyes	Textile workers
Methyl methacrylate	Healthcare workers
Drugs	
Penicillins, psyllium, cimetidine	Pharmaceutical industry, healthcare workers
Metals	
Platinum salts	Platinum-refining workers
Cobalt	Hard-metal grinders
Chromium, nickel	Metal-plating workers
Other	
Metal-working fluids	Machinists
Aluminum potroom emissions	Aluminum-refining workers
Colophony in solder flux	Electronics workers

Courtesy of National Institute of Environmental Health Sciences, Lombardo LJ, Balmes JR. Occupational asthma: a review. *Environ Health Perspect.* 2000;108(suppl 4):697-704.

'dust' is meant to be an aerosol composed of solid inanimate particles."[28] Pneumoconiosis can result in fibrosis of the lungs (development of fibrous tissues) and lung nodules. Substances that, when inhaled, may cause pneumoconiosis including the following materials:

- Asbestos (associated with asbestosis and mesothelioma)
- Cotton dust (byssinosis)
- Silica-containing dusts (silicosis)
- Coal dust (black lung disease, coal workers' pneumoconiosis)

Asbestosis

Asbestosis refers to a type of pulmonary fibrosis that is associated with exposure to asbestos. Asbestos is "[t]he name given to a group of six different fibrous minerals (amosite, chrysotile, crocidolite, and the fibrous varieties of tremolite, actinolite, and anthophyllite) that occur naturally in the environment."[29] Asbestos fibers are shown in **FIGURE 7.4**.

Asbestosis results from inhalation of large amounts of asbestos fibers over long time periods. This condition occurs mainly among workers exposed to asbestos and is uncommon among the larger population. Asbestosis is

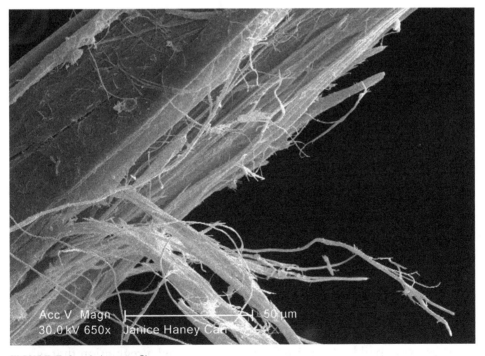

FIGURE 7.4   Asbestos fibers

Courtesy of Centers for Disease Control and Prevention, Public Health Image Library/John Wheeler, Ph.D., DABT, Janice Haney Carr, 2009.

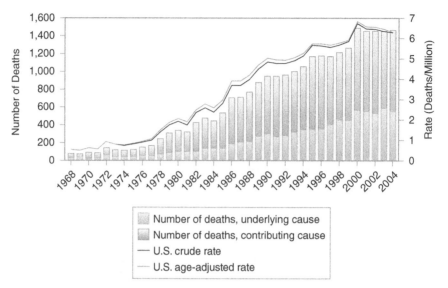

FIGURE 7.5   Asbestosis: Number of deaths, crude and age-adjusted death rates, U.S. residents age 15 and over, 1968–2004

Courtesy of Centers for Disease Control and Prevention, National Institute for Occupational Safety and Health, Work-related lung disease surveillance report 2007. 2008. DHHS (NIOSH) Publication No. 2008–143a.

associated with declines in pulmonary function and increased risk of lung cancer, especially among smokers. From 1968 to 1999, this condition was responsible for more than 18,000 deaths in the United States (**FIGURE 7.5**). Asbestos-associated mesothelioma is a rare form of cancer that invades the chest lining.

Irving Selikoff, a famous epidemiologist, and his associates identified hazards of asbestos exposure during the 1950s. In 1964, a classic publication that summarized the researchers' findings regarding linkages between asbestos exposure and cancer appeared in the *Journal of the American Medical Association*.[30] Although the use of asbestos has declined greatly since the publication of such reports on its dangers, asbestos-containing products were incorporated for many years into materials for motor vehicle brakes as well as for fireproofing and insulation. Consequently, exposure to residual asbestos from the latter two sources is possible during renovation and demolition of older buildings.

Asbestos has many useful attributes as a building material, such as fire resistance and insulating ability. In 1973, however, the U.S. Environmental Protection Agency (EPA) banned the spraying of materials that contained asbestos on buildings; in 1989, the agency issued a regulation that would prohibit most other uses of asbestos. The EPA's 1989 regulation was overturned in 1991 by a court action that continued to permit many uses of

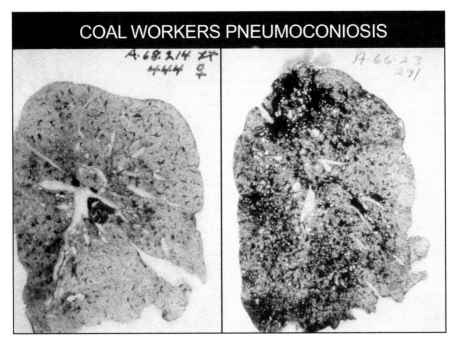

FIGURE 7.6   Coal workers' pneumoconiosis

Courtesy of Centers for Disease Control and Prevention, Public Health Image Library.

asbestos.[31] Currently asbestos is banned from six categories of products, including certain types of construction materials, certain paper goods, and all new applications of asbestos. The majority of car manufacturers have adopted substitutes for asbestos-containing brake linings.

Coal Workers' Pneumoconiosis (Black Lung Disease)

Coal workers' pneumoconiosis (CWP; black lung disease) is the most common disease in the world caused by mineral dusts.[32] This serious lung disease is caused by breathing coal dust over an extended time period (FIGURE 7.6). Often, the beginning phases of CWP are asymptomatic, but later stages may cause disability and premature mortality among miners.[33] The most severe form of coal workers' pneumoconiosis is called progressive massive fibrosis.

During earlier eras of coal mining (FIGURE 7.7), miners were exposed to heavy concentrations of dust associated with frequent cases of CWP. As a result of subsequent improvements in working conditions and reductions in exposures to coal dusts, rates of CWP declined substantially. Nevertheless, during the early 2000s, severe coal workers' pneumoconiosis continued to be a problem among coal miners in parts of Appalachia and in the smaller mines.[34]

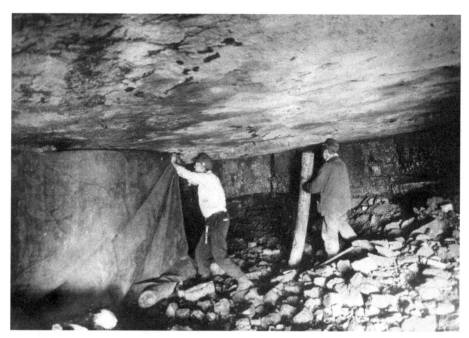

FIGURE 7.7   Historical image of a coal mine

Courtesy of Centers for Disease Control and Prevention, Public Health Image Library/Barbara Jenkins, NIOSH.

One of the outcomes studied in relation to excessive exposure to coal dust is premature deaths among miners. Mortality studies indicate that miners' contact with dust in coal mines leads to increased death rates.[35] Not all of the increased mortality is attributable to CWP. A cohort life-table analysis of mortality followed 8899 coal miners over more than two decades from their initial examination in 1969 to 1971. In a detailed review of causes of mortality among the cohort, researchers found that in addition to mortality from coal-mine dust exposure, mortality was elevated for non-violent causes, nonmalignant respiratory disease, and unintentional injuries.[35] FIGURE 7.8 shows age-adjusted death rates of CWP by U.S. states; note the high rates for coal-mining states such as Pennsylvania.

The National Institute for Occupational Safety and Health (NIOSH) collects surveillance data for mortality from work-related respiratory diseases.[36] From 1968 to 2006, deaths from CWP declined 73%, from 1106.2 deaths per year to 300.0 deaths per year among persons 25 years of age and older. The annual years of potential life lost (YPLL) from CWP decreased by more than 90% between 1968 and 2006. However, since 2006, the YPLL from CWP have trended upward among miners younger than 65 years of age. FIGURE 7.9 provides annual data on YPLL from CWP before age 65 years.

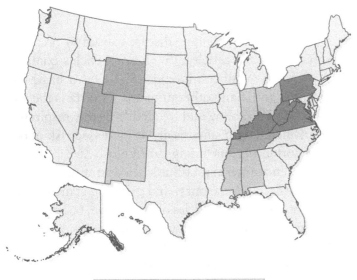

Deaths/Million/Year	No. of States
■ >9.56	4
■ >4.78–9.56	3
■ >2.39–4.78	6
□ ≤2.39	38

FIGURE 7.8   Coal workers' pneumoconiosis: Age-adjusted death rates by state, U.S. residents age 15 and over, 1995–2004

Reproduced from Centers for Disease Control and Prevention, National Institute for Occupational Safety and Health, Work-related lung disease surveillance report 2007. 2008. DHHS (NIOSH) Publication No. 2008–143a.

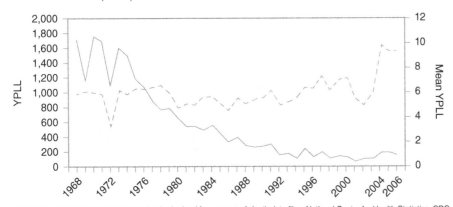

*Based on annual underlying cause of death obtained from cause-of-death data files, National Center for Health Statistics, CDC.

——— YPLL
- - - Mean YPLL

FIGURE 7.9   Years of potential life lost (YPLL) before age 65 years and mean YPLL per decedent for decedents age ≥ 25 years with coal workers' pneumoconiosis as the underlying cause of death—United States, 1968-2006

Reproduced from Centers for Disease Control and Prevention, Coal workers' pneumoconiosis-related years of potential life lost before age 65 years—U.S., 1968–2006. *MMWR.* 2009;58(50).

Silicosis

The term silicosis describes "a lung disease caused by breathing dust containing respirable silica particles."[32] These particles contain crystalline silica. Crystalline silica (silicon dioxide, SiO_2) "is a basic component of soil, sand, granite, and many other minerals. Quartz is the most common form."[37] Silicosis is a disabling and frequently deadly respiratory disease.[38] Also, persons afflicted with silicosis are at increased risk of or susceptibility to other comorbidities, including tuberculosis.[11,39]

Workers may encounter crystalline silica during activities such as sandblasting, cutting tiles and masonry, and grinding cement. The dangers of silica dust are not limited to particles of visible size, because very fine, invisible silica particles also may be drawn into the lungs. **FIGURE 7.10** shows a lung that has been damaged by silicosis.

Silicosis presents in three major forms: chronic silicosis, accelerated silicosis, and acute silicosis.[40] *Chronic silicosis* (associated with long-term exposures to silica at low levels) takes many years to develop and starts to emerge after 10 to 20 years. Early in the course of the disease, few symptoms may be present or, if observable, may consist of coughing and

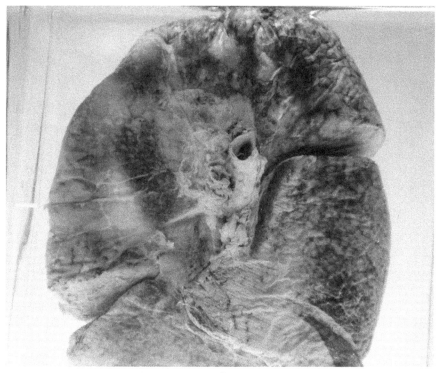

FIGURE 7.10   Silicosis-damaged lung
© Photopat/Alamy

shortness of breath. Long after initial exposure to silica (e.g., 10 or more years), nodules may develop on the lobes of the lungs. More severe cases, designated as complicated silicosis, may result in pulmonary fibrosis and loss of lung function.

Accelerated silicosis (a rapidly progressing form that is associated with exposure to large amounts of silica during short time periods) has an onset after 5 to 10 years. *Acute silicosis* (caused by very heavy exposures to silica during short time periods) begins within a period of several weeks up to 5 years following exposure.

Potentially, silicosis can be a fatal disease. EXHIBIT 7.3 describes a case report of a U.S. death from silicosis.

Occupational exposure to silica-containing dusts occurs in many occupations. TABLE 7.4 gives a few examples of these occupations.

Byssinosis

Byssinosis (brown lung disease) is a lung disorder characterized by reduced lung function and other adverse pulmonary effects associated with breathing

---

EXHIBIT 7.3   Case Report of a Death from Silicosis

In November 1988, a physician in western Texas reported three cases of sandblaster's silicosis to the Ector County Health Department. All three patients had been employed at a facility where they sandblasted oil-field drilling pipes. One of the workers, a 34-year-old man, subsequently died as a result of acute silicosis. Following a later report by the physician in January 1989, the Ector County Health Department and the Texas Department of Health contacted local physicians and identified 7 additional sandblasters who had suffered from silicosis since 1985. Of the 10 workers identified, 9 had worked at the same facility, which employed approximately 60 persons.

Each of the 10 workers had a history of occupational exposure to silica and a chest X-ray consistent with pneumoconiosis; 8 had a lung tissue pathology report of silicotic nodules or acute silicosis. All were Hispanic males aged 24 to 50 at the time of diagnosis. Seven workers were younger than age 30. Although tuberculosis was considered in all of the reported patients (three of whom had reactive tuberculin skin tests), all sputum and tissue samples from all patients were negative for *Mycobacterium tuberculosis*.

All 10 workers had used sandblasting machinery. Their duration of exposure to sandblasting ranged from 18 months to 8 years (mean: 4.5 years). Nine workers reported no previous silica exposure; the remaining worker had sandblasted oil-field drilling equipment for 3 years before working at the originally identified facility for 5 years. Supplied-air respirators had not been used during sandblasting, and workers reported wearing only disposable particulate respirators.

Modified from Centers for Disease Control and Prevention (CDC). National Institute for Occupational Safety and Health (NIOSH). Preventing silicosis and deaths from sandblasting. http://www.cdc.gov/niosh/docs/92-102/. Accessed October 15, 2013.

TABLE 7.4 Examples of Occupations that Expose Workers to Silica or Silica-Containing Dusts

Abrasive blasting/ tunnel construction	Construction activities in tunnels expose workers to dust from rock drilling, grinding, blasting, and spraying concrete.[41]
Agriculture	Soil preparation exposes agricultural workers to dusts that may contain silica particles.[42]
Construction	Power tools (e.g., grinders, masonry saws, and jackhammers) used frequently in construction often stir up clouds of silica-containing dusts.
Fracking	Hydraulic fracturing operations ("fracking") expose workers to health hazards from inhalation of silica, which can cause silicosis, lung cancer, and other pulmonary diseases. The sand used in fracking is laden with silica. Workers at oil extraction sites can be exposed to large amounts of silica.[43]
Mining	Underground mining involves blasting and excavating that produce silica-laden dusts.[44]
Pottery manufacture	Mortality was examined among more than 74,000 Chinese workers exposed to silica dust in metal mines and pottery factories (**FIGURE 7.11**). The workers were employed in these settings for approximately 15 years. Exposure to silica dust was associated with increased all-cause mortality and mortality from respiratory diseases and lung cancer. Increased risk of mortality also was found for cardiovascular disease.[44]

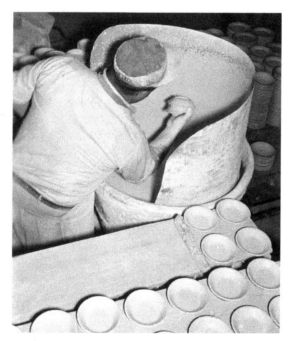

FIGURE 7.11 Application of slip (liquefied clay) to ceramic pieces can produce airborne silica particles

Courtsy of the Centers for Disease Control and Prevention. Public Health Image Library/Barbara Jenkins, NIOSH, 1936.

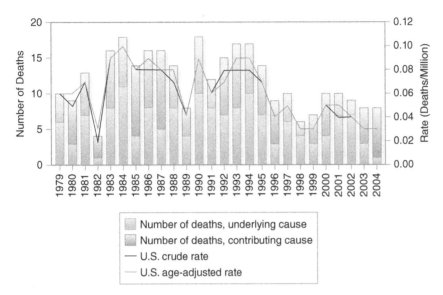

FIGURE 7.12   Byssinosis: Number of deaths, crude and age-adjusted death rates, U.S. residents age 15 and over, 1979–2004

Reproduced from Center for Disease Control and Prevention, National Institute for Occupational Safety and Health, Skin exposures and effects, http://www.cdc.gov/niosh/topics/skin/. Accessed August 16, 2013.

cotton dust; it is a form of pneumoconiosis and is both an underlying cause of and a contributing cause to mortality (**FIGURE 7.12**). Byssinosis develops among textile workers and others who inhale cotton dust because they do not wear face masks and personal protective equipment. One notable symptom of byssinosis is the development of chest tightness when returning to work after the weekend. Smoking adds to the deleterious effects of exposure to cotton dust in its association with byssinosis.[45] Surprisingly, some studies have reported a reduced risk of lung cancer among persons exposed to cotton dust. This result is thought to stem from the protective effect of bacterial endotoxins, which can contaminate cotton fibers as demonstrated among female textile workers.[46]

Synthetic Mineral Fibers

Synthetic mineral fibers are "fibrous inorganic substances made primarily from rock, clay, slag, or glass. These fibers are classified into three general groups: fiberglass (glass wool and glass filament), mineral wool (rock wool and slag wool), and refractory ceramic fibers (RCF)."[47] According to OSHA, 225,000 U.S. workers currently have exposures to synthetic mineral fibers in manufacturing and other applications.[47]

Fiberglass comprises "a silicate fiber made from very fine strands of glass." This human-made material is used for insulation and creating light-weight materials.[48] Inhalation of fiberglass is associated with reduced lung function, inflammation, and skin, eye, and throat irritation.[48] As an example of the health effects of working with synthetic mineral fibers, the respiratory health of workers exposed to glass dust from glass fiber–reinforced plastic was studied. The workers demonstrated changes in the cellular and enzymatic components deep in their lungs.[49] A Brazilian man who used glass wool fibers and coating materials in the speed boat industry developed pulmonary lesions.[50]

Occupationally Associated Cancers

The development of occupationally associated cancers reflects increased risks of cancer from exposure to carcinogens in the work environment. Both the American Cancer Society[51] and the CDC have implicated exposures to such occupational carcinogens as risk factors for cancer. According to the CDC, "Based on well-documented associations between occupational exposures and cancer, it has been estimated that 4% to 10% of U.S. cancers (48,000 incident cases annually) are caused by occupational exposures."[52] The estimates from the American Cancer Society are at the lower end of this range.[51] Job-related exposures to carcinogens are commonplace. According to Landrigan, based on estimates from the National Institute for Occupational Safety and Health, "over seven million American workers have the potential for regular occupational exposure to proven human carcinogens."[53(p. 67)]

Percival Pott published the first report of workplace exposures associated with human cancers. In 1775, he described cases of scrotum cancer among London chimney sweeps and asserted that this form of cancer was associated with contact with soot. Pott's observation has held up over time, and it is now known that the chemicals in soot include polycyclic aromatic hydrocarbons, which are considered to be carcinogens.

Examples of Occupational Carcinogens

A carcinogen is a substance that causes cancer in mammals, including humans. Examples of chemical exposures associated with cancer include perchloroethylene (perc), asbestos, benzene, and arsenic.[51] Widespread exposure to carcinogenic substances persists in many industries and is an especially problematic issue for developing countries.[54] In addition, "[m]illions of U.S. workers are exposed to substances that have tested as carcinogens in animal studies. However, less than 2% of chemicals manufactured or processed in the United States have been tested for carcinogenicity."[51]

The International Agency for Research on Cancer (IARC), a branch of the World Health Organization (WHO), has developed one of the most widely used classification systems for carcinogens.[55] The IARC organizes carcinogens into the following groups:

- Group 1: Carcinogenic to humans
- Group 2A: Probably carcinogenic to humans
- Group 2B: Possibly carcinogenic to humans
- Group 3: Unclassifiable as to carcinogenicity in humans
- Group 4: Probably not carcinogenic to humans

Childhood Cancer and Parents' Occupations

One line of research has investigated the relationship between parents' occupational exposures and the development of cancer among their children. Some researchers hypothesize that such exposures could result in genetic changes in human eggs and sperm cells. These genetic changes might then affect children born to exposed parents. Another possibility is that carcinogens might be transported across the placenta. However, researchers have not obtained definitive findings regarding these kinds of associations. Parental exposures to occupational agents might produce other adverse reproductive outcomes as well as cancer.[56]

Environmental Factors

EXHIBIT 7.4 provides information on the role of environmental factors in cancer.

Forms of Cancer Linked with Occupational Exposures

Researchers have explored associations between occupational exposures and several types of cancer, as shown in **TABLE 7.5**. The identification of relationships between occupational exposures and cancer is a challenging problem for several reasons. One issue is the difficulty of exposure assessment—measuring the levels of exposure in the workplace and differentiating occupational exposures to potential carcinogens from other environmental exposures. Another issue is the long latency period between exposures to possible carcinogens and subsequent development of cancer. A third issue is researchers' increasing awareness of the complex interactions between genetic influences and exposures to carcinogens.

> **EXHIBIT 7.4** **The Role of Environmental Factors in Cancer**
>
> Environmental factors (as opposed to hereditary factors) account for an estimated 75%–80% of cancer cases and deaths in the United States. Exposure to carcinogenic agents in occupational, community, and other settings is thought to account for a relatively small percentage of cancer deaths—about 4% from occupational exposures and 2% from environmental pollutants (human-made and naturally occurring). Although the estimated percentage of cancers related to occupational and environmental carcinogens is small compared to the cancer burden from tobacco smoking (30%) and the combination of poor nutrition, physical inactivity, and obesity (35%), the relationship between such agents and cancer is important for several reasons. First, even a small percentage of cancers can represent many deaths: 6% of cancer deaths in the United States in 2011 corresponds to approximately 34,320 deaths. Second, the burden of exposure to occupational and environmental carcinogens is borne disproportionately by lower-income workers and communities, contributing to disparities in the cancer burden across the U.S. population. Third, although much is known about the relationship between occupational and environmental exposure and cancer, some important research questions remain. These include the role of exposures to certain classes of chemicals (such as hormonally active agents) during critical periods of human development and the potential for pollutants to interact with each other, as well as with genetic and acquired factors.
>
> Reprinted from American Cancer Society. Cancer Facts and Figures 2014. Atlanta, GA: American Cancer Society; 2014, 55-56.

The *Hazards from Chemicals and Toxic Metals* chapter explored examples of relationships between several types of cancer and exposures to chemicals and metals. One topic covered there was the association between nasal cancer and exposure to nickel and chromium. Other potential relationships noted in that chapter were the link between benzene and leukemia and the association between vinyl chloride and angiosarcoma of the liver. The relationship between ultraviolet radiation and skin cancer was identified in the *Physical Hazards in the Workplace* chapter. Some of the hypothesized associations of occupational exposures with other forms of cancer shown in Table 7.5 are reviewed in the following sections. Other forms of occupationally associated cancer not shown in the table but discussed in this chapter are bone cancer, female breast cancer, and brain cancer.

Bone Cancer

Bone cancer is an uncommon form of cancer that originates in the bone (primary bone cancer).[57,58] It is not called cancer of the bone if the cancer has metastasized from other sites in the body—for example, the breast or lung. Studies have identified increased death rates from bone cancer among former employees of nuclear facilities.[57]

TABLE 7.5   Cancers Associated with Various Occupations or Occupational Exposures

Cancer	Examples of Substances or Processes Encountered in an Occupational Setting
Lung	Arsenic, asbestos, beryllium, cadmium, coke oven fumes, chromium compounds, coal products, nickel refining, foundry substances, radon, soot, tars, silica, vinyl chloride, diesel exhaust, radioactive ores like uranium
Bladder	Paint/dyeing products; printing processes; benzidine; beta-naphthylamine; arsenic; chemicals used in rubber, leather, and textile industries
Nasal cavity and sinuses	Formaldehyde, textile industry, mustard gas, nickel refining, chromium dust, leather dust, wood dust, baking, flour milling, radium
Larynx	Asbestos; wood dust; paint fumes; chemicals used in metal working, petroleum, plastics, and textile industries
Mesothelioma	Asbestos
Lymphatic and hematopoietic (*Lymphatic*: pertaining to the lymphatic system; lymphomas are cancers of the lymph nodes. *Hematopoietic*: pertaining to the formation of blood or blood cells; an example of a hematopoietic cancer is leukemia.)	Benzene, herbicides, insecticides, radiation
Skin	Arsenic, coal tars, paraffin, certain oils, sunlight
Soft-tissue sarcoma (a type of cancer that develops in the soft tissues of the body, such as muscles, nerves, and fatty tissues)	Radiation
Liver	Arsenic, vinyl chloride
Lip	Sunlight (association not confirmed)

Female Breast Cancer

Information on the role of occupational exposures in female breast cancer tends to be lacking.[59] This topic will become increasingly important as greater numbers of women continue to enter the workforce. Among the occupational exposures studied in relationship to breast cancer are ionizing and non-ionizing radiation, endocrine disruptors, and chemical carcinogens. Some evidence suggests an association exists between breast cancer and employment in the pharmaceutical field, in cosmetology, in the chemical industry, and in occupations in which women are exposed to extremely low-frequency electromagnetic fields.[59]

A representative example of research in this field was a case-control study of female breast cancer conducted by Italian researchers. They compared more than 10,000 incident breast cancer cases with 25,000 controls in Lombardy, Italy.[60] Regarding the occurrence of breast cancer, their findings suggested a potential role for occupational exposures in industries involved with the manufacture of electrical products, textiles, paper, and rubber. Brophy et al. reported that a case-control study of Canadian women supported hypotheses regarding associations between exposures thought to include endocrine disruptors (and also carcinogens) and breast cancer risk.[61]

Lung Cancer

According to WHO statistics, 10% of lung cancer deaths worldwide are related to workplace risks.[62] About half of the burden of occupational cancer is from lung cancer.[63] Furthermore, many of these lung cancer deaths come from exposure to asbestos. Lung cancer from asbestos exposure, asbestos-related mesothelioma (a rare form of cancer that invades the chest lining), and asbestosis—all as a result of occupational exposures—account for more than 107,000 deaths globally.

In the United States, lung cancer is the most important cause of cancer mortality for both men and women. Cigarette smoking is a leading risk factor for lung cancer mortality. However, occupational exposures to carcinogens may increase risks of lung cancer mortality and sometimes act synergistically with lifestyle factors, which include cigarette smoking and alcohol consumption.[52]

The Environment and Genetics in Lung Cancer Etiology (EAGLE) case-control study probed the relationship between occupation and lung cancer among workers in the Lombardy region of northern Italy.[64] Consonni et al. concluded that past occupational exposure to carcinogens was important in lung cancer occurrence. These researchers estimated that 4.9% of male lung cancers could be ascribed to occupation.

Other examples of occupational carcinogens associated with lung cancer include the following substances and exposures:[65]

- Ionizing radiation from radioactive materials and gases (e.g., radon, alpha particles, and X-rays)
- Metals and related materials (e.g., arsenic, asbestos, and heavy metals such as cadmium and beryllium)

- Polycyclic aromatic hydrocarbons (PAHs) (e.g., coal tar, soot)
- Diesel exhaust
- Nonsmokers' workplace exposure to second-hand cigarette smoke

Brain Cancer

Brain cancer is a very uncommon type of cancer with a high case-fatality rate.[66] Research has examined the association between brain cancer (brain tumors) and employment in different types of occupations.[67] However, no consensus has been reached regarding the role of occupational risk factors in development of brain cancer, as research on this front has been inconclusive.[68] Some of the occupational exposures (selected as representative examples) that have been studied in this extensive field of investigation are as follows:

- Magnetic fields, such as from electrically powered tools[66,69]
- Carcinogenic chemicals, pesticides, and neurotoxic substances, such as organic solvents[68,70]
- Chemicals used in work settings, such as in the Finnish INTEROCC study[71]

Bladder Cancer

Globally, bladder cancer is the ninth most common cause of cancer when the data for men and women are combined.[72] Use of tobacco is the leading risk factor for bladder cancer. However, occupational exposures are believed to have a role in the etiology of this form of cancer. Associations have been found between bladder cancer and occupational exposures to amines (e.g., in aniline dyes and other dyes containing amines), polycyclic hydrocarbons, and perchloroethylene (used in dry cleaning and metal cleaning solvents). Exposure to ionizing radiation is also related to bladder cancer.[73] Kellen et al. reported that occupational exposures to amines increased the risk of bladder cancer in their case-control study conducted in Belgium.[72]

Prevention of Occupational Exposures to Potential Carcinogens

Occupational exposures to carcinogenic substances are highly preventable, and implementing measures to guard against such exposures would aid in reducing the burden of occupationally associated cancers.[52] Insights into cancer prevention will come about as a result of well-designed research programs. According to the National Occupational Research Agenda Team, "Focus on occupational cancer research methods is important both because occupational factors play a significant role in a number of cancers, resulting in significant morbidity and mortality, and also because occupational cohorts (because of higher exposure levels) often provide unique opportunities to evaluate health effects of occupational toxicants and understand the carcinogenic process in humans… . Progress in occupational cancer will require interdisciplinary research involving epidemiologists, industrial hygienists, toxicologists, and molecular biologists."[74(p. 1)]

Occupational Skin Diseases (Occupational Dermatoses)

The term *dermatoses* pertains to skin diseases. Although a standard definition of occupational dermatoses is lacking, the European Agency for Safety and Health at Work (EU-OSHA) states that they may defined as "those [dermatoses] for which the cause can be found partly or wholly in the conditions in which the work is carried out."[75] Dermatoses can be classified into the three subtypes shown in **TABLE 7.6**.

Significance of Occupational Dermatoses

Occupational skin diseases rank as the second most frequent type of occupational disease.[76] They are responsible for approximately half of all occupational illnesses and one-fourth of all days of lost work. Failure to recognize their linkage with work-related exposures has resulted in undercounting of occupational dermatoses.[77]

One reason for the high prevalence of occupational skin diseases is the widespread use of chemicals in job settings. According to NIOSH, approximately 13 million U.S. workers each year come into contact with chemicals that might be absorbed through the skin. These dermal exposures can be the cause of occupational diseases, which include occupational skin diseases and systemic toxicity.[76]

TABLE 7.6   Categories of Dermatoses

Exclusively occupational	"[T]he relationship with the occupational activity is clearly established."
Aggravated by occupational activity	"This implies pre-existing skin conditions that are reactivated or aggravated during the occupational activity."
Non-occupational	"[N]o relationship with occupational activity has been shown."

Modified from De Craecker W, Roskams N, op de Beeck R. Occupational skin diseases and dermal exposure in the European Union (EU-25): policy and practice overview. Brussels, Belgium: EU-OSHA; 2008, p. 16.

Dermal Effects of Occupational Exposures

The two types of dermal effects of occupational exposures are local effects and systemic effects, which occur when a chemical is absorbed by the skin and is circulated throughout the body, respectively. **FIGURE 7.13** identifies types of exposures associated with skin diseases in the work environment. Examples of effects of occupational exposures to the skin include the following:

- Irritation/burning/urticaria (hives): Caused by numerous products and exposures such as chemicals (e.g., acids, pesticides, and solvents) and contact with animals (e.g., caterpillars and jellyfish) and plants (e.g., nettles)
- Sensitization/allergy/phototoxicity[75]

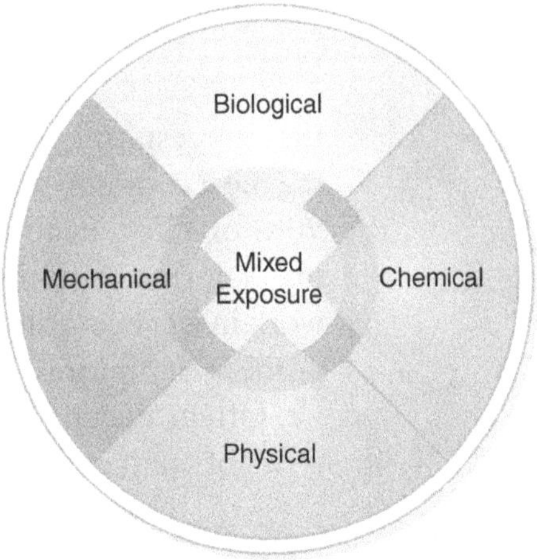

Types of Occupational Skin Diseases

FIGURE 7.13 Exposures associated with skin diseases in the work environment

Reproduced from Disease Control and Prevention, National Institute for Occupational Safety and Health, Skin exposures and effects, http://www.cdc.gov/niosh/topics/skin/. Accessed August 16, 2013.

Occupational skin diseases include contact dermatitis (both irritant and allergic) and skin cancer (**FIGURE 7.14**). Other work-related skin conditions include skin infections and injuries,[76] which are not covered in this chapter.

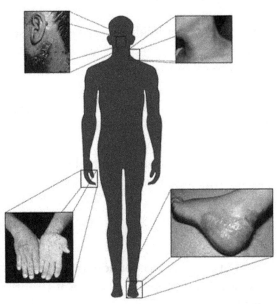

FIGURE 7.14 Examples of occupationally associated skin diseases

Reproduced from Centers for Disease Control and Prevention, National Institute for Occupational Safety and Health, Skin exposures and effects, http://www.cdc.gov/niosh/topics/skin/. Accessed August 16, 2013.

Contact Dermatitis

"Contact dermatitis, also called eczema, is defined as an inflammation of the skin resulting from exposure to a hazardous agent."[76] This condition is the most common occupational skin disease, accounting for approximately 90% of all occupational skin disease cases. Hand dermatitis is one of the major forms of skin-related morbidity among hairdressers.[78] People who work in wet occupations (e.g., nursing, kitchen work, and cleaning) are also prone to dermatitis, which may be prevented through skin care programs.[79]

Often, occupational health dermatologists distinguish between two types of contact dermatitis—irritant and allergic:

- Irritant contact dermatitis is "a non-immunologic reaction that manifests as an inflammation of the skin caused by direct damage to the skin following exposure to a hazardous agent."[76] This form of contact dermatitis is the most common type. Substances implicated in contact dermatitis include primary irritants, such as pesticides, cement, and hair dyes.
- Allergic contact dermatitis is "an inflammation of the skin caused by an immunologic reaction triggered by dermal contact to a skin allergen."[76] Sometimes even minute exposures to allergens can cause acute contact dermatitis.[77] Common skin allergens include beauty products such as nail polish and certain antibiotics.

In many instances, when individuals are first exposed to an allergen, they may not experience any reaction; instead, sensitivity to the allergen develops over time with repeated exposure.[80] Skin sensitizers are substances that "may not cause immediate skin reactions, but repeated exposure can result in allergic reactions."[76] Two types of skin sensitizers are (1) chemicals (e.g., nickel and chromium, some resins and plastics, chemicals in rubber, and solvents) and (2) proteins from natural materials such as natural rubber latex, animal dander, and products from plants. Photosensitizers (e.g., coal tar products) are substances that cause a response after an individual has been exposed to the sun.

Allergies to Latex Gloves

Latex allergies are an important occupational health issue for the medical profession.[81] Latex gloves are the greatest source of airborne latex allergens in surgical settings.[82] Healthcare workers can experience serious health effects from latex allergies.[83] Patients who have latex allergies also are at risk from airborne latex allergens. Consequently, both patients and health professionals need to be protected from these allergens.[82] Workers need to wear gloves during medical procedures, however; thus persons who have latex allergies should be identified early in their careers so they can use alternatives to latex gloves.[83]

Skin and Lip Cancer

Skin cancers represent a noteworthy example of an occupational skin disease.[84] Among Caucasian populations worldwide, non-melanoma skin cancer is the most common tumor of any kind.[85] This type of cancer tends to be underreported but is also regarded as highly curable. Occupational skin cancers can result from exposures to chemical substances (e.g., polycyclic hydrocarbons found in coal tar products and arsenic compounds) and physical hazards including ionizing radiation and solar ultraviolet radiation.[77,84,85] A potential occupational risk factor for lip cancer is exposure to ultraviolet radiation from the sun when working outdoors, although this relationship has not been definitively proved.

Occupations and Reproductive Hazards

Workers' occupational exposures to reproductive hazards are a significant topic of growing concern because of the large number of employees who are of child-bearing age. As more and more chemicals are introduced into manufacturing processes, the potential for adverse effects on reproductive health from this source is increasing.

"Reproductive hazards are substances or agents that may affect the reproductive health of women or men or the ability of couples to have healthy children. These hazards may cause problems such as infertility, miscarriage, and birth defects."[86] This section reviews how reproductive hazards might affect the health of male and female workers.

Reproductive Hazards to Women

Reproductive hazards are salient for women because approximately three-fourths of all women employed in the workforce are of reproductive age.[87] Among the most common sources of hazardous workplace exposures for women are tobacco smoke, video display terminals, and indoor air quality; specific hazards include chemicals, ionizing radiation, tobacco smoke, alcohol, certain pharmaceuticals, and biohazards (FIGURE 7.15).[88] TABLE 7.7 and TABLE 7.8 list chemical and physical agents and disease-causing agents that are reproductive hazards for women in the workplace.[89] Another chemical agent is the anesthetic gas nitrous oxide (N_2O), which research has suggested can cause female workers to experience lessened fertility, spontaneous abortions, neurologic effects, and renal and liver disease. In one

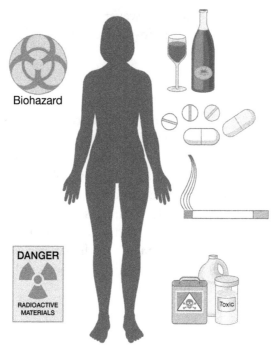

FIGURE 7.15 Reproductive hazards for female workers

Reproduced from Centers for Disease Control and Prevention, National Institute for Occupational Safety and Health, The effects of workplace hazards on female reproductive health. DHHS (NIOSH) Publication No. 99-104. Cincinnati, OH: 1999.

TABLE 7.7 Chemical and Physical Agents that Are Reproductive Hazards for Women in the Workplace

Agent	Observed Effects	Potentially Exposed Workers
Cancer treatment drugs (e.g., methotrexate)	Infertility, miscarriage, birth defects, low birth weight	Healthcare workers, pharmacists
Certain ethylene glycol ethers, such as 2-ethoxyethanol (2EE) and 2-methoxyethanol (2ME)	Miscarriages	Electronics and semiconductor workers
Carbon disulfide (CS_2)	Menstrual cycle changes	Viscose rayon workers
Lead	Infertility, miscarriage. low birth weight, developmental disorders	Battery makers, solderers, welders, radiator repairers, bridge repainters, firing range workers, home remodelers
Ionizing radiation (e.g., X-rays and gamma rays)	Infertility, miscarriage, birth defects, low birth weight, developmental disorders, childhood cancers	Healthcare workers, dental personnel, atomic workers
Strenuous physical labor (e.g., prolonged standing, heavy lifting)	Miscarriage late in pregnancy, premature delivery	Many types of workers

Courtesy of National Institute for Occupational Safety and Health, The effects of workplace hazards on female reproductive health. Cincinnati, OH: NIOSH; 1999. DHHS (NIOSH) Publication NO. 99-104.

TABLE 7.8 Disease-Causing Agents that Are Reproductive Hazards for Women in the Workplace

Agent	Observed Effects	Potentially Exposed Workers	Preventive Measures
Cytomegalovirus (CMV)	Birth defects, low birth weight, developmental disorders	Healthcare workers, workers in contact with infants and children	Good hygienic practices such as hand washing
Hepatitis B virus	Low birth weight	Healthcare workers	Vaccination
Human immunodeficiency virus (HIV)	Low birth weight, childhood cancer	Healthcare workers	Practice universal precautions
Human parvovirus B19	Miscarriage	Healthcare workers, workers in contact with infants and children	Good hygienic practices such as hand washing
Rubella (German measles)	Birth defects, low birth weight	Healthcare workers, workers in contact with infants and children	Vaccination before pregnancy if no prior immunity
Toxoplasmosis	Miscarriage, birth defects, developmental disorders	Animal care workers, veterinarians	Good hygiene practices such as hand washing
Varicella-zoster virus (chickenpox)	Birth defects, low birth weight	Healthcare workers, workers in contact with infants and children	Vaccination before pregnancy if no prior immunity

Courtesy of the National Institute for Occupational Safety and Health (NIOSH). The effects of workplace hazards on female reproductive health. Cincinnati, OH: NIOSH; 1999. DHHS (NIOSH) Publication NO. 99-104

study, female dental assistants developed reduced fertility associated with occupational exposure to N_2O.[90]

Reproductive Effects Associated with Occupational Exposures

Reproductive effects studied in relation to occupational exposures include preterm births and adverse live birth outcomes (**TABLE 7.9**). Specific examples of occupationally associated adverse reproductive effects among women include the following:

- *Adverse live-birth outcomes:* Exposure to heavy metals, pesticides, petroleum products, and chemicals were found to increase the risk of

TABLE 7.9   Reproductive Effects Studied in Relation to Women's Occupational Exposures

Reproductive Effect	Definition
Spontaneous abortion (miscarriage)	Loss of a fetus before the 20th week of pregnancy that is not due to a medical or surgical abortion[96]
Adverse live-birth outcomes	Adverse effects that include a number of conditions (e.g., preterm birth, low birth weight, and birth defects)
Preterm birth	Delivery of the newborn before 37 weeks' gestation
Low birth weight	Newborns with a birth weight of less than 2500 grams or 5.5 pounds
Birth defects (congenital malformations)	Structural defects present in the newborn at birth, such as cleft palate, heart defects, or hypospadias (abnormal location of the urethra in boys)

adverse live-birth outcomes. This effect was described among women in the U.S. Navy.[91]

- *Preterm birth:* Job classification—potentially a determinant of occupational exposures to injurious chemicals—was shown to be a possible risk factor for preterm birth. Los Angeles foreign-born Hispanic women who were employed in building and grounds cleaning and maintenance operations were found to have increased risks of preterm birth.[92] Also, mothers' occupational exposure to lead has been shown to be related to preterm birth.[93] For information on methodologic issues on environmental exposures and preterm births, consult Zeger's review of two epidemiologic studies.[94]
- *Spontaneous abortion (miscarriage):* Some metal smelters are known to emit arsenic, heavy metals, other metals, and sulfur dioxide into the environment. These emissions could jeopardize the pregnancies of female workers in these facilities. However, a Swedish study did not identify increased risk of spontaneous abortions among workers in a metal smelter or among women who resided near the smelter.[95]

Reproductive Hazards for Men

A reproductive hazard for men is infertility, which is an example of adverse male reproductive function. Male infertility is a condition caused by "low sperm production, misshapen or immobile sperm, or blockages that prevent the delivery of sperm."[97] Evidence from epidemiologic studies appears to provide strong evidence of a relationship between occupational and environmental exposures and adverse male reproductive function.[98] For example, researchers found that Canadian men who had heavy exposures to organic solvents tended to have fertility problems, as manifested by low active sperm counts.[99] Another study reported that firefighters have exposures that are suspected of affecting reproductive function.[100]

TABLE 7.10   Occupational Exposures with Possible Adverse Effects on Male Reproductive Function

- Heat (from occupations such as baking and foundry employment that have high heat levels; occupational sitting for long periods increases scrotal temperature)
- Heavy metals (e.g., inorganic lead, mercury)
- Ionizing radiation
- Microwave radiation
- Pesticides (e.g., ethylene dibromide, dibromochloropropane)
- Solvents (e.g., some glycol ethers [chemicals used in paint solvents], carbon disulfide)
- Volatile organic compounds (VOCs)
- Welding operations
- Xenoestrogens (a type of natural or human-made chemical that mimics the effects of the female sex hormone estrogen)

Data from Jensen TK, Bonde JP, Joffe M. The influence of occupational exposure on male reproductive function. *Occup Med.* 2006;56:544-553; Ten J, Mendiola J, Torres-Cantero AM, et al. Occupational and lifestyle exposures on male infertility: a mini review. *Open Reprod Sci J.* 2008; 1:16-21; Sheiner EK, Sheiner E, Hammel RD, et al. Effect of occupational exposures on male fertility: literature review. *Ind Health.* 2003;41:55-62.

Another potential effect of male (paternal) occupational exposures is adverse reproductive outcomes observed among exposed men's children.[56] TABLE 7.10 lists occupational exposures suspected of being related to impairment of male reproductive function.[98,101,102]

In conclusion, NIOSH states that "[a] number of workplace substances such as lead and radiation have been identified as reproductive hazards for men.... However, there is no complete list of reproductive hazards in the workplace. Scientists are just beginning to understand how these hazards affect the male reproductive system. Although more than 1,000 workplace chemicals have been shown to have reproductive effects on animals, most have not been studied in humans. In addition, most of the 4 million other chemical mixtures in commercial use remain untested."[103]

SUMMARY

Occupational illnesses, including workplace chronic diseases, account for a substantial burden of morbidity and mortality and have significant economic costs in the United States. Among the important occupationally associated illnesses are occupational cancer, dermatoses, lung diseases, and reproductive hazards. Exposures to a wide variety of substances and procedures found in the work setting are implicated in the etiology of these conditions. Examples of workplace exposures include toxic chemicals used in industrial processes, contact with heavy metals and metalloids, doses of ionizing radiation, and inhalation of dusts.

Four dust-related conditions (pneumoconioses) are asbestosis, silicosis, coal workers' pneumoconiosis, and byssinosis. Asbestosis and asbestos-related mesothelioma can result from exposures to asbestos in mining and production operations. Many occupations (e.g., construction, masonry, and sandblasting) produce high levels of silica dust, which are the cause of silicosis. Coal workers' pneumoconiosis stems from workers' unprotected exposure to high levels of coal dust.

Occupational cancers may include lung cancer, brain cancer, and bone cancer, among others. Because the skin is a large organ and one of the first points of contact with hazardous substances, contact dermatitis is one of the most common work-related dermatoses. Reproductive effects of occupational exposures have been hypothesized to include adverse birth outcomes and male infertility.

Employers, workers, policy makers, and stakeholders need to achieve greater awareness of the scope, significance, and economic impact of occupational illnesses to reduce their prevalence and prevent their occurrence.

STUDY QUESTIONS AND EXERCISES

1. Define the following terms:
   A. Occupational illnesses
   B. Work-aggravated asthma
   C. Occupational asthma
   D. Occupational dermatoses
   E. Adverse live-birth outcomes
2. Give three examples of illnesses and diseases associated with the occupational environment.
3. Which occupational exposures are believed to increase the risk of cancer? Give three examples of such exposures.
4. Describe at least four cancer diagnoses that have been linked to the work environment and, using your own ideas, discuss methods for their prevention.
5. Define the term *bone cancer* and describe work-related exposures associated with this condition.
6. How frequently do dermatoses occur in the work environment? What is the role of sensitizers in the occurrence of occupational dermatoses? Suggest methods for preventing skin diseases related to on-the-job exposures.
7. Give examples of adverse reproductive effects associated with occupational exposures. Include reproductive effects that occur (a) among men and (b) among women.
8. Describe the roles of occupational exposures in adverse respiratory health outcomes.
9. Define the term *crystalline silica*. How might workers be exposed to silica? How does silicosis develop? What are three potential health effects of exposure to silica? Are workers always aware of their exposure to silica?
10. Describe the major risk factors for occupationally associated lung cancer. Using your own ideas, discuss methods for the prevention of work-related lung cancer.

REFERENCES

1. International Labour Organization. *The prevention of occupational diseases*. Geneva, Switzerland: International Labour Organization; 2013.
2. Leigh JP. Economic burden of occupational injury and illness in the United States. *Milbank Q.* 2011;89(4):728–772.

3. Lax MB, Grant WD, Manetti FA, Klein R. Recognizing occupational disease: taking an effective occupational history. *Am Fam Physician*. 1998;58(4):935–944.

4. Markowitz G, Rosner D. "The street of walking death": silicosis, health, and labor in the Tri-State region, 1900–1950. *J Am Hist*. 1990;77(2):525–552.

5. Key MM, Henschel AF, Butler J, et al., eds. *Occupational diseases: a guide to their recognition*. Revised ed. Washington, DC: U.S. DHEW, CDC, NIOSH; 1977.

6. Centers for Disease Control and Prevention, National Institute for Occupational Safety and Health. Occupational health disparities. n.d. http://www.cdc.gov/niosh/programs/ohd/. Accessed March 4, 2014.

7. Healey BJ, Walker KT. *Introduction to occupational health in public health practice*. San Francisco, CA: Jossey-Bass; 2009.

8. American Lung Association. Occupational lung disease. In: *State of lung disease in diverse communities*. Washington, DC: American Lung Association; 2010:63–68.

9. Frew AJ. Advances in environmental and occupational disorders. *J Allergy Clin Immunol*. 2003;111:S824–S828.

10. Astarita C, Gargano D, Manguso F, et al. Epidemiology of allergic occupational diseases induced by *Tetranychus urticae* in greenhouse and open-field farmers living in a temperate climate area. *Allergy*. 2001;56(12):1157–1163.

11. Bonura E, Rom WN. Occupational lung diseases. In: Schraufnagel DE, ed. *Breathing in America: diseases, progress, and hope*. New York, NY: American Thoracic Society; 2010:131–144.

12. Speizer FE, Horton S, Batt J, Slutsky AS. Respiratory diseases of adults. In: Jamison DT, Breman JG, Measham AR, et al., eds. *Disease control priorities in developing countries*. 2nd ed. Washington, DC: World Bank; 2006:681–694.

13. Web MD. Obstructive and restrictive lung disease. n.d. http://www.webmd.com/lung/obstructive-and-restrictive-lung-disease. Accessed February 28, 2014.

14. American Lung Association. What are occupational lung diseases? n.d. http://www.lung.org/assets/documents/publications/lung-disease-data/ldd08-chapters/ldd-08-old.pdf. Accessed February 9, 2014.

15. Uuksulainen SO, Heikkilä PR, Olkinuora PS, Kiilunen M. Self-reported occupational health hazards and measured exposures to airborne impurities and noise in shoe repair work. *Int J Occup Environ Health*. 2002;8:320–327.

16. Hanna J, Hegeman R. Last victims of Kansas grain elevator blast found. *San Francisco Chronicle*. November 1, 2011. http://www.sfgate.com/nation/article/Last-victims-of-Kansas-grain-elevator-blast-found-2324654.php. Accessed August 16, 2013.

17. U.S. Department of Labor, Occupational Safety and Health Administration. Bartlett Grain in Atchison, Kan., cited for willful and serious violations by US Labor Department after 6 die, 2 injured in grain elevator explosion. n.d. https://www.osha.gov/pls/oshaweb/owadisp.show_document?p_table=NEWS_RELEASES&p_id=22161. Accessed August 16, 2013.

18. Magnier M. In India, toiling on the horns of a dilemma. *Los Angeles Times*. June 25, 2011:A7.

19. U.S. National Library of Medicine, National Institutes of Health, MedlinePlus. Hypersensitivity pneumonitis. n.d. http://www.nlm.nih.gov/medlineplus/ency/article/000109.htm. Accessed August 13, 2013.

20. Thefreedictionary.com. Sick building syndrome. n.d. http://www.thefreedictionary.com/sick+building+syndrome. Accessed March 7, 2014.

21. Centers for Disease Control and Prevention. Work-related asthma—38 states and District of Columbia, 2006–2009. *MMWR*. 2012;61(20):375–378.

22. Mapp CE, Boschetto P, Maestrelli P, Fabbri LM. Occupational asthma. *Am J Respir Crit Care Med.* 2005;172(3):280–305.

23. Goe SK, Henneberger PK, Reilly MJ, et al. A descriptive study of work aggravated asthma. *Occup Environ Med.* 2004;61:512–517.

24. Chan-Yeung M. Assessment of asthma in the workplace. *Chest.* 1995;108:1084–1117.

25. Lombardo LJ, Balmes JR. Occupational asthma: a review. *Environ Health Perspect.* 2000;108(4):697–704.

26. Kenyon NJ, Morrissey BM, Schivo M, Albertson TE. Occupational asthma. *Clinic Rev Allerg Immunol.* 2012;43:3–13.

27. Delclos GL, Gimeno D, Arif AA, et al. Occupational exposures and asthma in health-care workers: comparison of self-reports with a workplace-specific job exposure matrix. *Am J Epidemiol.* 2009;169:581–587.

28. David A. Pneumoconioses: definition. In: David A, Wagner GR, eds. Respiratory system. In: Stellman JM, ed. *Encyclopedia of occupational health and safety.* Geneva, Switzerland: International Labour Organization; 2011. http://www.ilo.org/oshenc /part-i/respiratory-system/item/415-pneumoconioses-definition?tmpl=componen t&print=1. Accessed February 27, 2014.

29. Agency for Toxic Substances and Disease Registry. ToxFAQs for asbestos. CAS#1332-21-4. September 2001; updated November 2004. http://www.atsdr .cdc.gov/toxfaqs/tf.asp?id=29&tid=4. Accessed February 26, 2014.

30. Selikoff IJ, Churg J, Hammond EC. Asbestos exposure and neoplasia. *JAMA.* 1964;188:22–26.

31. U.S. Environmental Protection Agency. Asbestos ban and phase-out *Federal Register* notices. n.d. http://www2.epa.gov/asbestos/asbestos-ban-and-phase-out-federal -register-notices. Accessed March 5, 2014.

32. U.S. Department of Labor, Mine Safety and Health Administration. Dust—what you can't see can hurt you! 1999. http://www.msha.gov/S&HINFO/blacklung/DUST99. PDF. Accessed March 3, 2014.

33. American Lung Association. Understanding pneumoconiosis. n.d. http://www.lung .org/lung-disease/pneumoconiosis/understanding-pneumoconiosis.html. Accessed February 26, 2014.

34. Laney AS, Petsonk EL, Hale JM, et al. Potential determinants of coal workers' pneumoconiosis, advanced pneumoconiosis, and progressive massive fibrosis among underground coal miners in the United States, 2005–2009. *Am J Public Health.* 2012;102(suppl 2):S279–S283.

35. Attfield MD, Kuempel ED. Mortality among U.S. underground coal miners: a 23-year follow-up. *Am J Ind Med.* 2008;51:231–245.

36. Centers for Disease Control and Prevention. Coal workers' pneumoconiosis-related years of potential life lost before age 65 years—United States, 1968–2006. *MMWR.* 2009;58(50):1412–1416.

37. U.S. Department of Labor, Occupational Safety and Health Administration (OSHA). OSHA factsheet: what is crystalline silica? n.d. https://www.osha.gov/OshDoc/data _General_Facts/crystalline-factsheet.pdf. Accessed February 27, 2014.

38. Centers for Disease Control and Prevention, National Institute for Occupational Safety and Health (NIOSH). *Silicosis: learn the facts!* Publication No. 2004-108. Cincinnati, OH: DHHS (NIOSH); 2004.

39. Nasrullah M, Mazurek JM, Wood JM, et al. Silicosis mortality with respiratory tuberculosis in the United States, 1968–2006. *Am J Epidemiol.* 2011;174(7):839–848.

40. Centers for Disease Control and Prevention, National Institute for Occupational Safety and Health. Preventing silicosis and deaths from sandblasting. n.d. http:// www.cdc.gov/niosh/docs/92-102/. Accessed October 15, 2013.

41. Bakke B, Stewart P, Eduard W. Determinants of dust exposure in tunnel construction work. *Appl Occup Environ Hyg.* 2002;17(11):783–796.

42. Schenker M. Exposures and health effects from inorganic agricultural dusts. *Environ Health Perspect.* 2000;108(suppl 4):661–664.

43. U.S. Department of Labor, Occupational Safety and Health Administration (OSHA). Silica exposure during hydraulic fracturing. OSHA 3622-12 2012. n.d. https://www.osha.gov/Publications/OSHA3622.pdf. Accessed March 3, 2014.

44. Chen W, Liu Y, Wang H, et al. Long-term exposure to silica dust and risk of total and cause-specific mortality in Chinese workers: a cohort study. *PLoS Med.* 2012;9(4):e1001206.

45. Su Y-M, Su J-R, Sheu J-Y, et al. Additive effect of smoking and cotton dust exposure on respiratory symptoms and pulmonary function of cotton textile workers. *Ind Health.* 2003;41:109–115.

46. Astrakianakis G, Seixas NS, Ray R, et al. Lung cancer risk among female textile workers exposed to endotoxin. *J Natl Cancer Inst.* 2007;99:357–364.

47. U.S. Department of Labor, Occupational Safety and Health Administration. Synthetic mineral fibers. n.d. https://www.osha.gov/SLTC/syntheticmineralfibers/. Accessed September 23, 2013.

48. American Lung Association. Fiberglass. n.d. http://www.lung.org/healthy-air/home/resources/fiberglass.html. Accessed September 23, 2013.

49. Abbate C, Giorgianni C, Brecciaroli R, et al. Changes induced by exposure of the human lung to glass fiber-reinforced plastic. *Environ Health Perspect.* 2006;114(11):1725–1729.

50. Ferreira AS, Moreira VB, Castro MCS, et al. Case report: analytical electron microscopy of lung granulomas associated with exposure to coating materials carried by glass wool fibers. *Environ Health Perspect.* 2010;118(2):249–252.

51. American Cancer Society. Occupation and cancer. n.d. http://www.cancer.org/acs/groups/content/@nho/documents/document/occupationandcancerpdf.pdf. Accessed February 24, 2014.

52. Centers for Disease Control and Prevention, National Institute for Occupational Safety and Health. Occupational cancer. n.d. http://www.cdc.gov/niosh/topics/cancer/. Accessed May 13, 2013.

53. Landrigan PJ. The prevention of occupational cancer. *CA Cancer J Clin.* 1996;46(2)67–69.

54. Boffetta P. Epidemiology of environmental and occupational cancer. *Oncogene.* 2004;23:6392–6403.

55. American Cancer Society. Known and probable human carcinogens. n.d. http://www.cancer.org/cancer/cancercauses/othercarcinogens/generalinformationabout-carcinogens/known-and-probable-human-carcinogens. Accessed March 2, 2014.

56. Savitz DA, Chen J. Parental occupation and childhood cancer: review of epidemiologic studies. *Environ Health Perspect.* 1990;(88):325–337.

57. JSI Center for Environmental Health Studies. Bone cancer and exposure to ionizing radiation. n.d. http://www.clarku.edu/mtafund/prodlib/jsi/Bone_Cancer_and_Exposure_to_Ionizing_Radiation.pdf. Accessed October 3, 2013.

58. Mayo Clinic. Bone cancer. n.d. http://www.mayoclinic.org/diseases-conditions/bone-cancer/basics/definition/con-20028192. Accessed February 28, 2014.

59. Goldberg MS, Labrèche F. Occupational risk factors for female breast cancer: a review. *Occup Environ Med.* 1996;53:145–156.

60. Oddone E, Edefonti V, Scaburri A, et al. Female breast cancer in Lombardy, Italy (2002–2009): a case-control study on occupational risks. *Am J Ind Med.* 2013;56(9):1051–1062.

61. Brophy JT, Keith MM, Watterson A, et al. Breast cancer risk in relation to occupations with exposure to carcinogens and endocrine disruptors: a Canadian case–control study. *Environ Health.* 2012;11:87.

62. World Health Organization. Environmental and occupational cancers. March 2011. http://www.who.int/mediacentre/factsheets/fs350/en/. Accessed March 2, 2014.

63. Straif K. The burden of occupational cancer. *Occup Environ Med.* 2008;65:787–788.

64. Consonni D, De Matteis S, Lubin JH, et al. Lung cancer and occupation in a population-based case-control study. *Am J Epidemiol.* 2010;171:323–333.

65. Field RW, Withers BL. Occupational and environmental causes of lung cancer. *Clin Chest Med.* 2012;33(4):681–703.

66. Coble JB, Dosemeci M, Stewart PA, et al. Occupational exposure to magnetic fields and the risk of brain tumors. *Neuro-Oncol.* 2009;11:242–249.

67. Zheng T, Cantor KP, Zhang Y, et al. Occupational risk factors for brain cancer: a population-based case-control study in Iowa. *J Occup Environ Med.* 2001;43(4):317–324.

68. El-Zein RA, Minn AY, Wrensch M, Bondy M. Epidemiology of brain tumors. In: Levin VA, ed. *Cancer in the nervous system.* New York, NY: Oxford University Press; 2002:252–266.

69. Villeneuve PJ, Agnew DA, Johnson KC, et al. Brain cancer and occupational exposure to magnetic fields among men: results from a Canadian population-based case-control study. *Int J Epidemiol.* 2002;31(1):210–217.

70. Samanic CM, De Roos AJ, Stewart PA, et al. Occupational exposure to pesticides and risk of adult brain tumors. *Am J Epidemiol.* 2008;167:976–985.

71. van Tongeren M, Kincl L, Richardson L, et al. Assessing occupational exposure to chemicals in an international epidemiological study of brain tumours. *Ann Occup Hyg.* 2013;57(5):610–626.

72. Kellen E, Zeegers M, Paulussen A, et al. Does occupational exposure to PAHs, diesel and aromatic amines interact with smoking and metabolic genetic polymorphisms to increase the risk on bladder cancer? The Belgian case control study on bladder cancer risk. *Cancer Lett.* 2007;245:51–60.

73. Kiriluk KJ, Prasad SM, Patel AR, et al. Bladder cancer risk from occupational and environmental exposures. *Urol Oncol.* 2012;30:199–211.

74. National Occupational Research Agenda Team. Priorities for development of research methods in occupational cancer. *Environ Health Perspect.* 2003;111(1):1–12.

75. De Craecker W, Roskams N, Op de Beeck R. *Occupational skin diseases and dermal exposure in the European Union (EU-25): policy and practice overview.* Brussels, Belgium: European Agency for Safety and Health at Work (EU-OSHA); 2008.

76. Centers for Disease Control and Prevention, National Institute for Occupational Safety and Health. Skin exposures and effects. n.d. http://www.cdc.gov/niosh/topics /skin/. Accessed August 16, 2013.

77. Peate WF. Occupational skin disease. *Am Fam Physician.* 2002;66(2):1025–1032.

78. Ling TC, Coulson IH. What do trainee hairdressers know about hand dermatitis? *Contact Dermatitis.* 2002;47(4):227–231.

79. Held E, Mygind K, Wolff C, et al. Prevention of work related skin problems: an intervention study in wet work employees. *Occup Environ Med.* 2002;59:556–561.

80. U.S. National Library of Medicine, MedlinePlus. Contact dermatitis. n.d. http:// www.nlm.nih.gov/medlineplus/ency/article/000869.htm. Accessed March 3, 2014.

81. Turjanmaa K, Alenius H, Reunala T, Palosuo T. Recent developments in latex allergy. *Curr Opin Allergy Clin Immunol.* 2002;2(5):407–412.

82. Elliott BA. Latex allergy: the perspective from the surgical suite. *J Allergy Clin Immunol.* 2002;110:S117–S120.

83. Chen Y-H, Lan J-L. Latex allergy and latex-fruit syndrome among medical workers in Taiwan. *J Formos Med Assoc.* 2002;101:622–626.

84. Gawkrodger DJ. Occupational skin cancers. *Occup Med.* 2004;54:458–463.

85. Suárez B, López-Abente G, Martínez C, et al. Occupation and skin cancer: the results of the HELIOS-I multicenter case-control study. *BMC Public Health.* 2007;7:180.

86. U.S. Department of Labor. Occupational Safety and Health Administration. n.d. Reproductive hazards. http://www.osha.gov/SLTC/reproductivehazards/. Accessed February 25, 2014.

87. Centers for Disease Control and Prevention, National Institute for Occupational Safety and Health. Women's safety and health issues at work. n.d. http://www.cdc.gov/niosh/docs/2001-123/pdfs/2001-123.pdf. Accessed February 25, 2014.

88. McElgunn B. Reproductive and developmental hazards in the workplace. *Clin Excell Nurse Pract.* 1998;2(3):140–145.

89. Centers for Disease Control and Prevention, National Institute for Occupational Safety and Health (NIOSH). *The effects of workplace hazards on female reproductive health.* DHHS (NIOSH) Publication No. 99-104. Cincinnati, OH: NIOSH; 1999.

90. Centers for Disease Control and Prevention, National Institute for Occupational Safety and Health. Controlling exposures to nitrous oxide during anesthetic administration. n.d. http://www.cdc.gov/niosh/docs/94-100/. Accessed June 23, 2014.

91. Hourani L, Hilton S. Occupational and environmental exposure correlates of adverse live-birth outcomes among 1032 US Navy women. *J Occup Environ Med.* 2000;42:1156–1165.

92. von Ehrenstein OS, Wilhelm M, Wang A, Ritz B. Preterm birth and prenatal maternal occupation: the role of Hispanic ethnicity and nativity in a population-based sample in Los Angeles, California. *Am J Public Health.* 2014;104(suppl 1):S65–S72.

93. Savitz DA, Whelan EA, Kleckner RC. Effects of parents' occupational exposures on risk of stillbirth, preterm delivery, and small-for-gestational-age infants. *Am J Epidemiol.* 1989;129(6):1201–1218.

94. Zeger SL. Invited commentary: Epidemiologic studies of the health associations of environmental exposures with preterm birth. *Am J Epidemiol.* 2012;175(2):108–110.

95. Wulff M, Högberg U, Stenlund H. Occupational and environmental risks of spontaneous abortions around a smelter. *Am J Ind Med.* 2002;41:131–138.

96. U.S. National Library of Medicine, MedlinePlus. Miscarriage. n.d. http://www.nlm.nih.gov/medlineplus/ency/article/001488.htm. Accessed March 6, 2014.

97. Mayo Clinic. Male infertility. n.d. http://www.mayoclinic.org/diseases-conditions/male-infertility/basics/definition/con-20033113. Accessed March 6, 2014.

98. Jensen TK, Bonde JP, Joffe M. The influence of occupational exposure on male reproductive function. *Occup Med.* 2006;56:544–553.

99. Cherry N, Labrèche F, Collins J, Tulandi T. Occupational exposure to solvents and male infertility. *Occup Environ Med.* 2001;58:635–640.

100. McDiarmid MA, Agnew J. Reproductive hazards and firefighters. *Occup Med.* 1995;10(4):829–841.

101. Ten J, Mendiola J, Torres-Cantero AM, et al. Occupational and lifestyle exposures on male infertility: a mini review. *Open Reprod Sci J.* 2008;1:16–21.

102. Sheiner EK, Sheiner E, Hammel RD, et al. Effect of occupational exposures on male fertility: literature review. *Ind Health.* 2003;41:55–62.

103. Centers for Disease Control and Prevention, National Institute for Occupational Safety and Health. The effects of workplace hazards on male reproductive health. n.d. http://www.cdc.gov/niosh/docs/96-132/. Accessed February 24, 2014.

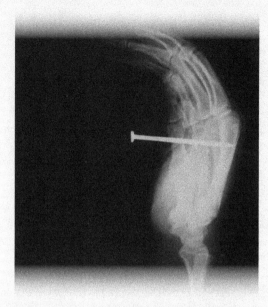

FIGURE 8.1   Nail from nail gun embedded in hand

One U.S. worker dies every 2 hours from a work-related injury.

—U.S. Department of Labor

Occupational injuries are important causes of morbidity and mortality for workers. Construction injuries are among the five leading causes of occupational mortality in the United States. **FIGURE 8.1** shows a nail gun injury.

CHAPTER 8

Work-Related Injuries and Fatalities

Learning Objectives

By the end of this chapter, you will be able to:

- Describe the personal, economic, and societal impacts of work-related injuries.
- Define terms used in occupational injury research.
- State risk factors for common occupational injuries and deaths.
- Compare and contrast four occupations with high risks for occupational injuries.
- Describe approaches to injury prevention.

Chapter Outline

- Introduction
- Terms Used in Occupational Injury Research
- Descriptive Epidemiology of Occupational Injuries
- Types of Occupational Injuries
- Occupations with High Risks for Injuries
- Workplace Violence
- Public Health and Epidemiologic Approaches to Injury Prevention
- Summary
- Study Questions and Exercises

Introduction

Occupational injuries are among the leading causes of work-related morbidity and mortality in the United States. The Bureau of Labor Statistics (BLS) estimates that work-related injuries accounted for 4690 deaths in the United States in 2010, the equivalent of 1 employee succumbing every 2 hours from this cause.[1] A similar number of deaths (4693) were reported in 2011. Workers' Memorial Day, held annually on April 28, commemorates the lives of workers killed from work-related causes; see **EXHIBIT 8.1** for more information.

In addition to their fatal consequences, work-related injuries are costly with respect to their societal and economic impacts. According to the U.S. Department of Labor (U.S. DOL), "Each year occupational injuries and illnesses cause employers, workers, and society to pay tremendous costs for workers' compensation and other insurance, medical expenses, lost wages and productivity, and the personal and societal costs associated with day to day living for injured and ill workers. In 2009, employers spent $74 billion on workers' compensation insurance alone."[2]

The Bureau of Labor Statistics, a unit of the U.S. DOL, is a federal agency that collects information on occupational injuries. Such data reveal epidemiologic characteristics of workplace injuries and occupations that have particularly high rates of morbidity and mortality from injuries. Among the more frequent types of injuries are musculoskeletal disorders, which incur high healthcare and other economic costs and can result in long-term disability. Another topic of concern for injury researchers is workplace violence, which in recent decades has become an increasingly

---

EXHIBIT 8.1   Workers' Memorial Day

Workers' Memorial Day recognizes workers who died or suffered from exposures to hazards at work. In 2011, a total of … [4693] U.S. workers died from work-related injuries…. Most fatalities from work-related illness are not captured by national surveillance systems, but an estimate for 2007 was 53,455 deaths…. Several national surveillance systems report new cases of nonfatal work-related injuries and illnesses, although no system captures all cases. In 2011, nearly 3 million injuries and illnesses to private industry workers and 821,000 to state and local government workers were reported by employers…. In the same year, an estimated 2.9 million work-related injuries were treated in emergency departments, resulting in 150,000 hospitalizations.

Reprinted from Centers for Disease Control and Prevention. Workers' Memorial Day—April 28, 2013. *MMWR*. 2013;62(16):301.

prominent contributor to injuries and fatalities. Through intervention programs, much can be done to reduce the frequency of all varieties of occupational injuries, which are largely preventable.

Many work settings are associated with specific injury hazards. Some examples discussed here are the fields of construction, fishing, mining, and transportation-related occupations. Less well known is the fact that reality TV crews face injury hazards, as described in **EXHIBIT 8.2**.

Terms Used in Occupational Injury Research

This section introduces some of the important terminology that researchers use to describe occupational injuries. One of the specialized fields that helps to identify the determinants of work-related injuries and leads to reduction of the incidence of such injuries is occupational injury epidemiology. To develop a complete picture of the scope of the problem, investigators require excellent data sources. At present, the full extent of job-associated injuries remains unknown, as many injuries go unreported.

How Occupational Injuries Are Defined

An occupational injury or work-related injury is "[a]ny damage inflicted to the body by energy transfer during work with a short duration between exposure and the health event (usually < 48 hrs)."[3(p. 110)] Occupational injuries include amputations, falls, musculoskeletal disorders, cumulative trauma disorders, repetitive motion disorders, and injuries caused by workplace violence. These kinds of occupational injuries are classified as either fatal or nonfatal. Many serious nonfatal injuries require that injured personnel take time off from work for recovery; hence they are referred to as injuries with days away from work.

Occupational injuries are categorized as being either unintentional or intentional. Unintentional injuries are those that occur when there is no deliberate intention for self-harm or harming other people.[4] Examples of unintentional injuries include falls, burns, animal bites, unintentional poisonings, and vehicle crashes. Intentional injuries are those that are caused willfully (on purpose). Causes of intentional injuries include workplace violence and assaults, deliberate ingestion of poisons, discharge of firearms, and suffocation. Associated injuries are homicides and suicides. Episodes of workplace violence command the attention of the media and are a noteworthy cause of death and injuries to workers.

Traumatic occupational injuries are those caused by traumatic events in the workplace. Trauma is defined as "an injury or wound to a living body caused by the application of external force or violence. Acute trauma can occur with the sudden, one-time application of force or violence that causes immediate damage to a living body."[5] These injuries often result in visits to emergency departments for treatment, as well as disability and death, and are very costly for employers, workers, and society.[2]

Epidemiology and Occupational Injuries

Occupational injury epidemiology is a field of research that seeks "to describe the distribution and determinants of occupational injuries and to make and test inferences about their prevention."[3(p. 106)] Later we will learn that such injuries are preventable. Hence, it is not appropriate to refer to them as accidents, which implies they are unpredictable. One of the essential prerequisites for conducting epidemiologic research is a source of high-quality data on work-related injuries. Unfortunately, epidemiologic data are often lacking because occupational injuries tend to be underreported.

Data Sources

Data sources for information on occupational injuries encompass statistical information systems for both fatal injuries and nonfatal injuries. This discussion focuses on initiatives organized by the U.S. Department of Labor. Two of the major systems for recording data on work-related fatalities and injuries are the Census of Fatal Occupational Injuries (CFOI) and the Survey of Occupational Injuries and Illnesses (SOII), both of which are conducted by the U.S. Bureau of Labor Statistics. **EXHIBIT 8.3** describes both programs.

EXHIBIT 8.3   Data Systems for Information on Occupational Injuries

The Bureau of Labor Statistics reports the number and frequency of work-related fatal injuries and nonfatal injuries and illnesses each year. The BLS also provides detailed information on the circumstances of the injuries and illnesses and on the characteristics of the affected worker. These data come from two programs: the Census of Fatal Occupational Injuries (CFOI) and the Survey of Occupational Injuries and Illnesses (SOII).

The CFOI, administered by the BLS in conjunction with the 50 states, the District of Columbia, and New York City, compiles detailed information on all work-related fatal injuries occurring in the United States. In an effort to compile counts that are as complete as possible, the CFOI uses diverse sources to identify, verify, and profile fatal work injuries. Source documents such as death certificates, news accounts, workers' compensation reports, and federal and state agency administrative records are cross-referenced to gather key information about each workplace fatality.

The SOII produces data on work-related nonfatal injuries and illnesses. These data identify the industrial, occupational, and worker groups having a relatively high risk of work-related injuries and illnesses. This survey is made possible through the cooperation of participating state agencies and nearly 200,000 business establishments that provide information on workplace injuries and illnesses to the BLS. State agencies collect and verify most of the data provided. BLS field offices collect and verify data from nonparticipating states.

Reprinted from U.S. Department of Labor, Bureau of Labor Statistics. Fatal occupational injuries and nonfatal occupational injuries and illnesses, 2008. http://www.bls.gov/iif/oshwc/osh/os/oshs2008.pdf. Accessed March 10, 2014.

Underreporting of Occupational Injuries

As noted, an unfortunate phenomenon is the failure to report many of the work-related injuries that occur in the United States:

> [E]xtensive evidence from academic studies, media reports and worker testimony shows that work-related injuries and illnesses in the United States are chronically and even grossly underreported. As much as 69 percent of injuries and illnesses may never make it into the Survey of Occupational Injuries and Illnesses (SOII), the nation's annual workplace safety and health "report card" generated by the Bureau of Labor Statistics (BLS). If these estimates are accurate, the nation's workers may be suffering three times as many injuries and illnesses as official reports indicate."[6(p. 2)]

Descriptive Epidemiology of Occupational Injuries

Although rates of fatal occupational injuries have stabilized in recent years, they remain at unacceptable levels. Consequently, occupational fatalities continue to be a pressing concern for officials from business and manufacturing, government, and unions. Also concerning is the fact that more

than 1 million workers sustained nonfatal injuries that necessitated taking time off from their jobs. The actual total is likely to be much higher,
as these data cover only the reported events.

Occupational injuries vary in systematic patterns according to the
descriptive epidemiologic variables of person, time, and place. Person variables related to injuries include demographic classifications such as age, gender, and race/ethnicity. Place variables include region and state of the United
States. The variable of time includes annual trends in the incidence of occupational injuries. One of the major determinants of occupational injuries is
the influence of health disparities. For example, fatal work-related injuries
are thought to reflect health disparities with respect to their recurrence.[7]

Fatal Injuries in the Work Environment

Using data from the Census of Fatal Occupational Injuries, the Bureau of
Labor Statistics indicated that in 2011 a total of 4693 fatal occupational
injuries were reported in the United States. This total corresponded to a
rate of 3.5 fatal work injuries per 100,000 full-time equivalent (FTE) workers.[8] Between 2006 and 2009, the fatality rate declined from 4.2 deaths
per 100,000 FTE workers to 3.5 deaths per 100,000 FTW workers. After
2009, the rate stabilized at approximately this level until 2011.

FIGURE 8.2 shows the numbers of fatal occupational injuries by major
event. The category "transportation incidents" is associated with the largest

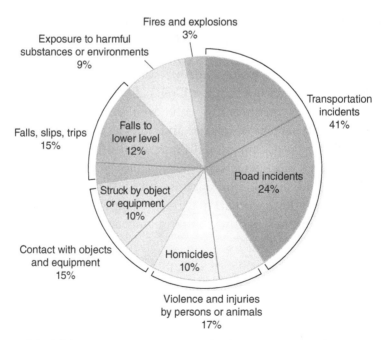

FIGURE 8.2   Fatal occupational injuries by major event, 2011

Courtesy of the U.S. Department of Labor, Bureau of Labor Statistics, Fatal occupational injuries in
2011. http://www.bls.gov/iif/oshwc/cfoi/cfch0010.pdf. Accessed March 20, 2014.

percentage (41%) of fatal injuries. Other major causes of fatalities include violence and injuries by persons or animals, contact with objects and equipment, and the category of falls, slips, and trips.

Nonfatal Injuries

Work-related injuries are common among the U.S. labor force.[9] In 2013, reports from employers demonstrated that nonfatal occupational injuries and illnesses affected about 3 million U.S. workers in private industry and 746,000 workers in state and local governments.[10] (Note that these totals includes both injuries and illnesses.) These numbers included both injuries that required time off from work and those that did not require time off from work. The rate of nonfatal injuries and illnesses in 2013 was 3.3 events per 100 full-time workers in private industry.[10] Full-time employment was defined as working for at least 2000 hours per year.

In 2013, a total of 1,162,210 cases (109.4 per 10,000 full-time workers) in all types of business ownerships—private industry, state government, and local government—were required to take time off from work as a result of injuries sustained.[11] The injury rates were higher in state government and local government than in private industry (**FIGURE 8.3**).[12]

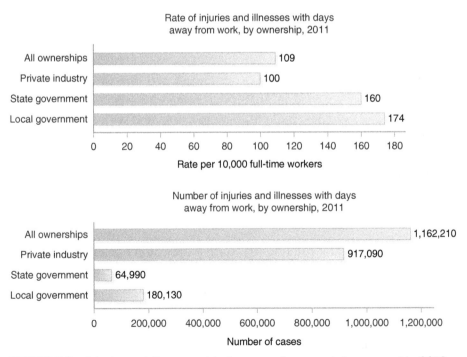

FIGURE 8.3 Injuries and illnesses with days away from work, by ownership, 2013 (Upper panel—rate; lower panel—number)

Reproduced from U.S. Department of Labor. Bureau of Labor Statistics (BLS). 2013 nonfatal occupational injuries and illnesses: cases with days away from work. http://www.bls.gov/iif/oshwc/osh/case/osch0053.pdf. Accessed January 29, 2015.

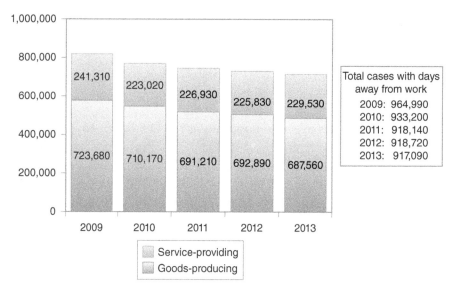

FIGURE 8.4 Number of injuries and illnesses with days away from work, private industry, 2009-2013

Reproduced from U.S. Department of Labor. Bureau of Labor Statistics (BLS). 2013 nonfatal occupational injuries and illnesses: cases with days away from work. http://www.bls.gov/iif/oshwc/osh/case/osch0053.pdf. Accessed January 29, 2015.

Between 2007 and 2011, the total number of injuries in private industry (goods-producing and service-providing industries combined) has shown a declining trend, decreasing from 1,158,870 in 2007 to 908,310 in 2011 (**FIGURE 8.4**).

The relative frequency of types of injuries and illnesses that required time off from work varied in 2013. Two categories—(1) sprains, strains, and tears and (2) soreness and pain—were associated with half of all such injuries and illnesses.[12] Other common types of injuries and illnesses were the categories of bruises and contusions; cuts, lacerations, and punctures; and fractures (**FIGURE 8.5**).

State Variation

FIGURE 8.6 reports the preliminary state-wide counts of fatal work injuries in the United States in 2012. The shading indicates states where the number of fatalities increased or decreased or did not change in comparison with the previous year.[13] According to the BLS, "Sixteen states and the District of Columbia had preliminary counts showing more fatal injuries in 2012 than in 2011. Thirty-two states had fewer fatal workplace injuries in 2012 compared to 2011. Two states saw no change between the two years."[13] The most populous states for which data are available

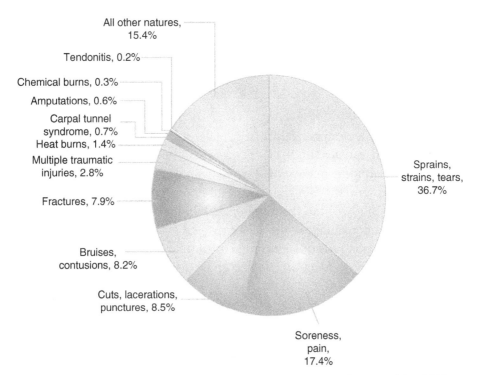

FIGURE 8.5   Distribution of injuries and illnesses by nature, all ownerships, 2013

Reproduced from U.S. Department of Labor. Bureau of Labor Statistics (BLS). 2013 nonfatal occupational injuries and illnesses: cases with days away from work. http://www.bls.gov/iif/oshwc/osh/case/osch0053.pdf. Accessed January 29, 2015..

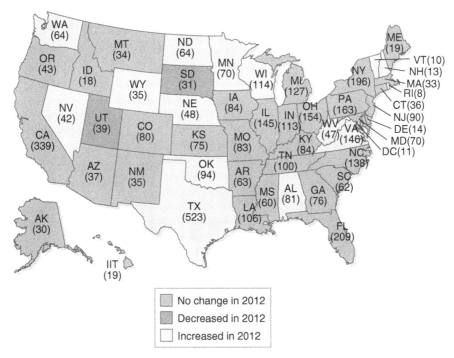

FIGURE 8.6   Number of fatal work injuries, by state, 2012

Reproduced from U.S. Department of Labor, Bureau of Labor Statistics. Fatal occupational injuries in 2011, http://www.bls .gov/iif/oshwc/cfoi/cfch0011.pdf. Accessed March 20, 2014.

tended to have the highest numbers of fatal work injuries. Given the available data from the BLS, it is not possible to compare states with respect to incidence of fatal injuries.

Gender

Both gender and race/ethnicity are associated with the distribution of occupational injuries. In 2011, the proportion of fatal work injuries was much higher among male workers than among female workers (92% versus 8%), despite the fact that the number of hours that men worked was only slightly higher than the number that women worked (**FIGURE 8.7**). In 2011, a higher percentage of men than women died from contact with objects and equipment and exposures to harmful substances or environments, whereas a higher percentage of women than men died in roadway incidents and homicides (**FIGURE 8.8**).

Race/Ethnicity

Researchers have observed racial and ethnic disparities in the occurrence of work-related fatalities. For example, from 2006 through 2008, Hispanic workers had the highest rate of fatal occupational injuries among all workers (irrespective of race and ethnicity).[14] During that time period, the mortality rate among Hispanics was 4.8 deaths per 100,000 FTE workers in comparison with 4.0 deaths per 100,000 among all workers. When Hispanic workers were compared based on foreign-born versus native-born status, their respective mortality rates were 5.7 and 3.6, indicating

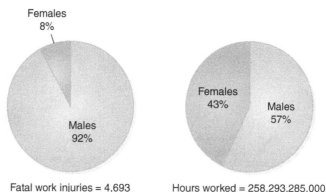

Fatal work injuries = 4,693   Hours worked = 258,293,285,000

FIGURE 8.7   Fatal work injuries and hours worked by gender of worker, 2011

Courtesy of the U.S. Department of Labor, Bureau of Labor Statistics, Fatal occupational injuries in 2011, http://www.bls.gov/iif/oshwc/cfoi/cfch0010.pdf. Accessed March 20, 2014.

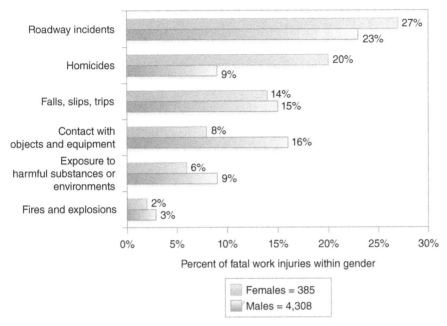

FIGURE 8.8   Distribution of fatal injury events, by gender of worker, 2011

Courtesy of the U.S. Department of Labor, Bureau of Labor Statistics, Fatal occupational injuries in 2011, http://www.bls.gov/iif/oshwc/cfoi/cfch0010.pdf. Accessed March 20, 2014.

that the work-related death rate among foreign-born Hispanics exceeded the rate for all workers combined; the rate for native-born Hispanics was lower than the rate for all workers combined.

Comparing 2011 data with preliminary 2012 data, one notes that non-Hispanic African American workers and non-Hispanic Asian workers had increasing rates of fatal work injuries in comparison with workers from other racial and ethnic groups.[15] However, the preliminary fatal injury rate in 2012 for Asian workers (1.8 deaths per 100,000 workers) was the lowest of all workers, who collectively had a rate of 3.2 work-related deaths per 100,000.

Disparities in Injuries

Disparities in occupational injuries seem to be dynamic, showing changes over time.[16] For 2005 through 2009, Hispanic workers had the highest rate of fatal injuries in comparison with persons from other ethnic and racial groups.[7] Foreign-born workers had higher mortality rates than persons born in the United States. In comparison with non-Hispanic white workers, non-Hispanic black individuals and workers from the racial/ethnic category of American Indian/Alaska Native/Asian/Pacific Islander

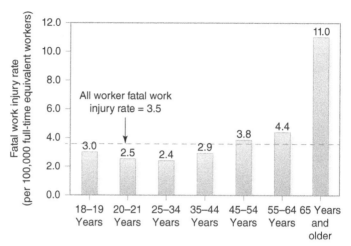

FIGURE 8.9 Fatal work injury rates by age group, 2011

Reproduced from U.S. Department of Labor, Bureau of Labor Statistics. Fatal occupational injuries in 2011, http://www.bls.gov/iif/oshwc/cfoi/cfch0010.pdf. Accessed March 20, 2014.

(AI/AN/A/PI) experienced work-related homicide deaths that were three times as high as the rates of their peers. In summary, programs for preventing health disparities should give increased attention to the needs of Hispanic and foreign-born workers and should conduct additional research into work-related homicides.

Age

FIGURE 8.9 shows the distribution of U.S. fatal work injuries according to age group in 2011. The overall fatal injury rate was 3.5 injuries per 100,000 FTE workers. Beginning at age 45, fatal injury rates for older workers exceeded the rate for all age groups. As age increased, the rate of fatal injuries increased. The highest rate occurred among the oldest age group (65 years and older); the rate in this group exceeded the rate for all workers by more than three times.

Older Workers

The U.S. workforce of the United States is aging, with the oldest age group of workers also being the fastest-growing group.[17] According to the CDC, older workers are defined as persons who are 55 years of age or older; they account for 19% of the nation's workers. With the exception of fatal injuries, the rates for all injuries and illnesses combined for older workers tend to be similar to or lower than the rates for younger workers. However, the length of absences and number of work-related illnesses due to injuries increase with age. In comparison with younger workers, older workers experience higher rates of falls, fractures, and hip injuries. Based on these data, the CDC concludes, "Public health and research agencies should conduct research to better understand the overall burden of occupational injuries and illnesses on older workers, aging-associated risks, and effective prevention strategies. Employers and others should take steps to address specific risks for older workers such as falls (e.g., by ensuring floor surfaces are clean, dry, well-lit, and free from tripping hazards)."[17](p. 503)

Younger Workers

Young workers (persons younger than 24 years of age) totaled 17.5 million individuals and accounted for 13% of the U.S. workforce in 2010.[18] In 2009, young workers experienced 359 fatal injuries, 27 of which occurred among persons who were younger than 18 years. The youngest members of this group are still developing and may not have attained their full adult strength levels as well as mature cognitive abilities. Consequently, they are vulnerable to injury hazards as a result of their inadequate physical and mental development and the situations that prevail in environments in which young workers often are employed. For example, hazards in these settings may include slippery floors and dangerous equipment in restaurants. Greater attention needs to be devoted to creating a safe work environment for young workers, providing adequate training, and tasking them with age-appropriate work assignments.

Types of Occupational Injuries

This review of occupational injuries concentrates on two categories of injuries that make a large contribution to worker morbidity: fall-related injuries and musculoskeletal disorders, which includes several related conditions.

Fall Injuries

Fall injuries affect workers in a broad cross-section of occupations. The economic costs of work-related falls in the United States total approximately $70 billion each year.[19] In 2009, the largest number of fatalities from falling occurred in the construction industry. The fields with the highest frequency of fall-related injuries were health services, wholesale industries, and retail industries. High-risk fields for falling are the following:

- Construction
- Healthcare support
- Transportation

- Moving of materials
- Cleaning and maintenance of buildings

Falls on the job can occur when there are slippery surfaces, cluttered walking areas, holes and openings in floor and walls, defective ladders, and building construction sites without protective barriers. **FIGURE 8.10** suggests methods for protecting construction workers against falls from rooftops. Use of safety harnesses can save a worker from a fall when other protections fail.[20]

Musculoskeletal Disorders

"Musculoskeletal disorders (MSDs) are injuries or disorders of the muscles, nerves, tendons, joints, cartilage, an[d] disorders of the nerves, tendons, muscles and supporting structures of the upper and lower limbs, neck, and lower back that are caused, precipitated or exacerbated by sudden exertion or prolonged exposure to physical factors such as repetition, force, vibration, or awkward posture."[21] Work-related musculoskeletal disorders (WRMSDs) are MSDs induced or made worse by occupational factors.[22(p. v)] They include upper limb disorders, conditions that affect the back, repetitive

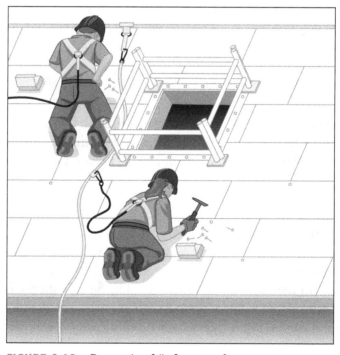

FIGURE 8.10 Preventing falls from rooftops

Reproduced from U.S. Department of Labor, Occupational Safety and Health Administration (OSHA), Fall prevention fact sheet, https://www.osha.gov/stopfalls/factsheet .html. Accessed March 20, 2014.

motion disorders, rotator cuff tendinitis, and carpal tunnel syndrome. For a MSD to be considered a WRMSD, it needs to meet the following criteria[23]:

- The MSD was caused substantially by an occupational environment or performance of work-related tasks. An example is a task that creates an ergonomic hazard.
- The MSD (i.e., an existing MSD) was exacerbated or made to last for a longer time as a result of working conditions.

In 2013, the rate of work-related MSDs requiring days away from work in private industry was 34 events per 10,000 full-time workers (**FIGURE 8.11**). The rates for state government workers and local government workers were substantially higher. The most common musculoskeletal disorder in 2008 was the category "sprains, strains, tears," which were responsible for approximately three-fourths of such disorders (**FIGURE 8.12**). The next most frequent category, accounting for almost 8% of MSDs, was "soreness, pain, hurt, except the back."

WRMSDs have very substantial economic, medical, and social impacts.[23] Some estimates place the economic costs of these conditions at $45 billion to $54 billion annually. They are believed to be responsible for 70 million annual physician office visits and a total of 130 million encounters with healthcare facilities such as hospitals and emergency rooms. Other impacts relate to loss of work time and worker disability, both temporary and permanent.

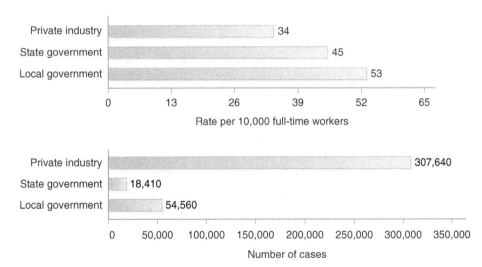

FIGURE 8.11   Musculoskeletal disorders with days away from work, by ownership, 2013 (Upper panel—rate; lower panel—number)

Reproduced from U.S. Department of Labor. Bureau of Labor Statistics (BLS). 2013 nonfatal occupational injuries and illnesses: cases with days away from work. http://www.bls.gov/iif/oshwc/osh/case/osch0053.pdf. Accessed January 29, 2015..

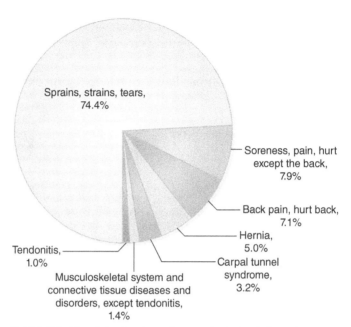

FIGURE 8.12   Distribution of musculoskeletal disorders by nature of injury or illness, 2008

Reproduced from U.S. Department of Labor, Bureau of Labor Statistics, Fatal occupational injuries and nonfatal occupational injuries and illnesses, 2008, May 2011. Report 1028. BLS; 2011.

Data for 2008 indicate that four occupations were linked with the highest frequency of days away from work from musculoskeletal disorders (**FIGURE 8.13**):

- Nursing aides, orderlies, and attendants
- Emergency medical technicians and paramedics
- Reservation and transportation ticket agents and travel clerks
- Laborers and freight, stock, and material movers

Evidence from epidemiologic research has identified associations between musculoskeletal disorders and particular types of work-related physical factors, such as hoisting, moving, dragging, carrying, and rotating burdensome objects, particularly when these activities occur in combination with uncomfortable postures.[24] The four occupations mentioned previously all share the propensity for workers to engage in such activities.

Cumulative trauma disorders (CTDs) are "chronic disorders involving connective tissue (muscles, tendons) and nerve, often resulting from work-related physical activities."[25] Synonyms for CTDs are repetitive strain injuries, repetitive motion disorders, overuse syndrome, and work-related musculoskeletal disorders.[26] However, the term CTD generally refers to disorders

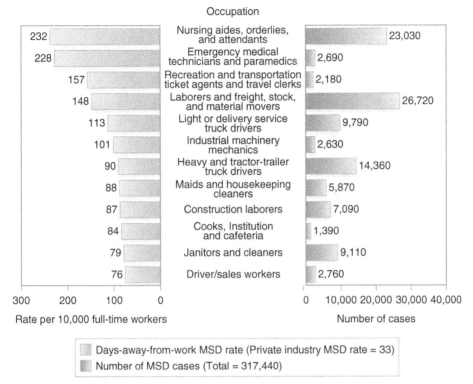

FIGURE 8.13   Incidence rate and number of musculoskeletal disorders, selected occupations, 2008

Reproduced from U.S. Department of Labor, Bureau of Labor Statistics, Fatal occupational injuries and nonfatal occupational injuries and illnesses, 2008. May 2011. BLS; Report 1028.

of the upper extremities—for example, the hands, neck, and shoulders.[22] Among the factors related to occurrence of CTDs at work are work tasks that require increased repetition, speed, and force. Management practices such as total quality management, self-directed work teams, and just-in-time inventory systems are believed to be related to the occurrence of cumulative trauma disorders.[27] A noteworthy example of a CTD is carpal tunnel syndrome, which is covered later in the chapter.

Work-Related Neck and Upper Limb Disorders

According to the European Agency for Safety and Health at Work (EU-OSHA), "Work-related neck and upper limb disorders are impairments of bodily structures such as muscles, joints, tendons, ligaments, nerves, bones and the localised blood circulation system."[28] This category of disorders results from (or is aggravated by) exposures that occur in the work environment. For example, risk factors for work-related neck and upper limb disorders include workers' exposure to repetitive hand and arm movements and vibrating tools.[28]

Repetitive Motion Disorders

"Repetitive motion disorders (RMDs) are a family of muscular conditions that result from repeated motions performed in the course of normal work or daily activities. RMDs include carpal tunnel syndrome, bursitis, tendonitis, epicondylitis, ganglion cyst, tenosynovitis, and trigger finger. RMDs are caused by too many uninterrupted repetitions of an activity or motion, unnatural or awkward motions such as twisting the arm or wrist, overexertion, incorrect posture, or muscle fatigue."[29]

Rotator Cuff Tendinitis

Problems with shoulders are a significant health issue for many groups of workers. One of the areas of the shoulder vulnerable to injury is the rotator cuff, a set of muscles and tendons that are attached to the bones of the shoulder joint (**FIGURE 8.14**). "Rotator cuff tendinitis refers to irritation of these tendons and inflammation of the bursa (a normally smooth layer) lining these tendons."[30] Risk factors for shoulder problems such as rotator cuff disorders include repetitive movements, heavy exertion, the need to maintain awkward positions, and high psychosocial job demands.[31]

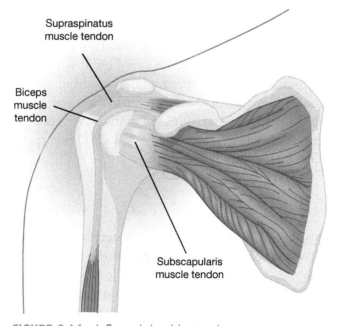

Supraspinatus muscle tendon

Biceps muscle tendon

Subscapularis muscle tendon

FIGURE 8.14 Inflamed shoulder tendons

Carpal Tunnel Syndrome

"Carpal tunnel syndrome occurs when the median nerve, which runs from the forearm into the palm of the hand, becomes pressed or squeezed at the wrist."[32] Workers with carpal tunnel syndrome develop symptoms that include burning, tingling, or itching of the palm of the hand. They may also experience pain, numbness, and weakness in the hand.

At present, researchers have not definitively proved a causative role for repetitive and forceful hand and wrist movements at work in development of carpal tunnel syndrome. However, risk of carpal tunnel syndrome is elevated among persons involved with assembly line work. This type of injury can be prevented by having workers wear splints that keep their wrists straight and encouraging them to maintain an erect, natural posture. Computer workstations can be designed so that computer monitors are positioned at eye level and wrists and hands are kept in line with the elbows.[33]

Low Back Pain, Back Injuries, and Hurt Back

Low back pain (LBP) is a very significant form of morbidity and is responsible for substantial lost work time. As many as 85% of workers globally experience LBP during their careers. Of this group, 10% will develop chronic back issues. Thus, LBP is one of the major occupationally associated causes of pain and impairment in developed countries.[34]

According to the Occupational Safety and Health Administration (OSHA), "Back disorders are one of the leading causes of disability for people [in the United States] in their working years and afflict over 600,000 employees each year with a cost of about $50 billion annually in 1991."[35] More than 38% of the U.S. general population experienced pain in the lower back in 2011, according to the National Health Interview Survey.[36] Work-related back problems (the BLS category of "back pain and hurt back") accounted for more than 7% of employment-associated musculoskeletal disorders in 2008 (Figure 8.12). The BLS includes back injuries within the global category of sprains, strains, and tears. According to this federal agency, "In 2010, sprains, strains, and tears accounted for 40 percent of total injury and illness cases requiring days away from work in all ownerships [incidence rate = 47 cases per 10,000 full-time workers]...In 36 percent of the sprain, strain, and tear cases, the back was injured,...Although the back is the most frequently injured part of the body in sprain, strain, and tear cases, the number of such cases has fallen faster over time than for most other parts of the body"[37]

Two occupations with especially high risks of back issues are construction work, particularly for male construction laborers, and health care, most significantly among female nursing aides.[38] Persons employed as carpenters, mechanics, hairdressers, truck drivers, maids, and janitors also are at high risk for back pain. Risk behaviors for back injuries include lifting heavy objects, especially on a repetitive basis, and not maintaining a good posture (e.g., sitting for long periods and slouching). Also prone to back problems are smokers who are overweight and under stress.[39] Additional factors for such injuries include poor body mechanics while lifting (e.g., lifting from an awkward position and lifting over barriers), working on slippery floors, and inadequacies in design of work procedures that involve lifting.

Occupations with High Risks for Injuries

FIGURE 8.15 compares the number and frequency of fatal occupational injuries in the United States according to industry sector for 2011. The category

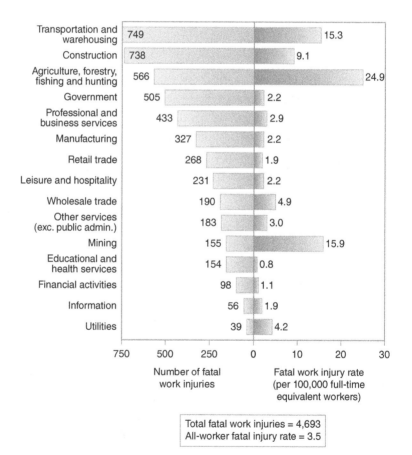

FIGURE 8.15   Number and rate of fatal occupational injuries, by industry sector, 2011

Reproduced from U.S. Department of Labor, Bureau of Labor Statistics, Fatal occupational injuries in 2011, http://www.bls.gov/iif/oshwc/cfoi/cfch0010.pdf. Accessed March 20, 2014.

of transportation and warehousing had the highest number of fatal injuries (749; rate = 15.3 deaths per 100,000 FTE workers), followed closely by construction (738; rate = 9.1 per 100,000). The highest rate of fatal injuries (24.9 per 100,000) was associated with the category of agriculture, forestry, fishing, and hunting. Rounding out the top five occupations with the highest rate of fatal injuries was mining (15.9 per 100,000).

The statistics for nonfatal injuries for 2008 indicated that transportation and warehousing was the private-industry sector with the highest incidence rate of occupational injuries (5.7 injuries per 100 workers; FIGURE 8.16). Healthcare and social assistance and the category of agriculture, forestry, fishing, and hunting had the second and third highest

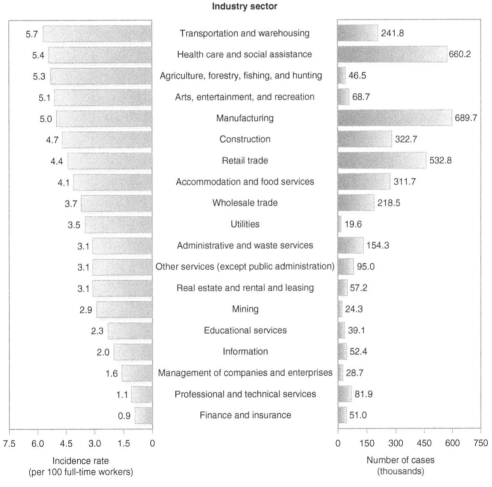

Industry sector

Incidence rate (per 100 full-time workers)	Industry sector	Number of cases (thousands)
5.7	Transportation and warehousing	241.8
5.4	Health care and social assistance	660.2
5.3	Agriculture, forestry, fishing, and hunting	46.5
5.1	Arts, entertainment, and recreation	68.7
5.0	Manufacturing	689.7
4.7	Construction	322.7
4.4	Retail trade	532.8
4.1	Accommodation and food services	311.7
3.7	Wholesale trade	218.5
3.5	Utilities	19.6
3.1	Administrative and waste services	154.3
3.1	Other services (except public administration)	95.0
3.1	Real estate and rental and leasing	57.2
2.9	Mining	24.3
2.3	Educational services	39.1
2.0	Information	52.4
1.6	Management of companies and enterprises	28.7
1.1	Professional and technical services	81.9
0.9	Finance and insurance	51.0

FIGURE 8.16   Incidence rate and number of nonfatal occupational injuries and illnesses by private industry sector, 2008

Reproduced from U.S. Department of Labor, Bureau of Labor Statistics, Fatal occupational injuries and nonfatal occupational injuries and illnesses, 2008. BLS; May 2011, Report 1028.

> **EXHIBIT 8.4   Cerebral Concussions among Participants in Collision Sports**
>
> Collision sports include soccer and American football. An investigation of more than 2500 retired football players reported that more than 60% had experienced at least one concussion during their careers; almost one-fourth had sustained three or more concussions. The researchers linked recurrent concussions with mild cognitive impairment and significant memory impairments. However, concussions were unrelated to Alzheimer's disease.[40]
>
> In 2009, the National Football League (NFL) acknowledged the long-term adverse neurologic consequences of concussions among players, with one of the associated disorders being termed chronic traumatic encephalopathy. In recognition of the potential harm from concussions, the NFL changed its policies regarding management of concussions. The NFL now requires players with signs of concussions to discontinue participation in practice or a game until they have been cleared by brain-injury specialists.[41]

incidence rates with 5.4 and 5.3 per 100, respectively. Together, these three sectors accounted for almost half of all cases of occupational injuries reported by private industry. Another hazardous occupational category is professional sports, which can subject athletes to high risks for injuries such as concussions (**EXHIBIT 8.4**).

Transportation and Warehousing

Highway transportation crashes contribute to the greatest number of fatal injuries among U.S. workers: 8173 deaths (24% of all fatal occupational injuries) during 2003–2008. The average rate per year was 0.9 death per 100,000 workers. The trucking industry sustained the highest number (2320) and rate (19.6 per 100,000 workers) of deaths from this cause.[42] **FIGURE 8.17** displays the statewide distribution of highway transportation deaths and shows concentrations of deaths in the southern, mountain, and northwest central states. Data for 2003 through 2010 indicated that the highest rates of fatal crashes (3.1 per 100,000 FTE workers) occurred among employees who were 65 years of age or older.[43]

Agriculture

According to the CDC, "Agriculture ranks among the most hazardous industries. Farmers are at very high risk for fatal and nonfatal injuries; and farming is one of the few industries in which family members (who often share the work and live on the premises) are also at risk for fatal and nonfatal injuries."[44] **EXHIBIT 8.5** describes injuries among agricultural workers.

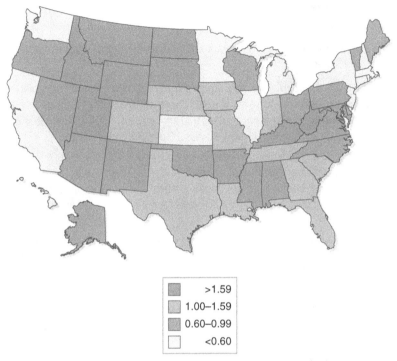

■	>1.59
■	1.00–1.59
■	0.60–0.99
□	<0.60

Note: Average annual deaths per 100,000 workers. Fatality rates exclude deaths to workers aged <16 years, volunteers, and resident military personnel.

FIGURE 8.17   Fatality rates for occupational highway transportation deaths—United States, 2003–2008

Reproduced from Centers for Disease Control and Prevention, Occupational highway transportation deaths—U.S., 2003–2008 MMWR. 2011;60(16):501.

Construction

In the United States during 2011, the field of construction had the highest number (*n* = 738) of fatal occupational injuries and the fourth highest rate (9.1 deaths per 100,000 FTE workers) by industry sector as defined by the Bureau of Labor Statistics. Construction-related hazards include collapses of cranes and walls of trenches, power tool injuries, asphyxiation in confined spaces, falls, and unique risks to female employees, who represent approximately 9% of construction workers. An example of an incident that killed six construction employees is the fatal tower crane collapse shown in **FIGURE 8.18** and described in **EXHIBIT 8.6**.

Injury Hazards from Tools

Examples of hazardous power tools used in construction are saws (table saws, hand-held saws, and chain saws), routers, nail guns, and many other tools designed to increase the speed and efficiency of construction projects. Power tools can cause grave injuries and amputations.

EXHIBIT 8.5   Agricultural Operations

Between 2003 and 2011, 5816 agricultural workers died from work-related injuries in the United States.

* In 2011, 570 agricultural workers died from work-related injuries. The fatality rate for agricultural workers was seven times higher than the fatality rate for all workers in private industry; agricultural workers had a fatality rate of 24.9 deaths per 100,000, while the fatality rate for all workers was 3.5 per 100,000.

* The leading cause of death for farm workers between 1992 and 2009 was tractor overturns, which accounted for more than 90 deaths each year. The most effective way to prevent tractor overturn deaths is the use of roll-over protective structures; however, in 2006 only 59% of tractors used on U.S. farms were equipped with these devices.

* Every day, approximately 243 agricultural workers suffer a serious lost-work-time injury. Five percent of these injuries result in permanent impairment.

* In 2011, the injury rate for agricultural workers was more than 40% higher than the rate for all workers. Crop production agricultural workers' injury rates were 5.5 events per 100 workers. Animal production agricultural workers' injury rates were 6.7 events per 100 workers. The rate for all workers was 3.8 events per 100 workers.

* Young workers who live and work on farms are also exposed to potentially dangerous farm-related hazards. Farm operators who hire youth to work on their farm should be aware of all applicable child labor laws.

* Approximately half of all U.S. farm workers are Hispanic. OSHA requires that employers conduct all required training of workers in a language and vocabulary workers can understand.

Modified from U.S. Department of Labor, Occupational Safety and Health Administration, Agricultural operations. https://www.osha.gov/dsg/topics/agriculturaloperations/. Accessed June 23, 2014.

Increasingly common are injuries from nail guns, which increase the speed of work, are easy to use, and are readily available to both workers and consumers.[45] According to the CDC, approximately 28,600 workers and 13,400 consumers incurred nail-gun injuries in 2005. Almost all of the injured persons were men. The most frequent types of nail-gun injuries were puncture wounds and lodgment of a foreign body (e.g., the nail) in an upper or lower extremity. Ocular, dental, and musculoskeletal injuries were among the other types of adverse effects.

Confined Spaces

A confined space is an area that limits the movement of workers (FIGURE 8.19). "A confined space has limited or restricted means for entry or

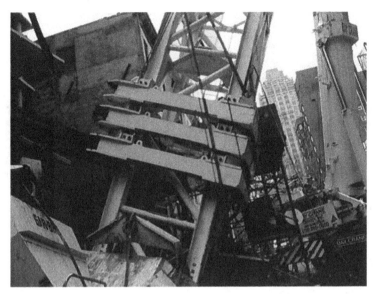

FIGURE 8.18   Fatal tower crane collapse, March 15, 2008,
New York.

Courtesy of the U.S. Department of Labor, Occupational Safety and Health Administration,
Investigation of the March 15, 2008 fatal tower crane collapse at 303 East 51st Street, New York, NY,
https://www.osha.gov/doc/engineering/2008_r_02.html. Accessed August 24, 2013.

EXHIBIT 8.6   Fatal Tower Crane Collapse, March 15, 2008, New York

On March 15, 2008, at approximately 2:30 p.m., a tower crane approximately 250 feet high
collapsed in uptown Manhattan, New York City, killing six construction employees. In addition, a civilian in a nearby apartment was killed when part of the crane struck the apartment building. The crane was being used in the construction of a 43-story concrete framed
building located at 303 E. 51st Street. At the time of the incident, employees were placing
lateral tie beams on the 18th floor of the building under construction to provide lateral
support to the crane. The crane was "jumped" about an hour earlier by adding four additional sections to the tower mast. ["Jumping a crane" is a procedure to raise its height.] The
jumping of the crane took place without any reported problems. The building under construction, a 43-story condominium, was framed in poured-in-place columns and beams/
slabs. The crane mast was located on the south side of the building under construction. . . .

The lack of lateral ties transformed the crane mast into a free-standing structure with
no lateral support above the third floor. The crane mast leaned a little toward the north and
then fell toward the south, pivoting near the base of the mast. . . . The crane boom
was facing toward the north and the counterweights [used to balance to boom] were
toward the south. The crane fell in one piece striking the building, known as 300–304 E.
51 Street, across the street. The crane mast was sheared off at the roof of the building,
with the top portion of the mast including the crane superstructure separating from
the lower portion of the mast. The top portion of the crane somersaulted and landed
one block away over another building.

Reprinted from U.S. Department of Labor. Occupational Safety and Health Administration
(OSHA). Investigation of the March 15, 2008 fatal tower crane collapse at 303 East 51st Street,
New York, NY. https://www.osha.gov/doc/engineering/2008_r_02.html. Accessed August 24, 2013.

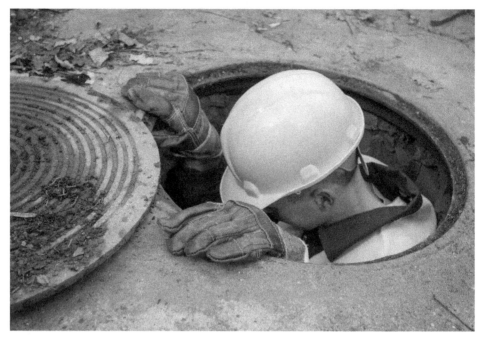

FIGURE 8.19 Working in confined spaces
© LightTheBox/Shutterstock

exit, and it is not designed for continuous employee occupancy."[46] Examples of confined spaces include underground utility vaults, manholes, pipes, tanks, and small storage bins. These work areas can pose a number of hazards, including asphyxiation, entrapment, electric shock, and high temperatures. OSHA applies the term "permit-required confined space" to a space that might have a hazardous atmosphere, could engulf the occupant (e.g., through collapse), or could trap or asphyxiate a worker because of downward-sloping walls or other physical configuration of the space.[47]

Female Construction Workers

As more women have become involved in construction work, awareness of the unique hazards for female workers in this industry has increased. Employment statistics for 2011 indicated that 164,000 women were employed in construction.[48] Approximately 9% of all construction workers in the United States are women.[49] Among the injury hazards for female construction workers are deaths from motor vehicle crashes, which are more common among women than men in the construction trades. Other injury hazards include cuts, falls, and musculoskeletal disorders, and injuries incurred while attempting to manipulate heavy objects. The types of injuries that occur among female construction workers suggest that more attention needs to be devoted to the design of safety and personal protective equipment to make sure that these devices are appropriate to the physical dimensions of women.

Fishing

The commercial fishing industry had the highest rate of occupational fatalities in the United States in 2011. Typical injuries include amputations, fractures, and asphyxiation caused by compression. One of the unique hazards associated with fishing is entanglement with winches, as described in **EXHIBIT 8.7**.[50]

Oil and Gas Operations

Between 2003 and 2010, industries specializing in the withdrawal of oil and gas from underground sources (oil and gas extraction) had a death rate that was seven times as high as that for all American workers (27.1 versus 3.8 deaths per 100,000 workers).[51] This figure includes mortality for onshore and offshore operations. In the Gulf of Mexico, the dramatic 2010 Deepwater Horizon explosion, which was accompanied by a massive oil spill, heightened societal awareness of the lethal hazards of offshore oil and gas extraction.

EXHIBIT 8.7   Fatal and Nonfatal Injuries Involving Fishing Vessel Winches—Southern Shrimp Fleet, United States, 2000–2011

Workers in the commercial fishing industry have the highest occupational fatality rate in the United States, nearly 35 times higher in 2011 than the rate for all U.S. workers....During 2000–2009, a total of 504 fishermen were killed in the U.S. fishing industry, most commonly by drowning as a result of vessels sinking (51%) and falls overboard (30%). Another 10% of fatalities (51 deaths) were caused by injuries sustained onboard vessels, such as entanglement in machinery.... This type of fatality occurred most often in the Gulf of Mexico.

During 2000–2011, 8 fatal and 27 work-related injuries involving deck winches occurred in the Southern shrimp fleet, which operates in the Gulf of Mexico and off the Atlantic coast from Florida to North Carolina.... Injuries involving the winch drum had a higher risk for fatal outcomes compared with injuries involving the winch cathead. Fatal outcomes also were associated with being alone on the vessel and being alone on deck. Interventions to prevent deck winch injuries might include guarding of winch drums and catheads, avoiding working alone on deck, not wearing baggy clothing, and improvements to cable winding guides. Training of deckhands in first aid and emergency procedures might reduce the severity of injuries when entanglements occur.

Reprinted from Centers for Disease Control and Prevention (CDC). Fatal and nonfatal injuries involving fishing vessel winches—Southern shrimp fleet, U.S., 2000-2011. *MMWR.* 2013;62(9):157

Despite the publicity accorded to this event, it accounted for only a small percentage of the total deaths in offshore activities. The most frequent cause of fatalities in offshore operations is helicopter crashes. EXHIBIT 8.8 provides more information about mortality associated with offshore oil and gas extraction.

Dental Professionals

Dental professionals experience unique risks associated with the necessity to maintain abnormal postures during clinical procedures. For example, dentists may be prone to harmful physiological changes in muscles and joints. In turn, these changes may be associated with joint injuries and nerve compression. Another adverse condition is carpal tunnel syndrome, a musculoskeletal disorder for which dentists are thought to have increased risks.[52] Dental hygienists are another professional group with increased risk of carpal tunnel syndrome.[53] In addition, dental hygienists can experience musculoskeletal disorders (e.g., of the neck, shoulder, and lower back), which may be associated with pain that can last for two or more days.[54]

Risk Factors for Occupational Injuries

Risk factors for occupational injuries encompass harmful exposures and events that take place within a worker's employment setting. Such risk factors include high-demand jobs and adverse physical health conditions such as overweight.

EXHIBIT 8.8   Fatal Injuries in Offshore Oil and Gas Operations—United States, 2003–2010

The 11 lives lost in the 2010 Deepwater Horizon explosion provide a reminder of the hazards involved in offshore drilling.... [F]or the period 2003–2010[,] ... 128 fatalities in activities related to offshore oil and gas operations occurred.... Transportation events were the leading cause (65 [51%]); the majority of these involved aircraft (49 [75%]). Nearly one fourth (31 [24%]) of the fatalities occurred among workers whose occupations were classified as "transportation and material moving." To reduce fatalities in offshore oil and gas operations, employers should ensure that the most stringent applicable transportation safety guidelines are followed. TABLE 8.1 presents data on the distribution of fatal injuries by event.

Reprinted from Centers for Disease Control and Prevention (CDC). Fatal injuries in offshore oil and gas operations—U.S., 2003-2010. *MMWR*. 2013;62(16):301-304

TABLE 8.1 Number and Percentage of Fatal Injuries among Workers Involved in Offshore Oil and Gas Operations, by Event—United States, 2003–2010

Event	Number	Percentage
Transportation events	65	50.8
Aircraft events [all involved helicopters]	49	38.3
Water vehicle events	16	12.5
Contact with objects and equipment	21	16.4
Fires and explosions	17	13.3
Exposure to harmful substances/environments	16	12.5
Other event types	9	7.0
Total	128	100.0

Reprinted from Centers for Disease Control and Prevention (CDC). Fatal injuries in offshore oil and gas operations—U.S., 2003-2010. *MMWR*. 2013;62(16):301-304.

High-Demand Jobs

High-demand jobs place heavy mental and physical burdens upon workers—burdens that may carry increased risks of injuries. For example, research has assessed the relationships among high cognitive ability and skill requirements required by occupations, physical hazards at the occupational level, and injury rates. Jobs that require high cognitive ability and skill levels have an increased potential for human error and, consequently, greater potential for injury from physical hazards.[55] A study of almost 3000 workers in France found that high-demand jobs—for example, those that required heavy physical workloads, the use of pneumatic and other vibrating tools, exposures to extreme temperatures, and the requirement to maintain awkward postures while performing tasks—tended to have high risks of injuries.[56]

Another example of a demanding job is one that requires working at night. Almost one-third of night-shift workers sleep only for six or fewer hours per day (called short sleep duration)—meaning that they are sleep deprived.[57] A total of 44% of all night-shift workers have short sleep duration. The prevalence is especially high (67%) among night-shift workers in the transportation and warehousing industry. Inadequate sleep contributes to lessened safety in the work environment in addition to adverse health effects among workers who do not obtain enough sleep. Drivers who are somnolent rather than well rested are prone to vehicle crashes.

Overweight

Overweight is hypothesized to be a risk factor for job-related injuries. Pollack et al. studied the relationship between body mass index and risk of occupational injury among hourly employees at a U.S. aluminum manufacturing company.[58] These researchers found that approximately 85% of workers who sustained injuries were overweight or obese. Very obese workers were especially prone to leg or knee injuries. Thus, these findings demonstrate an association between body mass index and traumatic workplace injuries.

Workplace Violence

The term workplace violence refers to "any act or threat of physical violence, harassment, intimidation, or other threatening disruptive behavior that occurs at the work site. It ranges from threats and verbal abuse to physical assaults and even homicide. It can affect and involve employees, clients, customers and visitors."[59]

In 2011, the category of fatal injuries caused by violence and other injuries by persons and animals was associated with 17% of fatal occupational injuries in the United States. (Refer to Figure 8.2.) During 2011, homicide was responsible for 10% of deaths. In 2010, it was the fourth-leading cause of fatal occupational injuries and resulted in 506 fatalities. Among women, homicide was the main cause of fatality in the workplace.[59]

The National Institute for Occupational Safety and Health (NIOSH) presents some alarming statistics on workplace violence. "According to the Bureau of Justice Statistics, an estimated 1.7 million workers are injured each year during workplace assaults; in addition, violent workplace incidents account for 18% of all violent crime in the United States."[60(p. 1)] In 1994, the number of workplace homicides reached a high of 1080, but subsequently declined to 551 homicides in 2004.

As shown in Figure 8.8, a larger percentage of female workers than male workers were killed by workplace homicides in 2011 (20% versus 9%). FIGURE 8.20 demonstrates that among women, in comparison to men, assailants responsible for homicides were most frequently relatives or domestic partners. This finding suggests that for women, workplace violence represents the carryover of domestic issues into the occupational environment. Among male victims, homicidal assailants were motivated most often by criminal intent (e.g., robbery).

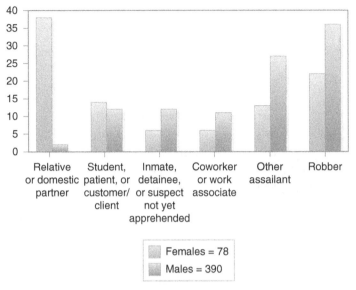

FIGURE 8.20   Work-related homicides by gender of decedent and assailant type, 2011

Reproduced from U.S. Department of Labor, Bureau of Labor Statistics, Fatal occupational injuries in 2011, http://www.bls.gov/iif/oshwc/cfoi/cfch0010.pdf. Accessed March 20, 2014.

Types of Workplace Violence

Workplace violence can be subdivided according to the typology shown in **TABLE 8.2**. The types of violence shown in the table include those arising from criminal intent, customer and client relationships, interactions among workers (worker-on-worker), and personal relationships.[59]

Venues for Violent Incidents

Employees who are at particular risk of workplace violence are delivery drivers, healthcare workers, law enforcement personnel, and individuals involved with monetary transactions. Persons who work alone or in small groups in public places have increased risk of violence. Examples of occupations and workplaces associated with violent happenings are the following:

- Taxi and for-hire drivers. The workers may carry large amounts of cash, work alone and at night, and travel to deserted areas where they are vulnerable to robberies.
- Postal workers. Media reports of workplace homicides that involved postal workers have given rise to the slang term "going postal."

TABLE 8.2   Typology of Workplace Violence

Type	Description
Criminal intent	The perpetrator has no legitimate relationship to the business or its employee, and is usually committing a crime in conjunction with the violence. These crimes can include robbery, shoplifting, trespassing, and terrorism. The vast majority of workplace homicides (85%) fall into this category.
Customer/client	The perpetrator has a legitimate relationship with the business and becomes violent while being served by the business. This category includes customers, clients, patients, students, inmates, and any other group for which the business provides services. A large portion of customer/client incidents occur in the healthcare industry, in settings such as nursing homes or psychiatric facilities; the victims are often patient caregivers. Police officers, prison staff, flight attendants, and teachers are some other examples of workers who may be exposed to this kind of workplace violence, which accounts for approximately 3% of all workplace homicides.
Worker-on-worker	The perpetrator is an employee or past employee of the business who attacks or threatens another employee(s) or past employee(s) in the workplace. Worker-on-worker fatalities account for approximately 7% of all workplace homicides.
Personal relationship	The perpetrator usually does not have a relationship with the business but has a personal relationship with the intended victim. This category includes victims of domestic violence assaulted or threatened while at work, and accounts for about 5% of all workplace homicides.

Reprinted from Centers for Disease Control and Prevention. National Institute for Occupational Safety and Health (NIOSH). Workplace violence prevention strategies and research needs. Cincinnati, OH: DHHS (NIOSH); 2006. DHHS (NIOSH) Publication No. 2006-144.

An analysis of fatal injuries among postal workers conducted more than two decades ago found that motor vehicle–related events and homicides were the leading causes of occupational fatalities. Nevertheless, the overall occupational fatality rate for postal workers was lower than that of all workers in the United States. The homicide rate for this group was not higher than that reported for other occupational categories.[61]

- Healthcare settings. High-risk environments include psychiatric facilities, nursing homes, and emergency medical care centers. For example, workplace violence has become increasingly concerning for employees in the home health industry.[62] Other personnel at risk for violence are emergency medical technicians (EMTs) and paramedics, who frequently become the victims of violence. An important cause of work-related mortality among EMTs and paramedics is assaults.[63] Also, these workers are at risk of other forms of job-associated injuries. Maguire et al. reported that the injury rates among EMTs and paramedics are approximately three times the national average for all occupations.[63] The majority of fatal injuries are from transportation-related incidents. More research is needed on work-related injuries among EMTs and paramedics, as little information is available regarding this issue.

- Retail settings including late-night establishments. An example of a violent event was the shooting and massacre at a beauty salon in Seal Beach, California, on October 12, 2011 (**FIGURE 8.21**).[64] In this incident, eight people died and one other individual was injured. The alleged shooter was the estranged husband of one of the deceased employees.

Public Health and Epidemiologic Approaches to Injury Prevention

The public health approach to injury prevention focuses on primary prevention of injuries at the population level. Some goals of this approach are to examine the occurrence of work-related injuries in the general population of employed persons, identify work settings at high risk for injuries, and determine specific industries that may have a high prevalence and incidence of injuries.

Sometimes the term *unintentional injury* is used interchangeably with the word *accident*. In reality, unintentional injuries are not accidents. The field of injury prevention is premised on the concept that deaths and harm from unintentional injuries are preventable, particularly through implementation of public health and epidemiologic approaches. Consequently, the word "accident" is not in favor for use as a scientific term, as an accident

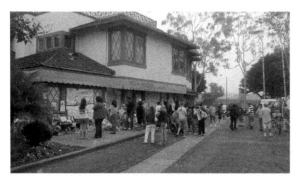

FIGURE 8.21　Seal Beach, California, site of a shooting alleged to be associated with a domestic conflict

implies an unpredictable and unpreventable event. According the World Health Organization (WHO),

> There is clear, scientific evidence that injury-related deaths can be avoided and the effect of injury mitigated. In high-income countries, injury-related deaths among children under the age of 15 years were reduced by half between 1970 and 1995. This reduction is attributed to a combination of research, development of data collection systems, the introduction of specific prevention measures such as improvements in the local environment, legislation, public education, product safety, and improvements in the level and quality of emergency care.[65]

One of the fundamental inputs into the public health aspects of injury prevention comes from the science of epidemiology.[66] This quantitative science develops information on person, place, and time variables associated with injuries and suggests interventions for improving worker safety. For example, surveillance data play a key role in helping researchers identify patterns of occupational injuries. Given the widespread occurrence of musculoskeletal injuries, interventions for improvement of workplace ergonomics are critical to reduce these types of injuries. A model for identification of risk factors for work-related injuries is also important.

Ergonomics

"Ergonomics is the scientific study of people at work. The goal of ergonomics is to reduce stress and eliminate injuries and disorders associated with the overuse of muscles, bad posture, and repeated tasks. This is accomplished by designing tasks, work spaces, controls, displays, tools, lighting, and equipment to fit the employee's physical capabilities and limitations."[67]

The nature of work organization is related to the ergonomics of the work environment.[68] Consequently, changes in organizational leadership that allow for input from employees can lead to improvements in the ergonomics of the work. For example, a participatory intervention program improved the health and safety of healthcare employees who were at risk of work-related injuries from lifting and transferring patients.[69] Participatory training programs for small workplaces were also able to improve the ergonomics in a work environment.[70] Stone et al. described a collaborative program among a research institution, a university, and an electric power utility to develop interventions to improve the ergonomics of tasks performed by underground utility workers.[71] This collaboration developed several interventions that improved the ergonomics of work processes.

The Haddon Matrix and Injury Prevention

The Haddon Matrix, developed by William Haddon, is applied widely to the prevention of unintentional injuries and is germane to work-related injuries. This matrix was used originally for categorizing highway safety phenomena, but it is applicable in more general terms to prevention of unintentional injuries. The two-dimensional Haddon Matrix shows factors associated with injuries along the columns of the matrix; the rows provide the time phases of an injury.[72,73] Factors associated with injuries are agent, host, and environment (social and physical environment) variables and time (pre-event, event, and post-event phases). The Haddon Matrix is useful for designing strategies for prevention of injuries from motor vehicle crashes by isolating the specific determinants from the triad of host, agent, and environmental factors that operate before, during, and after a crash (TABLE 8.3).[74]

Here are some examples of how the Haddon Matrix might be applied to the prevention of occupational injuries:

- Transportation and warehousing (intersection in the Haddon Matrix of the host characteristic, age, with post-event). Recall that transportation and warehousing is the occupational category with the largest percentage of fatal and nonfatal injuries. Transportation injuries include motor vehicle crashes. A host characteristic associated with vehicle crashes is being older than 65 years of age; a preventive intervention to reduce crashes might be to provide testing and driver safety programs for older drivers.

TABLE 8.3 Haddon Matrix Applied to Motor Vehicle Injuries

Type	Host	Agent	Environment
Pre-event	Alcohol use	Brake condition	Road curvature
	Fatigue	Load weight	Weather
	Driving experience	Vehicle visibility	Speed limit
	Defensive driving skill		
Event	Seat belt use	Speed at impact	Guard rails
	Bone density	Vehicle size	Median barriers
	Stature	Vehicle safety features	Recovery zones
Post-event	Age	Fuel tank integrity	911 access
	Sex		Triage protocols
	Frailty		Emergency medical services training

Reprinted from Sleet DA, Dahlberg LL, Basavaraju SV, et al. Injury prevention, violence prevention, and trauma care: building the scientific base. *MMWR.* 2011;60:80.

Truck drivers are another group at risk of vehicle crashes. Prevention of crashes might be accomplished by restricting the total number of hours driven each day and requiring rest breaks to reduce driver fatigue.

- Injuries from falling (intersection in the Haddon Matrix of environment with event). In this case, an entry in the cell might be safety rails on construction sites (not shown in Table 8.3). A preventive measure would be to ensure that safety rails are in place on top of buildings before allowing access to workers. Additional measures would be the use of safety harnesses and installation of secure scaffolding and secure and well-positioned ladders.

SUMMARY

Although the frequency of occupational injuries (work-related injuries) has shown a declining trend since the 1990s, work-related unintentional injuries continue to be significant causes of morbidity and mortality among U.S. workers. This chapter defined terms used in the context of work-associated injuries—for example, occupational injury, unintentional versus intentional injuries, traumatic injuries, cumulative trauma disorders, and occupational injury epidemiology.

The Bureau of Labor Statistics is a valuable resource for information regarding fatal and nonfatal occupational injuries. However, the full scope of such injuries is unknown because they tend to be underreported. Occupational injuries follow characteristic patterns according to descriptive epidemiologic variables. Falls and musculoskeletal disorders were two especially prevalent forms of occupational disorders. Musculoskeletal disorders include repetitive motion disorders such as rotator cuff tendinitis and carpal tunnel syndrome.

Some occupations have especially high risks for injuries and risk factors for work-related injuries. Workplace violence is also a concern. Public health and epidemiologic approaches can be applied to injury prevention, including use of the Haddon Matrix.

STUDY QUESTIONS AND EXERCISES

1. Define the following terms:
   A. Work-related injury
   B. Unintentional injury
   C. Musculoskeletal disorder
   D. Carpal tunnel syndrome
   E. Ergonomics
2. How important are nonfatal and fatal workplace injuries in terms of economic and social costs for the United States?
3. Describe common forms of occupational injuries, both fatal and nonfatal, in the United States.
4. To what extent do job-related injuries go unreported in the United States? Using your own ideas, discuss how reporting might be improved.

5. Identify three high-risk occupations for injuries. Compare and contrast them with respect to traumatic injury rates.
6. Describe variations in occupational injuries according to characteristics of person, such as gender and age.
7. Which occupations have the highest fatality rates? Give examples of factors associated with occupational fatalities.
8. Using your own ideas, suggest methods for preventing workplace injuries such as falling, back injuries, carpal tunnel syndrome, and traumatic injuries.
9. What is the toll from workplace violence? Describe factors associated with violence in the workplace and suggest methods for its prevention.
10. State the four typologies of workplace violence and give an example of each one.

REFERENCES

1. U.S. Department of Labor. Injuries, illnesses, and fatalities: fatal occupational injuries and Workers' Memorial Day. n.d. http://www.bls.gov/iif/oshwc/cfoi/worker_memorial.htm. Accessed August 16, 2013.
2. Centers for Disease Control and Prevention, National Institute for Occupational Safety and Health. Traumatic occupational injuries. n.d. http://www.cdc.gov/niosh/injury/. Accessed December 6, 2013.
3. Hagberg M, Christiani D, Courtney TK, et al. Conceptual and definitional issues in occupational injury epidemiology. *Am J Ind Med.* 1997;32:106–115.
4. Government of New Brunswick, Canada. Injury prevention. n.d. http://www.gnb.ca/0053/phc/injury_prevention-e.asp. Accessed January 22, 2013.
5. Centers for Disease Control and Prevention, National Institute for Occupational Safety and Health. Traumatic injury. http://www.cdc.gov/niosh/programs/ti/. Accessed December 6, 2013.
6. U.S. House of Representatives, Committee on Education and Labor. *Hidden tragedy: underreporting of workplace injuries and illnesses.* Washington, DC: U.S. House of Representatives; 2008.
7. Centers for Disease Control and Prevention. Fatal work-related injuries—United States, 2005–2009. *MMWR.* 2013;62(3):41–45.
8. U.S. Department of Labor. Revisions to the 2011 Census of Fatal Occupational Injuries (CFOI) counts. n.d. http://www.bls.gov/iif/oshwc/cfoi/cfoi_revised11.pdf. Accessed March 8, 2014.
9. Centers for Disease Control and Prevention. Nonfatal work-related injuries and illnesses—United States, 2010. *MMWR.* 2013;62(3):35–40.
10. U.S. Department of Labor, Bureau of Labor Statistics. *Employer-reported workplace injuries and illnesses—2013* [News release]. USDL-14-2183. December 4, 2014.
11. U.S. Department of Labor, Bureau of Labor Statistics. *Nonfatal occupational injuries and illnesses requiring days away from work, 2013* [News release]. USDL-14-2246. December 16, 2014.
12. U.S. Department of Labor, Bureau of Labor Statistics. 2011 nonfatal occupational injuries and illnesses: cases with days away from work. n.d. http://www.bls.gov/iif/oshwc/osh/case/osch0053.pdf. Accessed January 29, 2015.
13. U.S. Department of Labor. Bureau of Labor Statistics. Chart package.pdf. n.d. http://www.bls.gov/iif/oshwc/cfoi/cfch0011.pdf. Accessed December 22, 2013.

14. Byler CG. Hispanic/Latino fatal occupational injury rates. *Monthly Labor Rev.* 2013;136(2):14–23.

15. U.S. Department of Labor, Bureau of Labor Statistics. National Census of Fatal Occupational Injuries in 2012: preliminary results. n.d. http://www.bls.gov/news.release/pdf/cfoi.pdf. Accessed March 13, 2014.

16. Berdahl TA. Racial/ethnic and gender differences in individual workplace injury risk trajectories: 1988-1998. *Am J Public Health.* 2008;98(12):2258–2263.

17. Centers for Disease Control and Prevention. Nonfatal occupational injuries and illnesses among older workers—United States, 2009. *MMWR.* 2011;60(16):503–508.

18. Centers for Disease Control and Prevention, National Institute for Occupational Safety and Health. Young worker safety and health. n.d. http://www.cdc.gov/niosh/topics/youth/. Accessed March 21, 2014.

19. Centers for Disease Control and Prevention, National Institute for Occupational Safety and Health. Fall injuries prevention in the workplace. n.d. http://www.cdc.gov/niosh/topics/falls/. Accessed December 22, 2013.

20. U.S. Department of Labor, Occupational Safety and Health Administration. Fall prevention fact sheet. https://www.osha.gov/stopfalls/factsheet.pdf. Accessed February 1, 2015.

21. Centers for Disease Control and Prevention, National Institute for Occupational Safety and Health. Musculoskeletal disorders. n.d. http://www.cdc.gov/niosh/programs/msd/. Accessed March 15, 2014.

22. Centers for Disease Control and Prevention (CDC), National Institute for Occupational Safety and Health (NIOSH). *Cumulative trauma disorders in the workplace: bibliography.* Cincinnati, OH: U.S. DHHS, CDC, NIOSH; 1995.

23. Centers for Disease Control and Prevention. Work-related musculoskeletal disorders (WMSDs) prevention. n.d. http://www.cdc.gov/workplacehealthpromotion/evaluation/topics/disorders.html. Accessed March 15, 2014.

24. Bernard BP, ed. *Musculoskeletal disorders and workplace factors.* DHHS (NIOSH) Publication No. 97-141. Cincinnati, OH: DHHS (NIOSH); 1997.

25. mediLexicon.com. Cumulative trauma disorders (CTD). n.d. http://www.medilexicon.com/medicaldictionary.php?t=25986. Accessed March 15, 2014.

26. Connecticut Department of Public Health, Environmental and Occupational Health Assessment Program. Cumulative trauma disorders. n.d. http://www.ct.gov/dph/lib/dph/environmental_health/eoha/pdf/ctds_fact_sheet.pdf. Accessed March 15, 2014.

27. Brenner MD, Fairris D, Ruser J. "Flexible" work practices and occupational safety and health: exploring the relationship between cumulative trauma disorders and workplace transformation. *Ind Relations.* 2004;43(1):242–266.

28. European Agency for Safety and Health at Work (EU-OSHA). Work-related neck and upper limb disorders. n.d. https://osha.europa.eu/en/publications/factsheets/72. Accessed March 27, 2014.

29. National Institute of Neurological Disorders and Stroke. What are repetitive motion disorders? n.d. http://www.ninds.nih.gov/disorders/repetitive_motion/repetitive_motion.htm. Accessed October 6, 2013.

30. U.S. National Library of Medicine, MedlinePlus. Rotator cuff problems. n.d. http://www.nlm.nih.gov/medlineplus/ency/article/000438.htm. Accessed October 6, 2013.

31. van Rijn RM, Huisstede BMA, Koes BW, Burdoff A. Associations between work-related factors and specific disorders of the shoulder: a systematic review of the literature. *Scand J Work Environ Health.* 2010;36(3):189–201.

32. National Institute of Neurological Disorders and Stroke. Carpal tunnel syndrome fact sheet. n.d. http://www.ninds.nih.gov/disorders/carpal_tunnel/detail_carpal _tunnel.htm. Accessed October 6, 2013.

33. U.S. Department of Labor, Occupational Safety and Health Administration. Computer workstations. n.d. http://www.osha.gov/SLTC/etools/computerwork-stations/index.html. Accessed May 12, 2013.

34. Shaw WS, Linton SJ, Pransky G. Reducing sickness absence from work due to low back pain: how well do intervention strategies match modifiable risk factors? *J Occup Rehabil*. 2006;16:591–605.

35. U.S. Department of Labor, Occupational Safety and Health Administration (OSHA). OSHA Technical Manual (OTM): Section VII: Chapter 1: back disorders and injuries. n.d. https://www.osha.gov/dts/osta/otm/otm_vii/otm_vii_1.html. Accessed June 23, 2014.

36. Centers for Disease Control and Prevention (CDC), National Center for Health Statistics (NCHS). *Summary health statistics for U.S. adults: National Health Interview Survey, 2011*. DHHS Publication No. (PHS) 2013-1584. Hyattsville, MD: DHHS, CDC, NCHS; 2012.

37. U.S. Department of Labor, Bureau of Labor Statistics. *Nonfatal occupational injuries and illnesses requiring days away from work, 2010* [News release]. USDL-11-1612. November 9, 2011.

38. Guo HR, Tanaka S, Cameron LL, et al. Back pain among workers in the United States: national estimates and workers at high risk. *Am J Ind Med*. 1995;28(5):591–602.

39. Mayo Clinic. Back pain at work: preventing pain and injury. n.d. http://www.mayo-clinic.org/healthy-living/adult-health/in-depth/back-pain/art-20044526. Accessed March 17, 2014.

40. Guskiewicz KM, Marshall SW, Bailes J, et al. Association between recurrent concussion and late-life cognitive impairment in retired professional football players. *Neurosurgery*. 2005;57(4):719–726.

41. Schwarz A. N.F.L. acknowledges long-term concussion effects. *The New York Times*. December 21, 2009. http://www.nytimes.com/2009/12/21/sports /football/21concussions.html?pagewanted=all&_r=0. Accessed June 22, 2014.

42. Centers for Disease Control and Prevention. Occupational highway transportation deaths—United States, 2003–2008. *MMWR*. 2011;60(16):497–502.

43. Centers for Disease Control and Prevention. Occupational highway transportation deaths among workers aged ≥ 55 years—United States, 2003–2010. *MMWR*. 2013;62(33):653–657.

44. Centers for Disease Control and Prevention, National Institute for Occupational Safety and Health. Agricultural safety. n.d. http://www.cdc.gov/niosh/topics/aginjury/. Accessed June 23, 2014.

45. Centers for Disease Control and Prevention. Nail-gun injuries treated in emergency departments—United States, 2001–2005. *MMWR*. 2007;56(14): 329–332.

46. U.S. Department of Labor, Occupational Safety and Health Administration. Confined spaces. n.d. https://www.osha.gov/SLTC/confinedspaces/index.html. Accessed August 23, 2013.

47. U.S. Department of Labor (DOL), Occupational Safety and Health Administration (OSHA). *Permit-required confined spaces*. OSHA 3138-01R. U.S. DOL, OSHA; 2004.

48. Centers for Disease Control and Prevention, National Institute for Occupational Safety and Health. Women's safety and health issues at work. Job area: construction. n.d. http://www.cdc.gov/niosh/topics/women/construction.html. Accessed March 19, 2014.

49. U.S. Department of Labor, Occupational Safety and Health Administration. Women in construction. n.d. https://www.osha.gov/doc/topics/women/index.html. Accessed March 19, 2014.

50. Centers for Disease Control and Prevention. Fatal and nonfatal injuries involving fishing vessel winches—Southern shrimp fleet, United States, 2000–2011. *MMWR*. 2013;62(9):157–168.

51. Centers for Disease Control and Prevention. Fatal injuries in offshore oil and gas operations—United States, 2003–2010. *MMWR*. 2013;62(16):301–304.

52. Abichandani S, Shaikh S, Nadiger R. Carpal tunnel syndrome: an occupational hazard facing dentistry. *Int Dent J*. 2013;63(5):230–236.

53. Anton D, Rosecrance J, Merlino L, Cook T. Prevalence of musculoskeletal symptoms and carpal tunnel syndrome among dental hygienists. *Am J Ind Med*. 2002;42(3):248–257.

54. Hayes MJ, Smith DR, Taylor JA. Musculoskeletal disorders and symptom severity among Australian dental hygienists. *BMC Research Notes*. 2013;6:250.

55. Ford MT, Wiggins BK. Occupational-level interactions between physical hazards and cognitive ability and skill requirements in predicting injury incidence rates. *J Occup Health Psychol*. 2012;17(3):268–278.

56. Chau N, Bourgkard E, Bhattacherjee A, et al. Associations of job, living conditions and lifestyle with occupational injury in working population: a population-based study. *Int Arch Occup Environ Health*. 2008;81:379–389.

57. Centers for Disease Control and Prevention. Short sleep duration among workers—United States, 2010. *MMWR*. 2012;61(16):281–285.

58. Pollack KM, Sorock GS, Slade MD, et al. Association between body mass index and acute traumatic workplace injury in hourly manufacturing employees. *Am J Epidemiol*. 2007;166:204–211.

59. U.S. Department of Labor, Occupational Safety and Health Administration. Workplace violence. n.d. https://www.osha.gov/SLTC/workplaceviolence/. Accessed October 8, 2013.

60. Centers for Disease Control and Prevention, National Institute for Occupational Safety and Health (NIOSH). *Workplace violence prevention strategies and research needs*. DHHS (NIOSH) Publication No. 2006-144. Cincinnati, OH: DHHS (NIOSH); 2006.

61. Centers for Disease Control and Prevention. Occupational injury deaths of postal workers—United States, 1980–1989. *MMWR*. 1994;43(32):587–595.

62. Gross N, Peek-Asa C, Nocera M, Casteel C. Workplace violence prevention policies in home health and hospice care agencies. *Online J Issues Nurs*. 2013;18(1):1.

63. Maguire BJ, Smith S. Injuries and fatalities among emergency medical technicians and paramedics in the United States. *Prehosp Disaster Med*. 2013;28(4):1–7.

64. *Los Angeles Times*. Seal Beach salon reopens after shooting massacre. November 19, 2012. http://latimesblogs.latimes.com/lanow/salon-shooting/. Accessed March 20, 2014.

65. World Health Organization. How can injuries be prevented? n.d. http://www.who.int/features/qa/36/en/print.html. Accessed July 2, 2014.

66. Branche CM, Stout NA, Castillo DN, et al. Work-related unintentional injuries. In: Friis RH, ed. *The Praeger handbook of environmental health*. Vol. 4. Santa Barbara, CA: Praeger; 2012:163–184.

67. Centers for Disease Control and Prevention, National Institute for Occupational Safety and Health. Ergonomics and musculoskeletal disorders. n.d. http://www.cdc .gov/niosh/topics/ergonomics/. Accessed October 6, 2013.

68. Carayon P, Smith MJ. Work organization and ergonomics. *Appl Ergon*. 2000;31:649–662.

69. Evanoff BA, Bohr PC, Wolf LD. Effects of a participatory ergonomics team among hospital orderlies. *Am J Ind Med*. 1999;35:358–365.

70. Kogi K. Practical ways to facilitate ergonomics improvements in occupational health practice. *Hum Factors*. 2012;54(6):890–900.

71. Stone A, Usher D, Marklin R, et al. Case study for underground workers at an electric utility: how a research institution, university, and industry collaboration improved occupational health through ergonomics. *J Occup Environ Hyg*. 2006;3:397–407.

72. Haddon W, Jr. The changing approach to the epidemiology, prevention, and amelioration of trauma: the transition to approaches etiologically rather than descriptively based. *Am J Public Health*. 1968;58(8):1431–1438.

73. Haddon W, Jr. A logical framework for categorizing highway safety phenomena and activity. *J Trauma*. 1972;12(3):193–207.

74. Sleet DA, Dahlberg LL, Basavaraju SV, et al. Injury prevention, violence prevention, and trauma care: building the scientific base. *MMWR*. 2011;60:78–85.

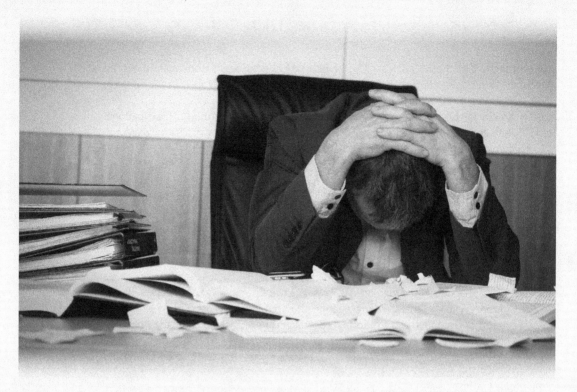

FIGURE 9.1 Job stress

© Lichtmeister/ShutterStock

In today's economic upheavals, downsizing, layoffs, mergers, and bankrupt-cies have cost hundreds of thousands of workers their jobs. Millions more have been shifted to unfamiliar tasks within their companies and wonder how much longer they will be employed. Adding to the pressures that workers face are new bosses, computer surveillance of production, fewer health and retirement benefits, and the feeling they have to work longer and harder just to main-tain their current economic status. Workers at every level are experiencing increased tension and uncertainty, and are updating their resumes.

Source: American Psychological Association. Stress in the workplace. n.d. http://www.apa.org/helpcenter /workplace-stress.aspx. Accessed September 11, 2013.

CHAPTER 9

Psychosocial Aspects of Work: Job Stress and Associated Conditions

Learning Objectives

By the end of this chapter you will be able to:

- Give alternative definitions of occupational stress.
- Describe environmental factors associated with occupational stress.
- Describe adverse physical and mental health outcomes associated with occupational stress.
- Discuss the relationship between the work environment and employee morale.
- Describe methods for preventing stress in the workplace.

Chapter Outline

- Introduction
- Psychological Stress
- Occupational Stress: A Theoretical Perspective
- The Work Environment and Job Stress
- Physical Health Effects of Occupational Stress
- Job Stress and Mental Health
- Employee Morale in the Occupational Setting
- Lifestyle and Work
- Interventions for Workplace Stress
- Summary
- Study Questions and Exercises

Introduction

Occupational stress is a universal predicament for workers in the 21st century and a noteworthy feature of contemporary life in general. Employees must confront numerous stressors that can have adverse effects on their mental and physical health. Many of the stresses that challenge today's workers result from economic downturns, downsizing, bankruptcies, mergers, and layoffs.[1] In a survey of almost 2000 workers conducted by the American Psychological Association in 2012, nearly two-fifths of respondents indicated that they felt stressed out during the workday; however, almost 60% said they believed they had the resources to manage stress (FIGURE 9.2).[2,3]

The National Institute for Occupational Safety and Health (NIOSH) has emphasized the broad scope of stress among the workforce:

> Stress is a prevalent and costly problem in today's workplace. About one-third of workers report high levels of stress, and high levels of stress are associated with substantial increases in health service utilization. Additionally, periods of disability due to job stress tend to be much longer than disability periods for other occupational injuries and illnesses.... . Attention to stress at work has intensified in the wake of sweeping changes in the organization of work that are feared to expose workers to heightened risk of stress.[4]

Both the characteristics of the physical environment—for example, biological, chemical, and physical hazards—and aspects of the psychosocial environment—influences that emanate from people—are salient dimensions of occupational settings and have important implications for the health of

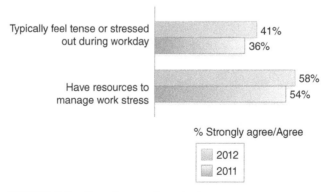

FIGURE 9.2   Prevalence of work stress

Reproduced from the American Psychological Association, Harris Interactive, Workplace survey, March 2012, http://www.apa.org/news/press/releases/phwa /workplace-survey.pdf. Accessed March 24, 2014.

workers. A growing body of evidence suggests that programs for employee wellness need to take into account how the physical and social environments jointly affect workers' health.[5] An additional consideration regarding employee well-being is the fit between the worker and the job environment.

One key component of the psychosocial environment is stress—a phenomenon that connotes an imbalance between demands originating from the environment and the person's capability to meet these demands. In addition, factors in the physical environment at work (for example, high noise levels) tend to exacerbate workers' sensations of being under stress.

Occupational stress is a complex area and the subject of a considerable body of research. With respect to occupational stress, important issues include the definition and prevalence of stress, mental and physical health effects, organizational consequences, risk factors, and moderating factors such as physical activity levels and other lifestyle variables in the workplace. TABLE 9.1 identifies a number of important topics and examples that pertain to occupational stress and are covered in more detail in this chapter.

Psychological Stress

Before defining the term "occupational stress," it is important to explore the more general concept of psychological stress, which has a venerable history in the behavioral sciences. The term psychological stress refers to "a particular relationship between the person and the environment that is appraised by the person as taxing or exceeding his or her resources and endangering his or her well-being."[6(p. 19)]

Stress research encompasses a broad area that explores how aversive environmental events control multiple response systems (verbal, physiological, and behavioral).[7] Clinical findings suggest that these aversive events produce negative health outcomes. Following are three examples of aversive events (couched in the language of experimental psychology) that may produce stress responses:

- Presentation of noxious or biologically damaging stimuli (either by actual presentation or by threat of presentation). An example is electric shock experimentation conducted with monkeys. The "executive monkey" experiments demonstrated that physiologic arousal linked to behavioral responses to remove the threat of electric shock was associated with the development of gastrointestinal lesions.
- Removal of reinforcements (either actual or threatened). In the work setting, reinforcements consist of rewards such as higher pay, promotions, and recognition. An example of the removal of reinforcement is the threat of layoff or docking a worker's pay.

TABLE 9.1   Some Important Topics and Examples Related to Occupational Stress

Topic	Examples
Psychological stress: definition	Lazarus and Folkman definition
Historical aspects of the stress concept	Walter Canon
	Hans Selye
	Joseph Brady
Theories of job stress	Definition of occupational stress
	Models of occupational stress
	Measurement of occupational stress
Prevalence of occupational stress	U.S. workers' stress levels
Stress and conditions in the work environment	Pathogenic work environment
	Job demands versus workers' resources
	Reduced decision latitude and control
	Effort–reward imbalance
	Person–environment fit
	Work overload
	Job insecurity
	Harassment and bullying
	Dysfunctional organizational structures
	Hazardous physical environment
Health effects of stress	Adverse physical and mental health outcomes
Physical health	Cardiovascular disease
	Hypertension
	Mortality
	Sleep disturbance
Mental health	Post-traumatic stress disorder
	Impaired cognitive functioning
	Depression and anxiety
	Sense of loneliness and isolation
Stress and employee morale	Absenteeism
	Lessened motivation
	Job dissatisfaction
Lifestyle and health	Physical activity on the job
Stress reduction interventions	Worksite mental health interventions

- Conflict situations. These situations refer to scenarios that require incompatible responses—for example, working longer hours to complete a task versus leaving on time at the end of the day to care for one's family.

History of the Stress Concept

The concept of stress has a lengthy history in psychology, the behavioral sciences, medicine, and allied fields, but often is regarded with scientific skepticism. However, many research findings have shown support for the stress concept. Some key historical developments were Canon's research on gastric function, Selye's formulation of the general adaption syndrome, and Brady's "executive monkey" experiments.

Several researchers in the 1800s and early 1900s had observed the gastrointestinal functioning of dogs and of human subjects who had gastric fistulas (holes in their stomachs that could be observed from outside the body).[8] This research suggested that changes in gastric secretions accompanied stressful events, such as pain, hunger, and major emotion. One of the interesting contributions in this area came from Walter Canon (1871–1945), who began studies of digestive function in cats and subsequently in a human subject "Tom," who had an open fistula in his stomach. Canon observed experiments under way with Tom and deduced that when Tom experienced frustration or conflict, his stomach secretions increased. One implication of this research finding was the possibility that stress could have adverse effects on the human body.

Hans Selye (1907–1982) postulated that stress has both negative and positive aspects, which he characterized through use of the words "eustress" and "distress." Eustress (good stress) denotes stress that has positive qualities[9]; distress refers to stress that has negative or undesirable consequences.[10] Distress can result from excessive demands placed upon the individual as in the case of an overworked assembly-line employee or professional worker. Ironically, a job that makes too few demands could also be stressful: a highly educated person forced to take an intellectually undemanding job might be under stress.

In contrast with distress, the term eustress denotes a worker's state that might occur when stresses exist but are kept at a moderate level. This view posits that certain levels of stress are desirable and that organizations should maintain some degree of stress among the workforce to optimize performance. Other researchers, however, have challenged this point of view.[11]

Selye specified in detail the stages of reaction to stress through the concept of the general adaptation syndrome.[12] He conceived of stress as a change in the environment of the organism and proposed that the organism's response consists of three stages: alarm reaction, stage of resistance, and stage of exhaustion. Activation of the general adaptation syndrome is associated with secretion of corticoids—that is, hormones produced by the adrenal gland and implicated in stress responses. Corticoid secretion may produce somatic disease, such as mineralocorticoid hypertension (hypertension caused by excessive activation of mineralocorticoid receptors) and cardiac necrosis (death of cardiac tissue).[13]

Selye's Concept of the General Adaptation Syndrome

1. Alarm reaction: physiologic responses associated with preparation to deal with stress and that lead the animal or person to fight or escape from the stressor.
2. Stage of resistance: return of physiologic responses to normal and resistance to further stressful stimuli.
3. Stage of exhaustion: failure of the organism to adapt to overwhelming stresses. "Adaptation energy" becomes exhausted, and, in the case of humans, severe bodily disease and death may result.

Executive Monkey Experiments

The term executive monkey refers to a monkey that is exposed to stress via the requirement to press a lever so as to avert an electric shock during an experiment (**FIGURE 9.3**). In the 1950s, Brady conducted a series of executive monkey experiments, which made an analogy between monkeys in a stressful experiment and executives at work. "The general context of Brady's study (1958) [reported in *Scientific American*] is stress, specifically, the effects of 'workplace stressors' and 'being in control.' Executives (in industry and business organisations), as an occupational group, face above-average stress levels (along with nurses, social workers, teachers, and those working in the emergency services). They constantly have to make important decisions, and are responsible for the outcomes. This is very stressful ('executive stress')."[14(p. 26)]

In Brady's experiments, several monkeys were tested in pairs consisting of an "executive monkey" and a "control monkey." The executive monkey was able to prevent an electric shock by pressing a lever. This phase, called the avoidance condition of the trial, was considered a form of psychological stress. The research team cued the executive monkey about an impending shock by turning on a red light during the avoidance period. The control monkey could press a similar-looking nonfunctional lever; that is, it was unable to prevent the shock by pressing the lever. Eventually the control monkey lost interest in pressing it.

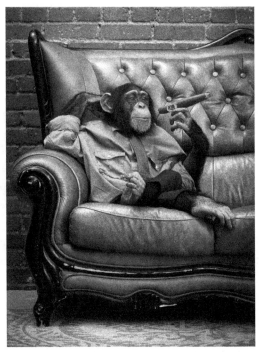

FIGURE 9.3   Executive monkey experiment

© lisegagne/iStockphoto.com

In the first pair, the executive monkey died after 23 days of participation in the experiment and, at autopsy, was found to have developed
severe gastrointestinal lesions.[15,16] The control monkey did not develop
such lesions. Other pairs of monkeys experienced a similar fate. This finding was consistent with the theory that high stress levels affect the gastrointestinal system via increases in secretion of stomach acids. One could
theorize that the control monkeys did not experience the high stress levels
that characterized the executive monkeys. Although considered unethical
in many respects when viewed in the light of contemporary standards for
experimentation, an implication of Brady's research was that stress could
have adverse and even fatal health consequences.

Occupational Stress: A Theoretical Perspective

According to one theoretical point of view, occupational stress results from
a mismatch between the capabilities of the worker and the demands of a
job. Several theoretical models have been developed to better conceptualize

the etiology of stress in the workplace and the health effects of exposure to occupational stress. Nevertheless, measurement of occupational stress remains a daunting methodologic challenge.

Definition of Job Stress (Occupational Stress)

For the purposes of this chapter, the terms "job stress," "occupational stress," "work stress," and "workplace stress" will be used as synonyms. Job stress (occupational stress) can be defined as "the harmful physical and emotional responses that occur when the requirements of the job do not match the capabilities, resources, or needs of the worker. Job stress can lead to poor health and even injury."[17(p. 6)] An employee may experience stress if he or she appraises (judges) the workplace as posing a challenge or a threat.[18] Job stress encompasses an extensive domain of environmental factors in the workplace that could be meaningful for workers' health and well-being.[19]

According to the American Psychological Association, job stresses are accompanied by a sense of powerlessness, coupled with helplessness and hopelessness.[1] Moreover, some levels and types of employment are prone to high stress levels—for example, providing secretarial services, waiting tables, working in law enforcement, holding middle management positions, and serving as a medical intern.[1]

Measurement of Stress in the Workplace

Some critics assert that the concept of job stress is ambiguous and poorly defined.[20] Also, the definition varies according to academic specialization—that is, whether the definition is taken from the psychological, environmental sciences, or biological disciplines.[21] The ambiguous nature of this concept detracts from our ability to construct reliable and valid measurement tools for it. The measurement of job stress would be facilitated by differentiating among several types of categories of measurement—for example, demands and stressors, healthy responses to stress, stress modifiers, and distress at the individual level.

One simple measure of job stress asks individuals, "Is your job stressful?" In fact, this or similar items are used in some national surveys of workplace stress. Although most of us could answer this question, the information obtained might not be helpful because the question is ambiguous and people define a "stressful job" in different ways. One possibility for improving the measurement of workplace stress is to use changes in biomarkers (e.g., cortisol) that occur in response to stress.[22]

Models of Job Stress

The NIOSH approach to job stress and model of job stress (**FIGURE 9.4**) are helpful for providing an overview of job stresses and associated health outcomes. Figure 9.4 includes stressful job conditions, individual and situational factors, and risk of injury and illness. **EXHIBIT 9.1** provides an explanation of the NIOSH approach.

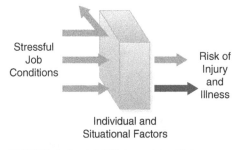

FIGURE 9.4   NIOSH model of job stress

Reproduced from Centers for Disease Control and Prevention, National Institute for Occupational Safety and Health, Stress…at work. DHHS (NIOSH) Publication No. 99-101. Cincinnati, OH: NIOSH; 1999.

In developing a model of job stress, one might include three classes of variables: independent variables or exposure factors (e.g., specific stressors), intermediate or modifying variables (e.g., individual responses, supportive relationships), and associated health outcomes (e.g., illnesses). Among the variables included in stress models is the concept of job strain. Job strain comprises employees' responses, both physiologic and mental, to exposures to stressors.[19] Outcomes associated with exposures to stressors and the strains they produce can include various psychological disorders and adverse physical health outcomes such as coronary heart disease.

The following models of job stress are reviewed here:

- Job demand–control model
- Effort–reward imbalance model
- Person–environment fit model

EXHIBIT 9.1   NIOSH Approach to Job Stress

On the basis of experience and research, NIOSH favors the view that working conditions play a primary role in causing job stress. However, the role of individual factors is not ignored. According to the NIOSH view, exposure to stressful working conditions (called job stressors) can have a direct influence on worker safety and health. But as shown [in Figure 9.4], individual and other situational factors can intervene to strengthen or weaken this influence…. Examples of individual and situational factors that can help to reduce the effects of stressful working conditions include the following:

- Balance between work and family or personal life
- A support network of friends and coworkers
- A relaxed and positive outlook

Reprinted from Centers for Disease Control and Prevention. National Institute for Occupational Safety and Health (NIOSH). Stress…at work. Cincinnati, OH: NIOSH; 1999. DHHS (NIOSH) Publication No. 99-101.

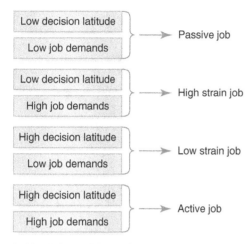

FIGURE 9.5   Job strain model

Data from Karasek RA, Jr. Job demands, job decision latitude, and mental strain: implications for job redesign. administrative science quarterly. 1979;24:288.

Job Demand–Control Model

The job demand–control (JD-C) model postulates an association between job strain and a combination of a high-demand job and low decision latitude (**FIGURE 9.5**). Robert Karasek is credited with developing and refining key aspects of this model,[23] which has been the focus of much empirical effort.

Decision latitude (job control) is the degree to which workers have authority to make decisions about the way in which a task is completed. It refers to "the level of skill and creativity required on the job and the flexibility the worker is permitted in deciding what skills to employ, and also the organisationally mediated possibilities for workers to make decisions about their work."[24(p. 296)] European studies have demonstrated large gender differences in perceived control decision latitude, with more men than women perceiving that they have decision latitude (job control).[25]

According to the JD-C model, job strain arises from work-related conditions of high demand (e.g., high workload and elevated levels of other job demands) and low control or decision latitude (e.g., constraints in alternative actions that can be taken to address these demands). Karasek's model (Figure 9.5) specifies four typologies of jobs that correspond to two levels (high and low) of demands and two levels of strains (high and low):

- High-strain job: low decision latitude and high demands
- Low-strain job: low demands and high decision latitude
- Passive job: low demands and low decision latitude
- Active job: high demand and high decision latitude

Another aspect of the JD-C model is that social support from associates and supervisors is hypothesized to mediate employees' responses to job demands and their own levels of decision authority.[26]

Effort–Reward Imbalance Model

The effort–reward imbalance (ERI) model, which was developed by Siegrist, proposes that the combination of high efforts at work with low rewards is likely to engender job stress.[27] It posits that such an imbalance between efforts and rewards in the work setting is associated with poor health.[28] In a review of 45 empirical studies of the ERI model, van Vegchel et al.

concluded that research supported an association between effort–reward imbalance at work and reduced employee health.[28] An example of an employee who is experiencing ERI is someone who is required to spend many hours working overtime to meet a deadline while simultaneously being confronted with the threat of layoff and few opportunities for alternative employment.[29]

Evaluation: Status of JD-C and ERI Models

Both the JD-C and ERI models have received empirical support. One example of supportive research for the models was a cross-sectional survey of more than 11,000 Dutch employees.[30] The researchers found that these models could account for adverse health symptoms, emotional exhaustion, and job dissatisfaction. The findings were supported for both male and female survey respondents.

Also, both models have been helpful in exploring the influence of work-related psychosocial influences on health inequalities. Jobs with high demands and low control, as well as those with high demands and low rewards, tend to be occupied by lower-status employees. The result may be health inequalities that reflect workers' sustained exposures to stress.[31]

A further elaboration of both the JD-C and ERI models is the job demands–resources model (JD-R) model, which includes two categories of work-related risk factors for job stress: job demands and job resources.[32] Thus, the JD-R model unites many of the features of the JD-C and ERI models and, according to Bakker and Demerouti, is more flexible and rigorous than either model by itself.[32] The JD-R model is applicable to many types of occupations and is helpful for enhancing employee well-being and performance.

Person–Environment Fit Model

The person–environment (P-E) fit model offers a theoretical perspective for characterizing such dimensions as the influence of work overload on worker strain and job dissatisfaction. This model takes into account the degree to which the characteristics of the person align with those of the environment. Adjustment (person–environment fit) of an individual is defined as "the goodness of fit between the characteristics of the person and the properties of his [or her] environment."[33(p. 316)]

In the context of the occupational environment, as person–environment fit decreases, adjustment decreases and the worker's situation becomes increasingly more stressful. One illustration of poor P-E fit is work overload, which refers to the inability of an employee to meet demands of the job setting. Work overload can be envisioned as a discrepancy between demands for work output and the capacity of an individual to meet those demands. The consequences of lack of adjustment to the work environment are the experience of a stressful state and accompanying strains that may culminate in adverse physical and mental health outcomes.

The Work Environment and Job Stress

Risk factors for job stress are identifiable conditions that involve the interpersonal environment and the design of the workspace. "These factors include a toxic work environment, negative workload, isolation, types of hours worked, role conflict, role ambiguity, lack of autonomy, career development barriers, difficult relationships with administrators and/or coworkers, managerial bullying, harassment, and organizational climate."[18(p. 89)]

The manner in which work is organized—for example, how work systems and procedures are designed—has implications for job stress.[34] Work-related stress arises when work demands and pressures are out of phase with workers' levels of knowledge and abilities. Stress also can occur when little support is available to workers from their supervisors and colleagues, and when workers have little control over the various processes that take place in the work environment.

The American Psychological Association has identified the top five factors for work stress: inadequate compensation, poor opportunity for advancement, work overload, long working hours, and uncertain work expectations (**FIGURE 9.6**). **EXHIBIT 9.2** presents additional examples of job

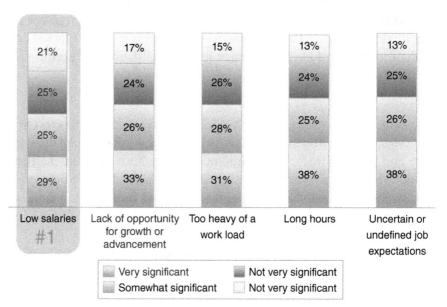

FIGURE 9.6   Top five work stress factors in 2012

EXHIBIT 9.2   Job Conditions that May Lead to Stress

* *Design of tasks*: Heavy workload, infrequent rest breaks, long work hours, and shift-work; hectic and routine tasks that have little inherent meaning, do not utilize workers' skills, and provide little sense of control

* *Management style*: Lack of participation by workers in decision making, poor communication in the organization, lack of family-friendly policies

* *Interpersonal relationships*: Poor social environment and lack of support or help from coworkers and supervisors

* *Work roles*: Conflicting or uncertain job expectations, too much responsibility, too many "hats to wear"

* *Career concerns*: Job insecurity and lack of opportunity for growth, advancement, or promotion; rapid changes for which workers are unprepared

* *Environmental conditions*: Unpleasant or dangerous physical conditions such as crowding, noise, air pollution, or ergonomic problems

Modified from Centers for Disease Control and Prevention. National Institute for Occupational Safety and Health (NIOSH). Stress…at work. DHHS (NIOSH) Publication No. 99-101. Cincinnati, OH: NIOSH; 1999, page 9.

---

stress risk factors, as identified by the National Institute for Occupational Safety and Health.

Work Overload/Long Working Hours

Both work overload and long working hours contribute to job stress. Work overload is the situation in which an employee is assigned more work than he or she is capable of finishing. Long working hours often require that employees remain on the job site even after they have become physically and mentally exhausted. Long working hours are implicated in chronic diseases such as coronary heart disease.[35]

Irregular Work Schedules/Shiftwork

Irregular work schedules and shiftwork are associated with adverse health outcomes that include temporary somatic disturbances and increased risks of chronic disease. "Shiftwork involves working outside the normal daylight hours … around 7 a.m. to 6 p.m."[36(p. 1)] Some irregular work schedules require that workers rotate between working during the day-time and at night. Among the health effects of shiftwork are sleep disturbance, disruption of the body's circadian rhythm (the normal rhythms tied to activity and sleep), tiredness, gastrointestinal conditions, and heart disease (**FIGURE 9.7**). In addition, shiftwork might exacerbate existing

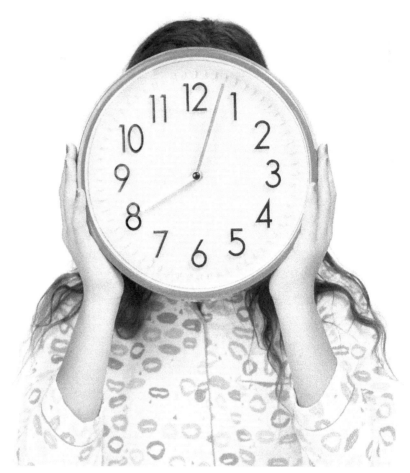

FIGURE 9.7   Sleep and shiftwork
© Kamira/Shutterstock

health problems. A study conducted at a German chemical factory suggested that shiftwork might have long-term adverse health effects such as overweight, diabetes, and circulatory conditions.[37] Another consequence of shiftwork is limitation of a worker's participation in family life.

Job Insecurity

Contemporary trends related to job insecurity are global competition and decreasing regulation of the workplace. Many workers feel insecure about the stability of their employment because of drastic changes in their places of employment. One of the most significant changes is the trend toward reducing the size of the workforce in the interest of profitability and efficiency (keeping production exactly in line with anticipated demand). Numerous companies employ temporary workers and independent contractors who have limited job security. These phenomena contribute to job insecurity, which is a growing problem both in the United States and internationally. For example, researchers in Taiwan found that job insecurity was related to poor health among a large representative sample of adult men and women workers in that country.[38]

Harassment and Workplace Bullying

Research has identified workplace harassment and bullying as important factors in psychological distress. Workplace harassment includes intimidation and the threat of physical violence, but may also involve sexual harassment—for example, comments of a sexual nature that an employee does not welcome. Harassment may originate from a worker's peers or supervisors. Related to harassment is workplace bullying, a form of intimidation that often originates from supervisors. Bullying can be a major source of job-related stress, has potential for causing psychological harm to the target of bullying, and may result in high costs for both the affected individual and the job site. One study that examined workplace bullying within the travel industry in New Zealand found that it was a frequent occurrence and a major determinant of employee stress.[39]

Organization of Work and Job Stress

The structure of an organization and the configuration of work-related procedures are related to levels of workers' stress.[34] In addition, organizational practices are determinants of workplace safety. Desirable organizational practices are inclusion of employees in the decision-making process and encouraging management to be concerned about occupational health and safety.[40]

The term organization of work (work organization) refers to "the work process (the way jobs are designed and performed) and to the organizational practices (management and production methods and accompanying human resource policies) that influence the job design."[41(p. 2)] In poorly designed organizational systems, workers lack control over processes.[34] In turn, this factor contributes to job stress.

Marchand et al. examined how pathogenic work organization conditions contribute to psychological distress among workers in Canada.[42] Examples of conditions associated with distress were demands (physical and psychological) made upon workers, use of irregular work shifts, and harassment. Also related to psychological distress were the worker's family situation and lack of social support outside of work. **EXHIBIT 9.3** describes the importance of organization of work.

> **EXHIBIT 9.3   Changing Organization of Work and Associated Risks of Stress, Illness, and Injury in the Workplace**
>
> The expressions "work organization" and "organization of work" refer to the nature of the work process (the way jobs are designed and performed) and to the organizational practices (e.g., management and production methods and accompanying human resources policies) that influence the design of jobs. Organizational downsizing and restructuring, dependence on temporary and contractor-supplied labor, and adoption of lean production practices are examples of recent trends in organizational practices that have been the subject of increased scrutiny in job stress research. Concerns have arisen that these trends may adversely influence aspects of job design (e.g., work schedules, work load demands, job security) that are associated with risk of job stress.
>
> ... [W]ork organization can have broader implications for the safety and health of workers—not just for stress-related outcomes. For example, long hours of work may increase exposures to chemical and physical hazards in the workplace, or night shifts may expose workers to heightened risk of violence. These causal pathways between work organization and worker safety and health are illustrated in [FIGURE 9.8, which] portrays a somewhat broader causal model, showing that new organizational practices of concern are the products of various background forces, including the growing global economy, changing worker demographics and the labor supply, and technological innovation.
>
> *Source:* Centers for Disease Control and Prevention, National Institute for Occupational Safety and Health. Work organization and stress-related disorders. n.d. http://www.cdc.gov/niosh/programs/workorg/. Accessed August 14, 2013.

Physical Work Environment and Stress

Conditions that exist in the physical work environment itself—for example, high noise levels, crowding, inadequate lighting, and lack of air conditioning— may exacerbate workers' stress levels. For instance, some hospital settings are noisy environments filled with beeping monitors and whirring surgical

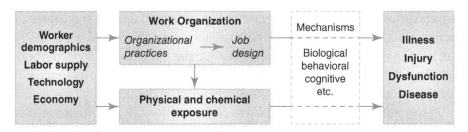

FIGURE 9.8   Causal pathways between work organization and worker safety and health

Centers for Disease Control and Prevention. National Institute for Occupational Safety and Health (NIOSH). Work organization and stress-related disorders. Program Description. http://www.cdc.gov/niosh/programs/workorg/. Accessed August 14, 2013.

instruments that can cause stress for patients and workers alike. High ambient temperature levels in work surroundings can cause heat stress. Inadequate lighting or harsh artificial lighting can interfere with work by causing eye strain. Crowded workspaces can be noisy and interfere with workers' concentration. The potential adverse psychosocial and physical health effects of the physical work environment are demonstrated by computer work, as described in **EXHIBIT 9.4**.

EXHIBIT 9.4   Computer Work

The potential adverse health effects of computer work have enormous public health implications, given the large percentage of employees who use computers routinely at work. Computer work can be highly stressful due to the conditions under which many workers must perform—for example, the need to work under time pressure and for long hours. Feelings of being under stress can contribute to mental health symptoms such as anxiety and depression. These stresses can be exacerbated by the ergonomics of computer work, such as the position of the monitor, the posture while typing, and the placement of the arms and wrists. Some of the specific adverse effects of computer work include the following:

- *Eye strain*: Staring at a computer screen can result in eye irritation, dry eyes, sore eye muscles, and headache.

- *Effects upon musculoskeletal system*: These effects can impact the neck, shoulders, and upper extremities and may result in soreness and lower back pain. Workers who remain stationary—sitting or standing—for long time intervals can experience leg swelling. Other examples of musculoskeletal disorders include the following conditions:

  o *Mouse arm*: Problems with the neck, shoulders, arms, and hands associated with use of a computer mouse.[1]

  o *Vulture neck*: An S-shaped curve in the neck caused when learning forward to better view the screen.[1]

Typing on a computer keyboard is a low-intensity and highly sedentary activity (called static work) that can produce prolonged strain on the shoulders, arms, wrists, hands, and back. The duration of work with visual display units is a risk factor for musculoskeletal disorders. Psychosocial risk factors proposed for such disorders include high job demands, time pressure, mental stress, and high workload.[2] Often computer work is associated with these risk factors even though it is an activity with low physical demands.

[1]Swedish Work Environment Authority. Computer work. n.d. http://www.av.se/dokument/inenglish/themes/computer_work.pdf. Accessed June 23, 2014.

[2]Wahlström J. Ergonomics, musculoskeletal disorders and computer work. *Occup Med.* 2005;55:168–176.

Physical Health Effects of Occupational Stress

The physical health effects associated with occupational stress are known also as health outcomes. Stress-related health outcomes are "the more enduring negative health states thought to result from exposure to job stressors."[19(p. 368)] Empirical research suggests that sustained job stress may incite biological reactions that culminate in reduced health status. Examples of such outcomes include cardiovascular disease and the conditions shown in TABLE 9.2, which lists several adverse physical health outcomes that are believed to be related to work-related stressors.

Cardiovascular Disease/Coronary Heart Disease

There appears to be a relationship between stress and heart disease (FIGURE 9.9). Coronary heart disease (CHD) is the leading cause of mortality in the United States for both men and women. This condition is responsible for major social and economic costs from lost work time due to absenteeism and medical care costs. Only a limited amount of research has been conducted on the role of occupational exposures and CHD, which is a topic worthy of additional investigation.

FIGURE 9.10 shows potential work-related risk factors for occupational heart disease. Environmental and physiological CHD risk factors include occupational exposures to toxic chemicals (e.g., carbon monoxide), extreme temperatures, environmental tobacco smoke, shiftwork, and level of physical activity on the job. In addition to the factors shown in Figure 9.10, job stress is an occupational exposure thought to be related to CHD. Accordingly, researchers have concluded that there is strong evidence that job strain is related to CHD and CHD risk factors.[45] However, the research literature reveals a body of inconsistent findings.

Examples of supportive studies for this relationship were published by Belkic et al., Virtanen et al., and Theorell et al. For example, Belkic et al.

TABLE 9.2   Hypothesized Physical Health Effects of Occupational Stress*

- Coronary heart disease/cardiovascular disease
- Hypertension
- Sleep disturbance
- Mortality: Increased among older workers with low job control[43]
- Health complaints, such as coughs, headaches, joint and muscle aches, abdominal pain[44]
- Musculoskeletal disorders
- Ulcers

*Outcomes suggested by research.

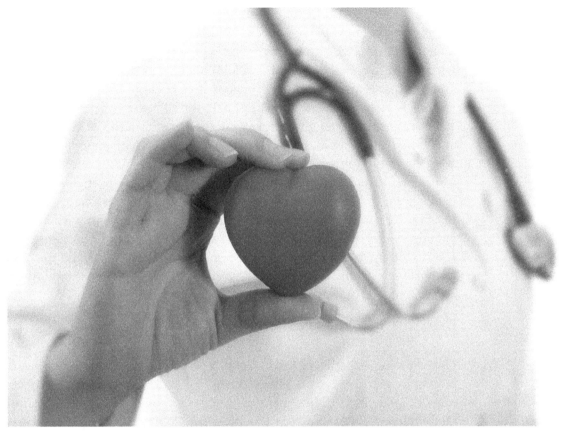

FIGURE 9.9   Stress and heart disease

© stockCe/Shutterstock

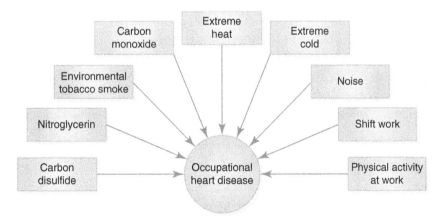

FIGURE 9.10   Potential work-related risk factors for occupational heart disease

Data from Centers for Disease Control and Prevention. National Institute for Occupational Safety and Health Administration (NIOSH). Occupational heart disease. http://www.cdc.gov/niosh/topics/heart disease/. Accessed October 2, 2013

reported that job strain is consistently related to cardiovascular disease among men but not among women.[46] Virtanen et al. published results from a meta-analysis, which indicated that long working hours are associated with a 40% increase in risk of developing CHD, as demonstrated by prospective observational studies.[35] Theorell et al. found that low decision latitude is associated with increased risk of first heart attack.[47]

Examples of nonconfirmatory findings came from the work of Hlatky et al. and Pelfrene et al. Hlatky et al. investigated whether employment in a high-demand job with low decision latitude is associated with the prevalence and severity of coronary artery disease.[48] Study participants were patients undergoing coronary angiography; they were classified according to three groups ranging from significant coronary disease to normal individuals. No relationship was found between job strain and prevalence and severity of coronary artery disease. Similarly, Pelfrene et al. did not find support for a strong relationship between high levels of occupational strain and coronary risk.[49]

Hypertension

Hypertension—that is, elevated blood pressure—is a risk factor for heart attacks and strokes, and is one of the hypothesized cardiovascular effects of work-related stress. In a meta-analysis, one group of researchers examined the relationship between job strain and ambulatory blood pressure. The researchers concluded that job strain increased the risk of elevated ambulatory blood pressure and that programs for work-site surveillance of ambulatory blood pressure are needed to promote cardiovascular risk factor reduction.[50]

Schnall et al. conducted a prospective study of 195 male workers that sought to examine the relationship between job strain and ambulatory blood pressure. The investigators found a relationship between job strain and elevated ambulatory blood pressure levels at follow-up. They concluded, "These results provide new evidence supporting the hypothesis that job strain is an occupational risk factor in the etiology of essential hypertension."[51(p. 697)]

Sleep Disturbances

Sleep disturbance is one of the reported adverse consequences of job stress. Workers who have disturbed sleep are vulnerable to work errors and unintentional injuries. Lallukka et al. surveyed middle-aged adult employees of the city of Helsinki, Finland.[52] Their research examined a range of psychosocial aspects of the employment environment, including job strain, physically strenuous working conditions, and work–family conflicts. All three variables were found to be related to complaints about sleep disturbances.

Job Stress and Mental Health

Potential consequences of occupational stress also include adverse mental health outcomes and behavioral disturbances. In the words of a NIOSH report, "Stress-related disorders encompass a broad array of conditions, including frank psychological disorders (depression, anxiety, post-traumatic stress disorder) and other emotional disturbances (dissatisfaction, fatigue, tension, etc.), maladaptive behaviors (aggression, substance abuse), and cognitive impairment. In turn, these conditions may lead to poor work performance or even injury."[4]

Methods for assessing employee mental health include analyses of consultation rates for mental health services and surveys of mental health issues among employees. A Japanese study of mental consultation rates found that computer systems engineers had higher consultation rates than other categories of white-collar jobs. This finding suggests that the occupation of computer systems engineer is stressful in Japan and can have adverse impacts on mental health.[53]

The National Opinion Research Center conducts the General Social Survey (GSS), which collects information on how frequently employees perceive their work as stressful. In 2002, the GSS included items addressing work organization and stress-related disorders such as poor mental health. Respondents were queried regarding the number of days during the past month that they experienced poor mental health. FIGURE 9.11 shows the mental health responses classified according to industry sector. The highest percentage (17%) of workers who reported 14 or more days of poor mental health in the past month were employed in the retail trade sector.[54]

The remainder of this section discusses the implications of job stress and related psychosocial phenomena for the mental health of workers. TABLE 9.3 provides some examples of adverse psychological effects of occupational stress covered here.

Impaired Cognitive Functioning

Cognitive functioning (e.g., difficulties with concentration, memory, decision making, and thinking) can be impaired by job stress. In one study, researchers examined the association between cognitive complaints and psychosocial work factors among representative samples of Swedish workers.[55] The investigators reported that a group of work-related characteristics— job demands, job conflicts, and being underqualified to perform specific

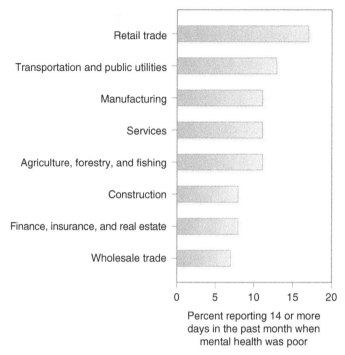

FIGURE 9.11   Employee reports of poor mental health (by industry sector)

Reprinted from Centers for Disease Control and Prevention. National Institute for Occupational Safety and Health (NIOSH). Work organization and stress-related disorders. Inputs: occupational safety and health risks. http://www.cdc.gov/niosh/programs/workorg /risks.html. Accessed August 14, 2013

TABLE 9.3   Examples of Adverse Psychological Effects of Occupational Stress

Name of Effect	Definition or Example
Impaired cognitive functioning	Difficulties with concentration, memory, decision making, and thinking
Depression and anxiety (Bureau of Labor Statistics classification: anxiety, stress, and neurotic disorders)	Generalized anxiety disorder, major depressive disorder
Loneliness	The result of workers' sense of isolation often due to organizational structures and norms
Post-traumatic stress disorder	A mental health condition triggered by a terrifying event*; symptoms include flashbacks, nightmares, and severe anxiety

* Mayo Clinic. Post-traumatic stress disorder (PTSD). n.d. http://www.mayoclinic.org /diseases-conditions/post-traumatic-stress-disorder/basics/definition/con-20022540. Accessed March 26, 2014.

work tasks—were positively related to cognitive complaints. Negatively associated factors included social support, being overqualified for a job, and having adequate work resources.

Anxiety, Stress, and Neurotic Disorders

The Bureau of Labor Statistics groups occupational illnesses stemming from adverse mental health states under the category of anxiety, stress, and neurotic disorders. The Survey of Occupational Injuries and Illnesses (SOII) collects information on this group of conditions from private industry.

Anxiety, stress, and neurotic disorders more frequently cause extended periods of lost work time than all other nonfatal injuries and illnesses.[54] **FIGURE 9.12**, which presents the most recently available data on this issue (for 2001), shows that beginning with 11 to 20 days away from work, a greater percentage of employees with anxiety, stress, and neurotic disorders were absent than workers afflicted with all nonfatal injuries and illnesses. Among injuries and illnesses that required more than 30 days off, 42% were from anxiety, stress, and neurotic disorders, in comparison with 22% for all nonfatal injuries and illnesses. The highest incidence rate of anxiety, stress, and neurotic disorders occurred among employees in the

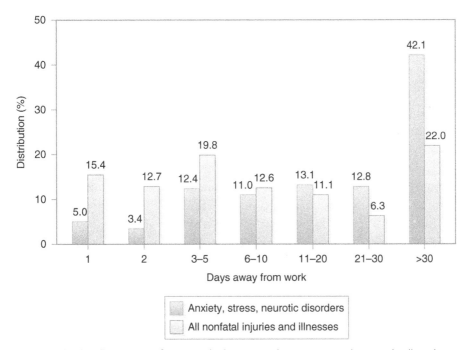

FIGURE 9.12   Days away from work due to anxiety, stress, and neurotic disorders compared to days lost for all injuries and illness

Reprinted from Centers for Disease Control and Prevention. National Institute for Occupational Safety and Health (NIOSH). Work organization and stress-related disorders. Inputs: occupational safety and health risks. http://www.cdc.gov/niosh/programs/workorg/risks.html. Accessed August 14, 2013.

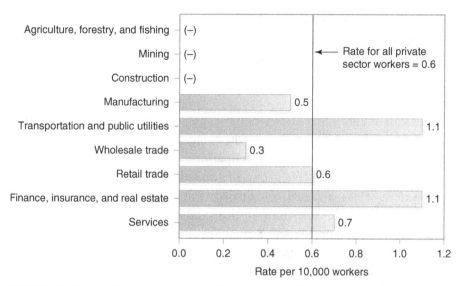

FIGURE 9.13   Incidence rates of anxiety, stress, and neurotic disorders (by industry sector)

Reprinted from Centers for Disease Control and Prevention. National Institute for Occupational Safety and Health (NIOSH). Work organization and stress-related disorders. Inputs: occupational safety and health risks. http://www.cdc.gov /niosh/programs/workorg/risks.html. Accessed August 14, 2013.

transportation and public utilities sector and in the finance, insurance, and real estate sector (**FIGURE 9.13**).

Anxiety and Depression

Several studies have examined the influence of the work-related psychosocial environment on anxiety and depression. As this area of research is quite extensive, a comprehensive review is beyond the scope of this text. In summary, the findings suggest that job strain and other psychosocial factors can play a role in development of both anxiety and depression. Two representative examples of studies are presented here; both were European investigations.

In a cross-sectional study of almost 8000 male and female workers randomly sampled from the French working population, anxiety and depression were studied in relationship to psychosocial work factors.[56] The investigators found that low decision latitude, over-commitment, and emotional demands were risk factors for generalized anxiety disorder and major depressive disorder.

In the Whitehall II study, Stansfield et al. reported that job strain was a risk factor for depression.[57] Their model of job strain involved high work demands combined with low control over work. Carried out between 1985 and 1988, the Whitehall II study included a cohort of 10,308 civil service workers in London.

Loneliness

The structure of an organization and the social climate within an organization may limit communication among employees and contribute to a sense of isolation and loneliness. In some organizations, employees may be expected to work independently without support and feedback from colleagues. Loneliness in the workplace is hypothesized to have a negative impact on work quality and the personal lives of employees.[58]

Post-Traumatic Stress Disorder

Traumatic events that occur at work are potential sources of occupational stress. Notably, first responders and other workers who experience job-related traumatic events such as those caused by motor vehicle crashes or mass casualties from disasters can be at increased risk of a condition known as post-traumatic stress disorder. "Post-traumatic stress disorder (PTSD) is a mental health condition that's triggered by a terrifying event. Symptoms may include flashbacks, nightmares and severe anxiety, as well as uncontrollable thoughts about the event."[59] Work-associated PTSD can lower productivity, result in absenteeism, and be a factor in loss of employment.[60] Categories of employees who have high rates of PTSD include disaster rescue workers, emergency service personnel, and police and fire department personnel.[61] Military veterans are also an affected group.

A term related to PTSD is traumatic incident stress. Traumatic incidence stress results from experience of a catastrophic event such as a terrorism-linked attack, natural disaster, or act of war (see **EXHIBIT 9.5**). This form of stress may be accompanied by intense emotional reactions and

---

EXHIBIT 9.5   Case Study of Responders to the September 11, 2011, Terrorist Attacks

First responders and disaster workers at the site of the September 11, 2001, terrorist attacks on the World Trade Center in New York witnessed events that could impact their mental health severely. Many workers who participated in the recovery operations at this site experienced psychological distress and were at increased risk of psychopathology. For example, Stellman et al. investigated the occurrence of psychological distress and psychopathology among workers involved with the 9/11 recovery operations and reported that some individuals developed chronic mental health and social impairments.[62]

Given the frequent occurrence of distress and adverse mental health outcomes, the 9/11 disaster highlights the need for an in-place comprehensive mental health treatment program that would be available for workers who respond to future disasters. Such a program should include ongoing post-disaster surveillance of mental health issues that need to be addressed by treatment programs.[63]

TABLE 9.4   Symptoms of Stress that May Be Experienced During or After a Traumatic Incident

Physical	Cognitive	Emotional	Behavioral
Chest pain	Confusion	Anxiety	Intense anger
Difficulty breathing	Nightmares	Guilt	Withdrawal
Shock symptoms	Disorientation	Grief	Emotional outburst
Fatigue	Heightened or lowered alertness	Denial	Temporary loss or increase of appetite
Nausea/vomiting		Severe panic (rare)	
Dizziness	Poor concentration	Fear	Excessive alcohol consumption
Profuse sweating	Memory problems	Irritability	Inability to rest, pacing
Rapid heart rate	Poor problem solving	Loss of emotional control	Change in sexual functioning
Thirst	Difficulty identifying familiar objects or people	Depression	
Headaches		Sense of failure	
Visual difficulties		Feeling overwhelmed	
Clenching of jaw		Blaming others or self	
Nonspecific aches and pains			

Source: Adapted from Centers for Disease Control and Prevention, National Institute for Occupational Safety and Health. Traumatic incidence stress: information for emergency response workers. 2002. http://www.cdc.gov/niosh/mining/UserFiles/works/pdfs/2002-107.pdf. Accessed March 26, 2014.

symptoms. It can affect disaster first responders—for example, emergency services personnel. **TABLE 9.4** lists symptoms of traumatic incident stress.

To examine this issue further, investigators studied volunteer emergency medical services personnel for their responses to chronic stress and coping techniques for managing stress.[64] Among these workers' responses were emotional exhaustion and a sense of depersonalization. Such findings highlight the need to include coping strategies for chronic stress in mental health programs for emergency medical services personnel.

Employee Morale in the Occupational Setting

Workplace stress is one of the determinants of employee morale. Employee morale is the "[d]escription of the emotions, attitude, satisfaction, and overall outlook of employees during their time in a workplace environment."[65] In work settings with high morale, employees are happy and hold their workplace in positive regard. The level of employee morale is correlated with job productivity and commitment to the workplace. In comparison with employees who are unhappy with their workplace, those with high morale are more likely to contribute productively to their work setting. Low employee morale translates into high levels of absenteeism, burnout, and job dissatisfaction, accompanied by reduced motivation.

Cultural influences can affect employee morale. As the U.S. workplace becomes increasingly diverse, cultural factors such as individualistic versus collective orientation become more relevant for the work environment. Workers from a culture that values a collective orientation may be uncomfortable in an environment that values independent, individualist performance. Employers need to take such influences into consideration.[66]

Worker Absenteeism

Worker absenteeism is a phenomenon of major significance for occupational health and public health. The term worker absenteeism refers to frequent or recurrent absences from a job, often without good cause. Sometimes absenteeism can result from specific factors, such as illness. Absenteeism as a result of illness is called sickness absence, which can be transitory or long term. When long term or recurrent, absenteeism can be grounds for dismissal from employment.

Absenteeism has deleterious effects for both employees and employers. For the worker, absenteeism can result in lost wages, social isolation, and reduced opportunity to become reemployed if poor attendance results in dismissal from work. Absenteeism, especially when long term, affects organizations through lost productivity, increased labor costs, and the need to constantly recruit and train new employees.

The following examples are representative of empirical studies that have shown a relationship between stressful working conditions and absenteeism:

- The Belstress study (1994–1998) followed more than 20,000 workers in 25 companies across Belgium.[67] High job strain accompanied by low social support at work predicted risk of sick leave for both male and female employees.
- The Maastricht (Netherlands) prospective cohort study examined sickness absence among 1271 employees of 45 companies and organizations.[24] The results indicated that workers who had at least one chronic disease and low levels of decision latitude were at risk of sickness absence.
- Another investigation of more than 35,000 employees found a significant relationship between behavioral health risks and worker absenteeism.[68] Examples of behavioral health risks were being under stress, having mental health issues, and being at risk of back problems.
- Sickness absence was associated with having a psychiatric disorder in the French GAZ and ELectricité (GAZEL) cohort study of almost 20,000 persons.[69] Sickness absence was also related to increased risk of mortality, particularly from cardiovascular disease and smoking-related cancer.

Coping is the term used to describe how individuals deal with and attempt to overcome difficulties such as stressful work environments. Active coping entails taking actions to focus on the problem at hand; passive coping focuses on withdrawal from a problem. Active and passive styles of coping with stress are hypothesized to have differential health and behavioral outcomes. For example, workers who are under stress and have active coping styles may experience continuous arousal of the autonomic nervous system, resulting in conditions such as high blood pressure. A German study, for example, examined middle managers employed in an automobile production facility.[70] Those managers who worked under low-reward conditions and showed high efforts at work (active coping styles) were at higher risk of hypertension than their counterparts. Those who worked under low-reward conditions and exhibited passive coping behaviors were more likely to experience sickness absence (which was regarded as a form of withdrawal behavior and, therefore, a passive coping style).

Bernaards et al. explored the relationship between sickness absence and general level of physical activity, which was found not to be associated with either sickness absence or work productivity.[71] Among computer workers, obesity was associated with sickness absence and lower work productivity.

Burnout

The concept of burnout refers to a syndrome that consists of emotional exhaustion, a sense of depersonalization (e.g., detachment and disengagement), and a feeling that one is less able to be effective in accomplishing goals. Often, burnout occurs in individuals who work in human services fields.[72] A study of three groups of workers involved with human services, industry, and transport demonstrated that the exhaustion component of burnout was related to high job demands; the lack of job resources was related to disengagement from a job.[73]

Job Dissatisfaction

Job satisfaction is one of the key dimensions of employee morale; employee stress is one of the factors correlated with employee dissatisfaction.[74] Workers with limited opportunities to influence the decision-making process are more likely to have negative attitudes about their job than employees who are allowed to make inputs into the operation of their place of work.[26] Research conducted in the United Kingdom found differences in job satisfaction scores (as well as scores for physical health and psychological well-being) across different types of jobs.[75] Occupations that were potentially stressful tended to have lower-than-average job satisfaction levels. These fields included the teaching profession, law enforcement, social services, soliciting customers via call centers, and emergency medical transport.

Lifestyle and Work

Job stressors, as noted elsewhere in this chapter, are predictive of adverse physical and mental health outcomes. Further, the relationship between job stressors and outcomes can be mediated through health behaviors, which include level of physical activity (ranging from vigorous exercise to being a sedentary "couch potato"), consumption of cigarettes and alcohol, and habitual dietary choices.[76] A meta-analysis examined the mitigating effects of lifestyle on the relationship between job strain and coronary artery disease.[77] The researchers found that adverse lifestyle characteristics (e.g., smoking, physical inactivity, heavy drinking, and obesity) in combination with job strain were related to increased risk of coronary artery disease. In comparison, persons who experienced job strain but maintained a healthy lifestyle did not have a similar risk of heart disease.

Another issue is whether work-related stress is associated with health risk behaviors. In a meta-analysis, researchers verified an association between work-related stress and unhealthy lifestyles (e.g., cigarette smoking, alcohol consumption, and lack of leisure-time exercise). In this study, job strain was an indicator of work-related stress.[78] However, Siegrist and Rödel reported low-level associations between work stress and health risk behavior[79]; in their study, overweight and men's heavy use of alcohol had the strongest associations with job stress.

Sedentary Occupations/Occupational Sitting

Evidence suggests that prolonged occupational sitting is linked with chronic diseases and all-cause mortality.[80] When Simons et al. examined data from more than 120,000 participants in the Netherlands Cohort Study, they concluded that workers who had fewer sitting hours of work and engaged in regular physical activity had a lower risk of colon cancer.[81] Interventions to reduce the duration of sitting times, such as providing an increased number of breaks from sitting, may reduce the risk of adverse health effects associated with excessive occupational sitting.

Interventions for Workplace Stress

The effects of workplace stress include both adverse physical and mental outcomes. As a function of radical alterations in the nature of employment, adverse outcomes from occupational stress are likely to remain a troubling

> **EXHIBIT 9.6   The World Health Organization's Definition of a Healthy Job**
>
> A healthy job is likely to be one where the pressures on employees are appropriate in relation to their abilities and resources, to the amount of control they have over their work, and to the support they receive from people who matter to them. As health is not merely the absence of disease or infirmity but a positive state of complete physical, mental and social well-being …, a healthy working environment is one in which there is not only an absence of harmful conditions but an abundance of health-promoting ones.
>
> *Source:* World Health Organization. Stress at the workplace. n.d. http://www.who.int/occupational_health/topics/stressatwp/en/index.html. Accessed August 24, 2013.

issue for our society. Which interventions could reduce job stresses? What should be the goals of such interventions?

Interventions for workplace stress should seek to create jobs that promote health—that is, "healthy jobs." **EXHIBIT 9.6** presents the World Health Organization's definition of a healthy job. The goal of creating healthy jobs will necessitate that organizations increase their commitment to the promotion of worker health and safety. Not only are these changes desirable from the standpoint of social justice, but they can also yield increased work productivity and greater cost-effectiveness.

Improvement of Mental Health in the Workplace

The workplace can be organized so as to reduce job stress and encourage protective factors for mental health by increasing social support for workers and fostering positive coping responses to stressful situations in the work environment. The European Agency for Safety and Health at Work (EU-OSHA) highlights the following factors as contributors to positive mental health at work:[82]

- "Social support;
- A feeling of inclusion and meaningful work;
- Finding sense in one's work;
- Being able to decide on a course of action during work;
- Being able to organise work according to your own pace."[82]

Primary, Secondary, and Tertiary Prevention of Adverse Mental Health Outcomes

As is true of many other occupational exposures, workplace stress is a preventable condition. Prevention of workplace stress can be aligned with the public health model of prevention, which includes three levels of intervention: primary, secondary, and tertiary prevention.[83] Cooper and Cartwright note that primary prevention would entail overall stress reduction in the workplace[83]; its goal would be to minimize stress so as to prevent stress-related disorders from ever developing. Secondary prevention might involve stress management in a stressful occupational environment among employees who are under stress. Finally, tertiary prevention would include the provision of employment assistance and counseling programs to employees who have already developed stress-related conditions to facilitate their recovery.

Surveillance Programs

Surveillance of work-related psychological disorders and their risk factors aids in elucidating the full extent of the problem of adverse mental health consequences of work.[84] Issues for surveillance should include workplace stressors, emotional demands upon workers, bullying and harassment, violence at work, and injustice.[85] Surveillance data might then be used to develop needed mental health programs and interventions. Often such data can be highly influential when they are collected at the national level. This comprehensive perspective aids researchers in developing a view of psychosocial risk factors for work-associated adverse employee mental health outcomes from the standpoint of an entire country.

Stress Management Training

Chronic occupational stress is associated with a variety of adverse consequences, such as absenteeism and increased risk of poor health for workers and, in turn, increased costs for employers. Given these relationships, it is imperative for employers to restructure the work environment to reduce stress and to develop programs for stress management. Stress management is defined as "[a] set of techniques and programs intended to help people deal more effectively with stress in their lives by analyzing the specific stressors and taking positive actions to minimize their effects. Most stress management programs deal with job stress and workplace issues.... Examples [of stress management methods] include progressive muscular relaxation, guided imagery, biofeedback, breathing techniques, and active problem solving."[86]

Stress management strategies should have comprehensive scope, addressing prevention and management of worker stress, supporting the needs of organizations and individual workers, and incorporating a plan for continuous review and evaluation.[87] Such approaches might include cognitive-behavioral interventions, relaxation training, and organization-focused interventions. Evaluations of interventions directed toward occupational stress demonstrate that they are effective; cognitive-behavioral approaches are among the most effective forms of stress management.[88] "Cognitive behavioral stress management (CBSM) is a short-term therapeutic approach that focuses on how people's thoughts affect their emotions and behaviors."[89] Brief stress management interventions can be effective in reducing stress levels and burnout. Researchers observed this outcome, for example, among social workers who were experiencing high stress levels.[90]

SUMMARY

Job stress (occupational stress) is a common occurrence in the workplace, especially in view of the rapidly evolving nature of work. Both the psychosocial work environment and the organizational structure affect workers' stress levels. Data from surveys of workers suggest that more than two-fifths of employees report being stressed out during the workday.

According to some theoretical perspectives, stress can be both a positive experience (eustress) and a negative occurrence (distress). The latter is related to adverse physical and mental health outcomes. For example, the executive monkey experiments demonstrated that stress can induce physical illness in experimental animals. Among the various models developed to describe work-related stresses are the job demand–control model, the effort–reward imbalance model, and the person–environment fit model. Some of the components of models for stress are decision latitude, job demands, work effort, rewards, and characteristics of workers. Models of occupational stress are used to characterize job strain and work overload and are helpful for improving the psychosocial work environment. Additional factors examined in relation to worker stress are shiftwork, irregular work schedules, and workplace bullying.

The mental health consequences of stress include impaired cognitive functioning and psychiatric disorders. Job stress can be a cause of worker absenteeism, job dissatisfaction, and job burnout. Stress management interventions, such as cognitive-behavioral stress management, have been developed in an effort to reduce job stress and avoid these negative consequences.

STUDY QUESTIONS AND EXERCISES

1. Define the following terms:
   A. Stress
   B. Occupational stress
   C. Job strain
   D. Job dissatisfaction
   E. Coping responses
2. Describe three physical health effects of occupational stress.
3. Describe three hypothesized associations between job stress and chronic disease. Are the effects of job-related stresses solely negative? Can job stress have beneficial aspects?
4. What are some barriers that limit the development of reliable and valid measures of occupational stress?

5. To what extent does work overload contribute to stress? Give examples of occupations in which work overload might occur.
6. Which conditions in the work environment contribute to burnout? Propose methods for preventing burnout.
7. Give examples of how job stress is associated with adverse mental health outcomes. Describe two types of mental disorders that might occur in the workplace.
8. How are low levels of physical activity at work related to adverse physical health outcomes?
9. In your opinion, which changes can be made in the organization of work to minimize the adverse consequences of occupational stress?
10. Which kinds of intervention programs have been created for stress management in occupational settings?

REFERENCES

1. American Psychological Association. Stress in the workplace. n.d. http://www.apa.org/helpcenter/workplace-stress.aspx. Accessed September 11, 2013.
2. American Psychological Association and Harris Interactive. Workplace survey. March 2012. http://www.apa.org/news/press/releases/phwa/workplace-survey.pdf. Accessed March 24, 2014.
3. HuffingtonPost.com. Work stress on the rise: 8 in 10 Americans are stressed about their jobs, survey finds. April 10, 2013. http://www.huffingtonpost.com/2013/04/10work-stress-jobs-americans_n_3053428.html. Accessed May 22, 2013.
4. Centers for Disease Control and Prevention, National Institute for Occupational Safety and Health. Work organization and stress-related disorders: program description. n.d. http://www.cdc.gov/niosh/programs/workorg/. Accessed August 14, 2013.
5. Stokols D, Pelletier KR, Fielding JE. The ecology of work and health: research and policy directions for the promotion of employee health. *Health Educ Q.* 1996;23(2):137–158.
6. Lazarus RS, Folkman S. *Stress, appraisal, and coping.* New York, NY: Springer; 1984.
7. Crider A. Experimental studies of conflict-produced stress. In: Levine S, Scotch NA, eds. *Social stress.* Chicago, IL: Aldine; 1970:165–188.
8. Wolf S. Psychosocial influences in gastrointestinal function. In: Levi L, ed. *Society, stress, and disease.* New York, NY: Oxford University Press; 1971:362–366.
9. Selye H. *From dream to discovery.* New York, NY: McGraw-Hill; 1964.
10. Selye H. *Stress without distress.* London, UK: Transworld; 1987.
11. Le Fevre M, Matheny J, Kolt GS. Eustress, distress, and interpretation in occupational stress. *J Manage Psychol.* 2003;18(7):726–744.
12. Selye H. *The stress of life.* New York, NY: McGraw-Hill; 1956.
13. Selye H. The evolution of the stress concept: stress and cardiovascular disease. In: Levi L, ed. *Society, stress, and disease.* New York, NY: Oxford University Press; 1971:299–311.
14. Gross R. The "executive monkey" experiment. *Psychol Rev.* April 2003:26–27.
15. Brady JV, Porter RW, Conrad DG, Mason JW. Avoidance behavior and the development of gastroduodenal ulcers. *J Exp Anal Behav.* 1958;1(1):69–72.
16. Brady JV. Ulcers in "executive" monkeys. *Sci Am.* 1958;199(4):95–100.
17. Centers for Disease Control and Prevention, National Institute for Occupational Safety and Health (NIOSH). *Stress … at work.* DHHS (NIOSH) Publication No. 99-101. Cincinnati, OH: NIOSH; 1999.

18. Colligan TW, Higgins EM. Workplace stress: etiology and consequences. *J Workplace Behav Health*. 2005;21(2):89–97.

19. Hurrell JJ Jr, Nelson DL, Simmons BL. Measuring job stressors and strains: where we have been, where we are, and where we need to go. *J Occup Health Psychol*. 1998;3(4):368–389.

20. Quick JC. Introduction to the measurement of stress at work. *J Occup Health Psychol*. 1998;3(4):291–293.

21. Kasl SV. Measuring job stressors and studying the health impact of the work environment: an epidemiologic commentary. *J Occup Health Psychol*. 1998;3(4):390–401.

22. Chandola T, Heraclides A, Kumari M. Psychophysiological biomarkers of workplace stressors. *Neurosci Biobehav Rev*. 2010;35:51–57.

23. Karasek RA Jr. Job demands, job decision latitude, and mental strain: implications for job redesign. *Admin Sci Q*. 1979;24:285–308.

24. Andrea H, Beurskens AJHM, Matsemakers JFM, et al. Health problems and psychosocial work environment as predictors of long term sickness absence in employees who visited the occupational physician and/or general practitioner in relation to work: a prospective study. *Occup Environ Med*. 2003;60:295–300.

25. de Smet P, Sans S, Dramaix M, et al. Gender and regional differences in perceived job stress across Europe. *Eur J Public Health*. 2005;15(5):536–545.

26. Baker E, Israel B, Schurman S. Role of control and support in occupational stress: an integrated model. *Soc Sci Med*. 1996;43(7):1145–1159.

27. Siegrist J. Adverse health effects of high-effort/low-reward conditions. *J Occup Health Psychol*. 1996;1(1):27–41.

28. van Vegchel N, de Jonge J, Bosma H, Schaufeli W. Reviewing the effort–reward imbalance model: drawing up the balance of 45 empirical studies. *Soc Sci Med*. 2005;60:1117–1131.

29. Hyvönen K, Feldt T, Tolvanen A, Kinnunen U. The role of goal pursuit in the interaction between psychosocial work environment and occupational well-being. *J Vocat Behav*. 2010;76:406–418.

30. de Jonge J, Bosma H, Peter R, Siegrist J. Job strain, effort–reward imbalance and employee well-being: a large-scale cross-sectional study. *Soc Sci Med*. 2000;50:1317–1327.

31. Siegrist J, Marmot M. Health inequalities and the psychosocial environment: two scientific challenges. *Soc Sci Med*. 2004;58:1463–1473.

32. Bakker AB, Demerouti E. The job demands–resources model: state of the art. *J Manage Psychol*. 2007;22(3):309–328.

33. French JRP Jr, Rodgers W, Cobb S. Adjustment as person–environment fit. In: Coehlo GV, Hamburg DA, Adams JE, eds. *Coping and adaptation*. New York, NY: Basic Books; 1974:316–333.

34. World Health Organization. Stress at the workplace. n.d. http://www.who.int/occupational_health/topics/stressatwp/en/index.html. Accessed August 24, 2013.

35. Virtanen M, Heikkilä K, Jokela M, et al. Long working hours and coronary heart disease: a systematic review and meta-analysis. *Am J Epidemiol*. 2012;176(7):586–596.

36. Rosa RR, Colligan MJ. *Plain language about shiftwork*. Cincinnati, OH: Centers for Disease Control and Prevention, NIOSH; 1997.

37. Oberlinner C, Ott MG, Nasterlack M, et al. Medical program for shift workers: impacts on chronic disease and mortality outcomes. *Scand J Work Environ Health*. 2009;35(4):309–318.

38. Cheng Y, Chen CW, Chen CJ, Chiang TL. Job insecurity and its association with health among employees in the Taiwanese general population. *Soc Sci Med.* 2005;61(1):41–52.

39. Bentley TA, Catley B, Cooper-Thomas H, et al. Perceptions of workplace bullying in the New Zealand travel industry: prevalence and management strategies. *Tourism Management.* 2012;33:351–360.

40. Geldart S, Smith CA, Shannon HS, Lohfeld L. Organizational practices and workplace health and safety: a cross-sectional study in manufacturing companies. *Safety Sci.* 2010;48:562–569.

41. Centers for Disease Control and Prevention, National Institute for Occupational Safety and Health (NIOSH). *The changing organization of work and the safety and health of working people.* DHHS (NIOSH) Publication No. 2002-116. Cincinnati, OH: DHHS (NIOSH); 2002.

42. Marchand A, Demers A, Durand P. Does work really cause distress? The contribution of organizational structure and work organization to the experience of psychological distress. *Soc Sci Med.* 2005;61:1–14.

43. Tobiasz-Adamczyk B, Brzyski P, Florek M, Brzyska M. Job stress and mortality in older age. *Int J Occup Med Environ Health.* July 15, 2013. [Epub ahead of print].

44. Lovell B, Moss M, Wetherell MA. Perceived stress, common health complaints and diurnal patterns of cortisol secretion in young, otherwise healthy individuals. *Hormones and Behavior.* 2011;60:301–305.

45. Schnall P. A brief introduction to job strain. May 1998. http://workhealth.org/strain /briefintro.html. Accessed August 15, 2013.

46. Belkic KL, Landsbergis PA, Schnall PL, Baker D. Is job strain a major source of cardiovascular disease risk? *Scand J Work Environ Health.* 2004;30(2):85–128.

47. Theorell T, Tsutsumi A, Hallquist J, et al. Decision latitude, job strain, and myocardial infarction: a study of working men in Stockholm. *Am J Public Health.* 1998;88(3)382–388.

48. Hlatky MA, Lam LC, Lee KL, et al. Job strain and the prevalence and outcome of coronary artery disease. *Circulation.* 1995;92:327–333.

49. Pelfrene E, Leynen F, Mak RP, et al. Relationship of perceived job stress to total coronary risk in a cohort of working men and women in Belgium. *Eur J Cardiovasc Prevention Rehab.* 2003;10:345–354.

50. Landsbergis PA, Dobson M, Koutsouras G, Schnall P. Job strain and ambulatory blood pressure: a meta-analysis and systematic review. *Am J Public Health.* 2013;103(3):e61–e71.

51. Schnall PL, Schwartz JE, Landsbergis PA, et al. A longitudinal study of job strain and ambulatory blood pressure: results from a three-year follow-up. *Psychosom Med.* 1998;60:697–706.

52. Lallukka T, Rahkonen O, Lahelma E. Sleep complaints in middle-aged women and men: the contribution of working conditions and work–family conflicts. *J Sleep Res.* 2010;19:466–477.

53. Soeda S, Hayashi T, Sugawara Y, et al. A comparison of white-collar jobs in regard to mental health consultation rates in a health care center operated by a Japanese company. *Ind Health.* 2003;41:117–119.

54. Centers for Disease Control and Prevention, National Institute for Occupational Safety and Health. Work organization and stress-related disorders. Inputs: occupational safety and health risks. n.d. http://www.cdc.gov/niosh/programs/workorg /risks.html. Accessed August 14, 2013.

55. Stenfors CUD, Hanson LM, Oxenstierna G, et al. Psychosocial working conditions and cognitive complaints among Swedish employees. *PLoS One.* 2013;8(4):e60637.

56. Murcia M, Chastang J-F, Niedhammer I. Psychosocial work factors, major depressive and generalised anxiety disorders: results from the French national SIP study. *J Affect Disord.* 2013;146:319–327.

57. Stansfeld SA, Shipley MJ, Head J, Fuhrer R. Repeated job strain and the risk of depression: longitudinal analyses from the Whitehall II study. *Am J Public Health.* 2012;102:2360–2366.

58. Erdil O, Ertosun ÖG. The relationship between social climate and loneliness in the workplace and effects on employee well-being. *Proc Soc Behav Sci.* 2011;24:505–525.

59. Mayo Clinic. Post-traumatic stress disorder (PTSD). n.d. http://www.mayoclinic.org/diseases-conditions/post-traumatic-stress-disorder/basics/definition/con-20022540. Accessed March 26, 2014.

60. Stergiopoulos E, Cimo A, Cheng C, et al. Interventions to improve work outcomes in work-related PTSD: a systematic review. *BMC Public Health.* October 31, 2011;11:838.

61. Javidi H, Yadollahie M. Post-traumatic stress disorder. *Int J Occup Environ Med.* 2012;3(1):2–9.

62. Stellman JM, Smith RP, Katz CL, et al. Enduring mental health morbidity and social function impairment in World Trade Center rescue, recovery, and cleanup workers: the psychological dimension of an environmental health disaster. *Environ Health Perspect.* 2008;116(9):1248–1253.

63. Bills CB, Levy NAS, Sharma V, et al. Mental health of workers and volunteers responding to events of 9/11: review of the literature. *Mt Sinai J Med.* 2008;75:115–127.

64. Essex B, Scott LB. Chronic stress and associated coping strategies among volunteer EMS personnel. *Prehosp Emerg Care.* 2008;12:69–75.

65. BusinessDictionary.com. Employee morale: definition. n.d. http://www.businessdictionary.com/definition/employee-morale.html. Accessed December 15, 2013.

66. Di Cesare J, Sadri G. Do all carrots look the same? Examining the impact of culture on employee motivation. *Manage Res News.* 2003;26(1):29–40.

67. Moreau M, Valente F, Mak R, et al. Occupational stress and incidence of sick leave in the Belgian workforce: the Belstress study. *J Epidemiol Community Health.* 2004;58:507–516.

68. Serxner SA, Gold DB, Bultman KK. The impact of behavioral health risks on worker absenteeism. *J Occup Environ Med.* 2001;43(4):347–354.

69. Melchior M, Ferrie JE, Alexanderson K, et al. Does sickness absence due to psychiatric disorder predict cause-specific mortality? A 16-year follow-up of the GAZEL occupational cohort study. *Am J Epidemiol.* 2010;172:700–707.

70. Peter R, Siegrist J. Chronic work stress, sickness absence, and hypertension in middle managers: general or specific sociological explanations? *Soc Sci Med.* 1997;45(7):1111–1120.

71. Bernaards CM, Proper KI, Hildebrandt VH. Physical activity, cardiorespiratory fitness, and body mass index in relationship to work productivity and sickness absence in computer workers with preexisting neck and upper limb symptoms. *J Occup Environ Med.* 2007;49(6):633–640.

72. Maslach C. Understanding burnout: definitional issues in analyzing a complex phenomenon. In Paine WS, ed. *Job stress and burnout.* Beverly Hills, CA: Sage; 1982:29–40.

73. Demerouti E, Bakker AB, Nachreiner F, Schaufeli WB. The job demands–resources model of burnout. *J Appl Psychol.* 2001;86(3):499–512.

74. Kakkos N, Trivellas P, Fillipou K. Exploring the link between job motivation, work stress and job satisfaction: evidence from the banking industry. 7th International Conference on Enterprise Systems, Accounting and Logistics; June 28–29, 2010. http://www.icesal.org/2010%20PROCEEDINGS/docs/P16.pdf. Accessed December 14, 2013.

75. Johnson S, Cooper C, Cartwright S, et al. The experience of work-related stress across occupations. *J Manage Psychol.* 2005;20(2):178–187.

76. LaMontagne AD. Invited commentary: job strain and health behaviors: developing a bigger picture. *Am J Epidemiol.* 2012;176(12):1090–1094.

77. Kivimäki M, Nyberg ST, Fransson EI, et al. Associations of job strain and lifestyle risk factors with risk of coronary artery disease: a meta-analysis of individual participant data. *CMAJ.* 2013;185(9):763–769.

78. Heikkilä K, Fransson EI, Nyberg ST, et al. Job strain and health-related lifestyle: findings from an individual-participant meta-analysis of 118,000 working adults. *Am J Public Health.* 2013:e1–e8.

79. Siegrist J, Rödel A. Work stress and health risk behavior. *Scand J Work Environ Health.* 2006;32(6):473–481.

80. Gilson N, Straker L, Parry S. Occupational sitting: practitioner perceptions of health risks, intervention strategies and influences. *Health Promot J Austr.* 2012;23:208–212.

81. Simons CCJM, Hughes LAE, van Engeland M, et al. Physical activity, occupational sitting time, and colorectal cancer risk in the Netherlands Cohort Study. *Am J Epidemiol.* 2013;177(6):514–530.

82. European Agency for Safety and Health at Work (EU-OSHA). *Mental health promotion in the workplace: a summary of a good practice report.* Facts 102. Bilbao, Spain: EU-OSHA; 2011.

83. Cooper CL, Cartwright S. An intervention strategy for workplace stress. *J Psychosom Res.* 1997;43(1):7–16.

84. Sauter SL, Murphy LR, Hurrell JJ Jr. Prevention of work-related psychological disorders. *Am Psychol.* 1990;45(10):1146–1158.

85. Dollard M, Skinner N, Tuckey MR, Bailey T. National surveillance of psychosocial risk factors in the workplace: an international overview. *Work Stress.* 2007;21(1):1–29.

86. TheFreeDictionary.com. Stress management. n.d. http://medical-dictionary.thefree-dictionary.com/stress+management. Accessed April 4, 2014.

87. Giga SI, Cooper CL, Faragher B. The development of a framework for a comprehensive approach to stress management interventions at work. *Int J Stress Manage.* 2003;10(4):280–296.

88. van der Klink JJL, Blonk RWB, Schene AH, van Dijk FJH. The benefits of interventions for work-related stress. *Am J Public Health.* 2001;91(2):270–276.

89. Schneiderman N, Antoni M, Ironson G. Updated by Kristina Rerucha. Cognitive behavioral stress management and secondary prevention in HIV/AIDS. n.d. http://www.apa.org/pi/aids/resources/research/schneiderman.aspx. Accessed April 4, 2014.

90. Brinkborg H, Michanek J, Hesser H, Berglund G. Acceptance and commitment therapy for the treatment of stress among social workers: a randomized controlled trial. *Behav Res Therap.* 2011;49:389–398.

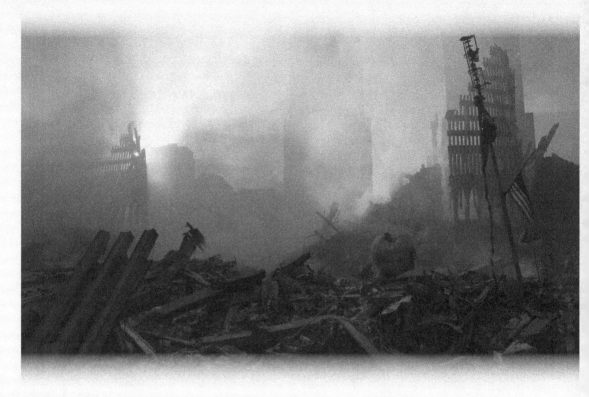

FIGURE 10.1 The World Trade Center after the September 11, 2001, attacks

Courtesy of Andrea Booher/FEMA

First responders and clean-up workers at the site of the World Trade Center after the September 11, 2011, terrorist attacks were confronted with a multitude of hazardous occupational exposures, many of which were unavoidable due to the urgent need to save the lives of the victims.

CHAPTER 10

Occupational Safety and the Prevention of Occupational Disease

Learning Objectives

By the end of this chapter, you will be able to:

- Describe the four steps used in risk assessment.
- Define the term *risk management* and give two examples of it.
- Describe occupational health surveillance.
- Give three examples of career opportunities in occupational health and safety.
- Discuss primary, secondary, and tertiary prevention in the work setting.

Chapter Outline

- Introduction
- Methods of Risk Assessment for Occupational Safety and Health
- Monitoring and Surveillance of Exposure to Occupational Hazards
- Careers in Occupational Health and Safety
- Some Concluding Topics
- Summary
- Study Questions and Exercises

Introduction

Each year, deaths, injuries, and illnesses from occupational causes exact a devastating toll globally and in the United States. These tragic deaths and injuries of workers are, for the most part, entirely preventable.[1] Safety in occupational settings is connected inextricably with workers' health and should focus on remediation of hazardous occupational environments and practices. Because occupational health services have traditionally been more concerned with treatment of occupationally associated conditions, however, a pressing need for the occupational health field is reduction of workplace risks.

Other chapters in this text have described the potential adverse health effects associated with workplace hazardous exposures and the frequent occurrence of such outcomes. Here, we explore occupational safety and offer additional information regarding methods for prevention of these conditions. Safety refers to "the quality of averting or not causing injury, danger, or loss."[2] Occupational safety involves the creation of a work environment that is free from exposures and conditions that are injurious to employees; prevention is the core focus of this field.

According to the Occupational Safety and Health Administration (OSHA), programs for the prevention of occupational injuries and illnesses "should include the systematic identification, evaluation and prevention or control of general workplace hazards and the hazards of specific jobs and tasks."[3(p. 1)] The requisites for an effective program include the following elements[3]:

- Management leadership
- Worker participation
- Hazard identification and assessment
- Hazard prevention and control
- Education and training
- Program evaluation and improvement

Techniques for maintenance and improvement of occupational safety include risk assessment programs, surveillance, and adoption of programs for promotion of a safe working environment. Consequently, the discussion here focuses on the important topics of risk assessment (which occurs in four phases), risk management, surveillance of occupational injuries and illnesses, and workplace health promotion. To create a work environment that is safer and healthier, tomorrow's occupational health experts will need to assume challenging career roles in the field. For readers interested in pursuing a career in occupational health and safety, this chapter offers information about career opportunities in this valuable and challenging field.

Methods of Risk Assessment for Occupational Safety and Health

Health risks refer to the chances of experiencing an adverse health effect if a person comes into contact with a harmful substance such as a carcinogen or toxic chemical.[4] The occupational environment has the potential for exposing workers to a variety of substances; such events could increase the likelihood of adverse health effects. In the field of environmental and occupational health, risk assessment is the procedure used to determine the risks associated with exposures to harmful materials. Risk assessment is defined as "the characterization of the potential adverse health effects of human exposures to environmental hazards."[5(p. 18)] Primarily a research and science-driven activity, risk assessment generally takes place in four steps: (1) hazard identification, (2) dose–response assessment, (3) exposure assessment, and (4) risk characterization (**FIGURE 10.2**).[6]

Hazard Identification

A hazard is defined as the "[i]nherent capability of an agent or a situation to have an adverse effect[; a] factor or exposure that may adversely affect health."[7]

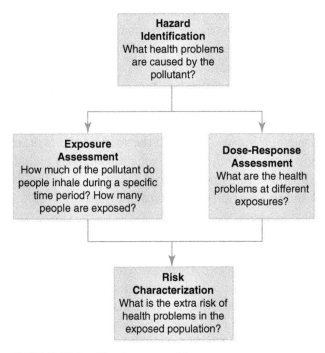

FIGURE 10.2   The four-step risk assessment process

Reproduced from U.S. Environmental Protection Agency, Risk assessment for toxic air pollutants: a citizen's guide, http://www.epa.gov/airquality/air_risc/3_90_024.html. Accessed April 16, 2014.

> **EXHIBIT 10.1   Examples of Occupational Hazards**
>
> Workplace hazards may originate from chemicals, biological agents, physical and mechanical energy and force, and psychosocial influences. Some physical hazards arise from ionizing radiation from medical X-rays and radioactive materials used in work settings. Other hazards originate from non-ionizing radiation, such as sunlight, infrared and ultraviolet radiation, and electromagnetic radiation from power lines and emissions from radio transmission towers. In urban and work environments, mechanical energy is associated with high levels of noise that can be hazardous for hearing and for psychological well-being. Other conditions in the work environment can cause falls, explosions and fires, electrical shocks, and muscle strains and sprains. Examples of psychosocial hazards are work-related stresses and post-traumatic stress disorder.

EXHIBIT 10.1 provides examples of workplace hazards, while summarizing and reviewing concepts presented elsewhere in the text.

Hazard identification is "the process of determining whether exposure to an agent can cause an increase in the incidence of a health condition (cancer, birth defect, etc.). It involves characterizing the nature and the strength of the evidence of causation."[5(p. 19)] Evidence of an association may be extrapolated from animal studies or derived from epidemiologic research with human beings.[8] These health effects may include dramatic outcomes such as mortality or cancer from contact with highly toxic chemicals or carcinogens. In many instances, however, information regarding the health effects of exposures may not be clear-cut.

Job hazard analysis is a procedure that can be applied to a specific work setting to control hazards and reduce risks. It is defined as "a technique that focuses on job tasks as a way to identify hazards before they occur. It focuses on the relationship between the worker, the task, the tools, and the work environment."[9(p. 1)] Priority jobs for analysis include those with high injury or illness rates or potential for causing such adverse effects. EXHIBIT 10.2 shows a sample job hazard analysis.

Dose–Response Assessment

Dose–response assessment is defined as "the process of characterizing the relation between the dose of an agent administered or received and the incidence of an adverse health effect in exposed populations and estimating the incidence of the effect as a function of human exposure to the agent."[5(p. 19)] According to Russell and Gruber, "Dose–response assessment examines the quantitative relation between the experimentally administered dose level of a toxicant and the incidence or severity or both of a response in test animals, and draws inferences for humans. The presumed human dosages

---

EXHIBIT 10.2   A Sample Job Hazard Analysis for Grinding Metal Parts

This example shows how a job hazard analysis can be used to identify the existing or potential hazards for each basic step involved in grinding iron castings.

Job Hazard Analysis Form

Job Location: *Analyst:*   *Date:*
Metal Shop   Joe Safety

Task Description: Worker reaches into metal box to the right of the machine, grasps a 15-pound casting, and carries it to grinding wheel. Worker grinds 20 to 30 castings per hour.

Hazard Description: When picking up a casting, the employee could drop it onto his or her foot. The casting's weight and height could seriously injure the worker's foot or toes.

Hazard Controls:
1. Remove castings from the box and place them on a table next to the grinder.
2. Wear steel-toe shoes with arch protection.
3. Change protective gloves that allow a better grip.
4. Use a device to pick up castings.

Reprinted from U.S. Department of Labor. Occupational Safety and Health Administration (OSHA). Job hazard analysis. OSHA 3071 2002 (Revised). Washington, DC: OSHA; 2002:9.

---

and incidences in human populations may also be used in cases where epidemiological studies are available."[8(p. 286)]

Exposure Assessment

Exposure assessment is defined as a procedure that "identifies populations exposed to the toxicant, describes their composition and size, and examines the routes, magnitudes, frequencies, and durations of such exposures."[8(p. 286)] The process of human exposure assessment is believed to be one of the weakest aspects of risk assessment. Quantitative information regarding how much humans are exposed to toxic substances as well as information on the specific kinds and patterns of exposure are lacking.[10] The quality of exposure assessment data determines the accuracy of risk assessments and, therefore, serves as a limiting factor in the risk assessment process. For this reason, high-quality data on exposure are necessary for making valid interpretations of the effects of exposures.

When referring to a toxic substance, exposure assessment must take into account where the exposure occurs, how much exposure occurs, and how the body absorbs the substance. The process of human exposure assessment examines "the manner in which pollutants come into actual contact with the human body—the concentration levels at the points of contact and the sources of these pollutants making contact. The key word here is 'contact'—the occurrence of two events at the same location and same time."[11(p. 449)]

Several methods of exposure assessment (e.g., personal exposure monitoring and use of biological markers) are used in environmental health disciplines such as toxicology and environmental and occupational health. In addition, occupational health providers may opt to assess occupational exposures during their routine and other medical evaluations of patients. For example, physicians should perform due diligence in collecting information on the history of exposures to chemicals and other hazards from patients being seen in occupational medicine practices.[12]

Yet another method of exposure assessment is review of the employment records of employees who are likely to have experienced exposures to chemicals and other substances. During an occupational health research program, an investigator may select a study population from personnel records maintained by a company. If the company has retained records of former and retired workers, a complete data set spanning long time periods may be available. Ideally, every previous and current worker exposed to the factor should be included. Selection bias may occur if some workers are excluded because their records have been purged from the company's database.[13] Data collected from employment records may include the following:

- Personal identifiers to permit individual records to be linked to Social Security Administration files and retrieval of death certificates
- Demographic characteristics, length of employment, and work history with the company
- Information about potential confounding variables, such as the employee's medical history, smoking habits, lifestyle, and family history of disease

Some environmental and occupational health studies use biomarkers that may be correlated with exposures to potential carcinogens and other chemicals. "Biomarkers are measurable substances or characteristics in the human body that can be used to monitor the presence of a chemical in the body, biological responses, or adverse health effects."[14] One type of biomarker involves genetic changes suspected to be the consequence of an exposure. For example, a biomarker used in occupational health studies is sister chromatid exchange (SCE)—that is, "reciprocal exchange of DNA between the two DNA molecules of a replicating chromosome."[15] In a study of workers' exposure to styrene gas (used in boat building and plastics manufacture), researchers examined the utility of SCEs in comparison with environmental monitoring as well as exhaled styrene levels as alternative measures of styrene exposure.[16]

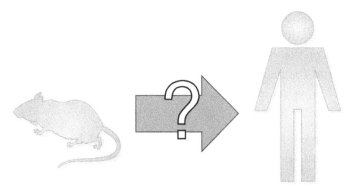

FIGURE 10.3   Uncertainty in risk estimates

Reproduced from U.S. Environmental Protection Agency, Risk assessment for toxic air pollutants: a citizen's guide, http://www.epa.gov/airquality/air_risc/3_90_024.html. Accessed April 16, 2014.

Risk Characterization

Risk characterization develops "estimates of the number of excess or unwanted health events expected at different time intervals at each level of exposure."[17(p. 38)] Risk characterization—the last of the four steps shown in Figure 10.2—integrates the information from hazard identification, dose–response assessment, and exposure assessment. The process of risk characterization yields "[a] synthesis and summary of information about a hazard that addresses the needs and interests of decision makers and of interested and affected parties. Risk characterization is a prelude to decision making and depends on an iterative, analytic-deliberative process."[18(p. 216)]

Of course, all risk estimates include some level of uncertainty, as suggested by FIGURE 10.3. For example, with respect to a chemical suspected of being a carcinogen, occupational health experts need to evaluate evidence from animal and human studies to confirm this relationship. Good evidence from human studies then strengthens the allegation that a substance or chemical has a high risk of carcinogenesis (FIGURE 10.4).

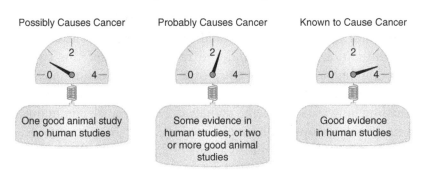

FIGURE 10.4   Weight of evidence for health problems of concern

Reproduced from U.S. Environmental Protection Agency, Risk assessment for toxic air pollutants: a citizen's guide. http://www.epa.gov/airquality/air_risc/3_90_024.html. Accessed April 16, 2014.

In conclusion, "[r]isk characterization presents the policy maker with a synopsis of all the information that contributes to a conclusion about the nature of the risk and evaluates the magnitudes of the uncertainties involved and the major assumptions that were used."[8(p. 286)]

Risk Management

Risk management is defined as "the process by which risk-assessment results are integrated with other information to make decisions about the need for, method of, and extent of risk reduction."[19(p. 28)] It includes actions "to reduce or eliminate ... [environmental] hazards or to reduce the harm that may result from their effects."[20(p. 105)] Suppose that a risk assessment has determined that there is a risk of adverse health outcomes associated with certain occupational exposures. Risk management involves making decisions to control these hazards.

Risk management is action oriented and follows a risk assessment. It involves risk evaluation, risk perception and communication, control of exposure, and risk monitoring.

Controlling Hazards

Control of workers' exposures to hazardous materials is a basic part of risk management. Risk control strategies include elimination, substitution, engineering controls, warnings, administrative controls, and personal protection.[21] These strategies represent a hierarchy in which elimination is the highest priority and personal protection is the lowest priority (TABLE 10.1).

Risk Communication

Related to the process of risk management is risk communication, which has been described by the noted authority Vincent Covello as follows:

> [T]he two-way exchange of information about risks, including environmental health risks associated with hazardous waste, water contamination, air pollution, and radiation. Numerous studies have highlighted the importance of effective risk communication in enabling people to make informed choices and participate in deciding how risks should be managed. Effective risk communication provides people with timely, accurate, clear, objective, consistent, and complete risk information.[22(p. 367)]

Risk communication is a difficult task, especially in emotionally charged situations in which people feel menaced. An example would be developing a measured response to an influenza epidemic that threatens the community,

TABLE 10.1   Compatible Risk Control Hierarchies

Control Level Step[a]	Description	Design Hierarchy[b]	Control[c]
Elimination	Remove exposure (e.g., replace asbestos in a workplace to prevent cancer-causing exposure)	Elimination	Prevent the exposure (passive control)
Substitution	Replace higher risk with lower risk (e.g., move power lines underground to remove the risk of overhead electrical contact)		
Engineering controls	Reinvent ways to control the hazard (e.g., vacuum wood dust away from saw blades)	Guarding	
Warnings (awareness)	Reveal all sources of the hazard (e.g., place audible and visible alarms in trucks to warn drivers of the proximity of other vehicles)	Warning	Mitigate the exposure (active control)
Administrative controls	Teach workers to be safe around the hazard (e.g., instruct miners of emergency procedures in the event of a mine fire)		
Personal protection	Reduce the risks of working with the hazard (e.g., fire fighters don respirators before entering a smoke-filled building)		

[a] Data from Allen PB. *Risk control hierarchy clarified electrical safety.* Davenport, IA: Grace Engineering Products; 2009. http://www.newark.com/pdfs/techarticles/GraceEngineered/riskControlHierarchy.pdf. Accessed June 19, 2011.

[b] Data from Wogather MS. Purposes and scope of warnings. In: Wogather MS, ed. *Handbook of warnings.* Mahwah, NJ: Lawrence Erlbaum Associates, 2006:3–9.

[c] Data from Haddon W. Strategies in preventive medicine: passive vs. active approaches to reducing human wastage. *J Trauma.* 1974;14(4):353–354.

Reprinted from Myers ML. Reducing hazards in the work environment. In: Friis RH, ed. *The praeger handbook of environmental health.* Vol 4. Santa Barbara, CA: Praeger; 2012:59.

but represents an unknown peril. Without careful planning and risk communication to the populace, the threat of an epidemic might lead to excessive stockpiling of vaccines.[23]

OSHA has developed a Hazard Communication Standard (HCS), which requires that the names of chemicals and their associated hazards must be made available to workers and stated in understandable language:

- "Chemical manufacturers and importers are required to evaluate the hazards of the chemicals they produce or import, and prepare labels and safety data sheets to convey the hazard information to their down-stream customers.

* All employers with hazardous chemicals in their workplaces must have labels and safety data sheets [SDSs] for their exposed workers, and train them to handle the chemicals appropriately."[24]

SDSs are described further in **EXHIBIT 10.3**.

Personal Protective Equipment

Table 10.1 notes that preferred risk control methods include the elimination of hazardous substances and implementation of engineering controls for preventing exposures. When these procedures are not feasible, personal protective equipment aids in minimizing hazardous exposures. Personal protective equipment (PPE) is defined as "equipment worn to minimize exposure to serious workplace injuries and illnesses. These injuries and illnesses may result from contact with chemical, radiological, physical, electrical, mechanical, or other workplace hazards."[25] PPE includes safety masks for inhalation hazards (**FIGURE 10.6**), laboratory safety suits (**FIGURE 10.7**), ear plugs for hearing protection, safety eyewear, and other equipment to prevent or limit workers' hazardous exposures.

Eye and Face Protection

Under OSHA regulations, employers are required to determine the risks of workplace exposure to hazards that may affect the eyes and face and to protect workers against the highest level of each type of hazard when multiple hazards are present.[26] **TABLE 10.2** presents an example of a hazard assessment for hazards to the eyes and face.

As shown in Table 10.2, dust is one of the occupational hazards to the eyes and face. Many types of dust-protection goggles are available, with the appropriate choice depending on the intended application. Goggles can provide a seal around the eyes to prevent dusts from entering. They can be equipped with corrective lenses. Some models can be worn over glasses and are ventilated so that the lenses will not fog up.

Another hazard is optical radiation: Specialized lenses are available for protection against optical radiation from lasers and welding procedures. Additional PPE for welders includes special hoods and face shields.

The range of options for PPE for the eyes and face is extensive. Refer to the link to OSHA (https://www.osha.gov/SLTC/etools/eyeandface/ppe/selection.html) for more information on this topic.

EXHIBIT 10.3   Hazard Communication Safety Data Sheets

The Hazard Communication Standard (HCS) requires chemical manufacturers, distributors, or importers to provide safety data sheets (SDSs) (formerly known as material safety data sheets [MSDSs]) to communicate the hazards of hazardous chemical products. (See FIGURE 10.5 for a sample SDS.) As of June 1, 2015, the HCS will require new SDSs to be in a uniform format, and include the section numbers, the headings, and associated information under these headings:

Section 1, Identification: includes the product identifier; manufacturer or distributor name, address, and phone number; emergency phone number; recommended use; and restrictions on use.

Section 2, Hazard(s) Identification: includes all hazards regarding the chemical and required label elements.

Section 3, Composition/Information on Ingredients: includes information on chemical ingredients and trade secret claims.

Section 4, First-Aid Measures: includes important symptoms/effects, both acute and delayed, as well as the required treatment.

Section 5, Firefighting Measures: lists suitable extinguishing techniques and equipment, as well as chemical hazards from fire.

Section 6, Accidental Release Measures: lists emergency procedures, protective equipment, and proper methods of containment and clean-up.

Section 7, Handling and Storage: lists precautions for safe handling and storage, including incompatibilities.

Section 8, Exposure Controls/Personal Protection: lists OSHA's permissible exposure limits (PELs); threshold limit values (TLVs); appropriate engineering controls; and personal protective equipment (PPE).

Section 9, Physical and Chemical Properties: lists the chemical's characteristics.

Section 10, Stability and Reactivity: lists chemical stability and possibility of hazardous reactions.

Section 11, Toxicological Information: includes routes of exposure; related symptoms, including both acute and chronic effects; and numerical measures of toxicity.

Section 12, Ecological Information

Section 13, Disposal Considerations

Section 14, Transport Information

Section 15, Regulatory Information

Section 16, Other Information: includes the date of preparation or last revision.

Modified from U.S. Department of Labor. Occupational Safety and Health Administration (OSHA). Hazard communication safety data sheets. 2012. Washington, DC: OSHA; 2012. OSHA 3493-02

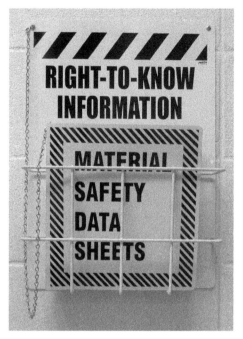

FIGURE 10.5   Material safety data sheets (now called safety data sheets)

© Travis Klein/ShutterStock

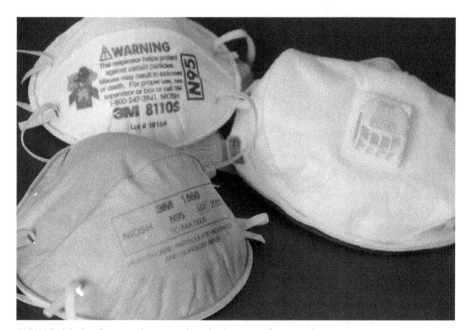

FIGURE 10.6   Personal protective devices—safety masks

Courtesy of Centers for Disease Control and Prevention, Public Health Image Library/Debora Cartagena.

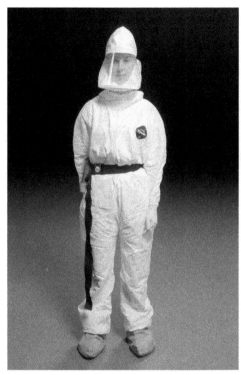

FIGURE 10.7 Personal protective devices for laboratory workers

Courtesy of Centers for Disease Control and Prevention, Public Health Image Library/James Gathany.

TABLE 10.2 Hazard Assessment for Eye and Face Hazards

Hazard Type	Examples of Hazard	Common Related Tasks
Impact	Flying objects such as large chips, fragments, particles, sand, and dirt	Chipping, grinding, machining, masonry work, wood working, sawing, drilling, chiseling, powered fastening, riveting, and sanding
Heat	Anything emitting extreme heat	Furnace operations, pouring, casting, hot dipping, and welding
Chemicals	Splash, fumes, vapors, and irritating mists	Acid and chemical handling, degreasing, plating, and working with blood
Dust	Harmful dust	Woodworking, buffing, and general dusty conditions
Optical radiation	Radiant energy, glare, and intense light	Welding, torch-cutting, brazing, soldering, and laser work

Courtesy of the U.S. Department of Labor, Occupational Health and Safety Administration, Eye and face protection eTool: selecting PPE for the workplace, https://www.osha.gov/SLTC/etools/eyeandface/ppe/selection.html. Accessed July 14, 2014.

Respiratory Protection

Respiratory hazards include airborne particles (dusts, mists, and fumes) and gases and vapors. Two types of respirators designed to protect against respiratory hazards are air purifying respirators (particulate; gas and vapor) and atmosphere-supplying respirators (those supplied with clean air and self-contained breathing apparatuses). These respirators have applications in a variety of occupational settings. For example, a self-contained breathing apparatus is used for short time periods (about half an hour) to enter atmospheres that are or may be immediately dangerous to life and health. Refer to the link to OSHA (https://www.osha.gov/SLTC/etools/respiratory/index.html) for considerations regarding PPE for respiratory protection and some of the available options.

Safety Procedures for Workers Who Use Chemicals

Chemical hygiene plans and specialized storage cabinets protect employees who use dangerous chemicals. The *NIOSH Pocket Guide*, described in a later section, is an invaluable resource for information about chemical safety.

Chemical Hygiene Plans

OSHA requires that laboratories maintain a chemical hygiene plan (CHP) for protection of workers against hazardous chemicals. "The CHP is a written program stating the policies, procedures and responsibilities that protect workers from the health hazards associated with the hazardous chemicals used in that particular workplace."[27] OSHA's Occupational Exposure to Hazardous Chemicals in Laboratories standard sets forth the mandatory requirements for a CHP. This standard includes the required elements described in **EXHIBIT 10.4**. Also there are requirements for training workers in the detection of hazardous chemicals, the hazards of chemicals in use, and protective measures. Medical examinations and consultations must be available for all workers who handle hazardous chemicals in the course of their duties.

Safe Storage of Chemicals

The material safety data sheet (MSDS) identifies the characteristics of chemicals and provides recommended safe storage methods. A variety of safety cabinets are manufactured for chemical storage. The customary colors of cabinets used by industry for chemical storage are as follows: yellow—flammable liquids; red—paints and combustible liquids; gray/white—waste materials; blue—corrosive materials; and green—pesticides.[28] In addition

EXHIBIT 10.4   Laboratory Safety Chemical Hygiene Plan (CHP)

1. Standard operating procedures relevant to safety and health considerations for each activity involving the use of hazardous chemicals.
2. Criteria that the employer will use to determine and implement control measures to reduce exposure to hazardous materials [i.e., engineering controls, the use of personal protective equipment, and hygiene practices] with particular attention given to selecting control measures for extremely hazardous materials.
3. A requirement to ensure that fume hoods and other protective equipment are functioning properly and identify the specific measures the employer will take to ensure proper and adequate performance of such equipment.
4. Information to be provided to lab personnel working with hazardous substances include:
   * The contents of the laboratory standard and its appendices
   * The location and availability of the employer's CHP
   * The permissible exposure limits (PELs) for OSHA-regulated substances or recommended exposure limits for other hazardous chemicals where there is no applicable OSHA standard
   * The signs and symptoms associated with exposures to hazardous chemicals used in the laboratory
   * The location and availability of known reference materials on the hazards, safe handling, storage and disposal of hazardous chemicals found in the laboratory including, but not limited to, the material safety data sheets received from the chemical supplier
5. The circumstances under which a particular laboratory operation, procedure, or activity requires prior approval from the employer or the employer's designee before being implemented.
6. Designation of personnel responsible for implementing the CHP, including the assignment of a chemical hygiene officer and, if appropriate, establishment of a chemical hygiene committee.
7. Provisions for additional worker protection for work with particularly hazardous substances. These include "select carcinogens"—that is, reproductive toxins and substances that have a high degree of acute toxicity. Specific consideration must be given to the following provisions and shall be included where appropriate:
   * Establishment of a designated area
   * Use of containment devices such as fume hoods or glove boxes
   * Procedures for safe removal of contaminated waste
   * Decontamination procedures
8. The employer must review and evaluate the effectiveness of the CHP at least annually and update it as necessary.

Reprinted from U.S. Department of Labor. Occupational Safety and Health Administration (OSHA). OSHA FactSheet. Laboratory Safety Chemical Hygiene Plan (CHP). Washington, DC: OSHA; 2011.

EXHIBIT 10.5   Chemical Storage

Requirements for hazardous material storage (general requirements, storage cabinets and shelves) include:

* Segregate incompatible chemicals (e.g., storing oxidizing acids and flammable solvents in separate locations). This is to prevent inadvertent mixing of incompatible chemicals that can produce harmful gases/vapors, heat, fire and explosions.

* Store hazardous materials away from heat and direct sunlight. Heat and sunlight may alter and degrade chemicals, and can cause storage containers and labels to deteriorate.

* Do not store hazardous materials (except cleaners) under sinks.

* Ensure caps and lids are securely tightened on containers. This prevents leaks and evaporation of contents.

* Use approved flammable storage lockers or flammable storage containers to store flammable and combustible liquids exceeding 10 gallons in one room. Flammable and combustible liquids kept in squeeze bottles and other secondary containers may be kept on counter and bench tops provided they do not exceed the 10-gallon limit and are kept in secondary containment.

* Store inorganic acids in corrosive or acid storage cabinets. Their interiors and hardware (door hinges and shelf brackets) are corrosion resistant. Corrosive storage cabinets can be located under fume hoods or exist as stand-alone units. Flammable storage cabinets are not corrosion resistant and shall not be used for inorganic acid storage.

* Install Plexiglas lips or use equivalent means to prevent materials from falling off open storage shelves. (Placing bottles on trays arranged on shelves of cabinets aids in secondary containment of spilled liquids.)

Modified from Earnest Orlando Lawrence Berkeley National Laboratory. Chemical hygiene and safety plan. Chemical storage. http://www2.lbl.gov/ehs/chsp/html/storage.shtml. Accessed June 24, 2014.

---

to cabinets, specially designed refrigerators are used for chemical storage. Conventional household refrigerators are inappropriate for this application. Also, foods and beverages should not be kept in refrigerators used for chemical storage.[29]

EXHIBIT 10.5 outlines procedures developed at the Ernest Orlando Lawrence Berkeley National Laboratory for chemical storage.

NIOSH Pocket Guide to Chemical Hazards

The introduction to the *Pocket Guide* explains the purposes of this publication:

> The *NIOSH Pocket Guide to Chemical Hazards* provides a concise source of general industrial hygiene information for workers,

employers, and occupational health professionals. The *Pocket Guide* presents key information and data in abbreviated tabular form for 677 chemicals or substance groupings commonly found in the work environment (e.g., manganese compounds, tellurium compounds, inorganic tin compounds, etc.). The industrial hygiene information found in the *Pocket Guide* assists users to recognize and control occupational chemical hazards. The chemicals or substances contained in this revision include all substances for which the National Institute for Occupational Safety and Health (NIOSH) has recommended exposure limits (RELs) and those with permissible exposure limits (PELs) as found in the Occupational Safety and Health Administration (OSHA) Occupational Safety and Health Standards."[30(p. vii)]

One category of chemicals described in the *Guide* are those that are immediately dangerous to life or health (IDLH). "The purpose for establishing an IDLH value ... was to determine the airborne concentration from which a worker could escape without injury or irreversible health effects from an IDLH exposure in the event of the failure of respiratory protection equipment."[30(p. x)]

Monitoring and Surveillance of Exposure to Occupational Hazards

The term disease surveillance refers to "monitoring distributions and trends of morbidity and mortality data."[31(p. 625)] Surveillance involves the "[s]ystematic and continuous collection, analysis, and interpretation of data, closely integrated with the timely and coherent dissemination of the results and assessments to those who have the right to know so that action can be taken."[7] As public health tools, surveillance data are used for health promotion and the control and prevention of diseases, but also are relevant to occupational health.

Disease surveillance has a long history in public health.[32] For example, it has been used in public health practice as a method for controlling communicable diseases such as polio and smallpox as well as some noninfectious conditions. Environmental public health tracking is the application of surveillance to environmental health issues.

With respect to the occupational environment, surveillance is a means for identifying hazardous conditions and introducing methods for improving health and preventing occupational diseases in the workplace. Surveillance data can assist in the detection of unusual clusters of illnesses.[33] An occupational example would be a cluster of specific cancer diagnoses among workers who are using a new and previously unknown carcinogenic chemical in an industrial process.

Occupational health surveillance, as an essential tool for prevention of occupational illnesses and injuries, provides the following benefits:[34]

- Aid in determining the magnitude of work-related injuries and illnesses
- Identify employees at high risk
- Formulate priorities for prevention
- Determine the effectiveness of preventive measures
- Identify issues that require further research

The insights provided by surveillance data can be enhanced by linking these data with data contained in national environmental health, occupational health, and other databases. By drawing upon several data sources, comprehensive surveillance systems at the national level can provide insights into relationships among exposures in different domains such as the environment, work settings, and food-related contamination.[35] For example, use of pesticides might cause environmental pollution, pesticide exposures among agricultural workers, and increased levels of pesticides in foods. At present, U.S. national surveillance systems for occupational injuries and illnesses are capable of providing only limited and fragmented information.[34] Surveillance of morbidity from job-associated exposures would be facilitated by development of improved national databases for occupational illnesses and injuries.

Two types of surveillance used in the work setting are hazard surveillance and health surveillance. *Hazard surveillance* refers to "the assessment of secular trends in exposure to toxic chemical agents in the workplace and to other hazards responsible for disease and injury. In a public health context, hazard surveillance identifies work processes or individual workers exposed to high levels of specific agents in particular industries and job categories. This enables timely intervention that will prevent occupational illness and its attendant morbidity and mortality." [36(p. 26)] Employers can implement strategies for reducing exposures to hazards that are present in sufficient quantities and sufficient magnitudes to affect health. For example, the Occupational Health Branch of the California Department of Public Health has developed an exemplary program for identifying workplace chemical hazards and protecting workers against such hazards.[37]

Health surveillance, in contrast, is concerned with the health of individual workers or groups of workers. The rationale for health surveillance is to "detect adverse health effects resulting from occupational exposures at as early a stage as possible, so that appropriate preventive measures can be instituted promptly. This is a form of secondary prevention."[38(p. 706)]

Related to heath surveillance is the concept of the sentinel health event, whose development is attributed to Rutstein and colleagues. The term sentinel health event (SHE) denotes "a preventable disease, disability, or untimely death whose occurrence serves as a warning signal that the quality of preventive and/or therapeutic medical care may need to be improved."[39(p. 1054)] Examples of occupational disease sentinel health events include infectious diseases (e.g., hepatitis, which is transmitted by blood-borne pathogens) acquired in an occupational setting, cancers (e.g., mesothelioma), and occupational lung diseases (e.g., silicosis). Sentinel health events can be included in surveillance programs for occupational health. Occupational SHEs signal that epidemiologic investigations are needed to elucidate the occurrence of these events and give warning signs about needed interventions (e.g., increased use of PPE such as dust masks and ear plugs, substitution of less hazardous materials, and improved design of equipment and manufacturing procedures).

Rutstein et al.'s original list of sentinel health events published in 1983 contained 50 disease conditions; this list was expanded to 64 disease conditions in 1991. Generally, sentinel health events fall into two categories: those that are inherently occupationally related (e.g., pneumoconiosis) and those that may be occupationally related but also could occur outside of occupational settings (e.g., lung cancer).[40]

In addition to tracking sentinel health events, occupational health statisticians may use occupational health indicators to assist in prevention of occupational injuries and illnesses. The Council of State and Territorial Epidemiologists (CSTE) defines occupational health indicators as "measures of health (work-related disease or injury) or factors associated with health (workplace exposures, hazards, or interventions) that allow a state to compare its health or risk status with that of other states and evaluate trends over time. These data can help guide priorities for prevention and intervention efforts."[41] Data from health indicators are the initial step in reducing the toll of occupational injuries and illnesses, many of which are highly preventable.[42] The CSTE has published a list of 20 indicators, which include these three examples:

- Nonfatal work-related injuries and illnesses reported by employers (indicator 1)
- Work-related hospitalizations (indicator 2)
- Fatal work-related injuries (indicator 3)

Careers in Occupational Health and Safety

TABLE 10.3 gives an overview of some of the many careers in the field of occupational health and safety. Three fields are covered here in more detail: occupational medicine, industrial hygiene, and occupational health nursing.

TABLE 10.3 Careers in Occupational Health and Safety

Occupation	Required Training and Education	Job Functions
Construction and building inspectors	High school diploma, or associate's degree in inspection technology. Inspectors may receive certification by the International Code Council (ICC).	Construction and building inspectors ensure that construction meets local and national building codes and ordinances, zoning regulations, and contract specifications.
Environmental scientists and specialists	Varies: bachelor's degree to doctoral degree, depending on the work setting.	Environmental scientists and specialists use their knowledge of the natural sciences to protect the environment and human health. They may clean up polluted areas, advise policy makers, or work with industry to reduce waste.
Fire inspectors and investigators	Usually a minimum of a high school diploma or equivalent; postsecondary education related to fire inspection.	Fire inspectors examine buildings to detect fire hazards and ensure that federal, state, and local fire codes are met. Fire investigators determine the origin and cause of fires and explosions.
Health and safety engineers	Bachelor's degree.	Health and safety engineers develop procedures and design systems to prevent people from getting sick or injured and to keep property from being damaged. They combine knowledge of systems engineering and knowledge of health and safety to make sure that chemicals, machinery, software, furniture, and other consumer products will not cause harm to people or buildings.
Industrial hygienists: Certified Industrial Hygienist (CIH)	Bachelor's degree in biology, chemistry, engineering, or physics; additional education related to occupational medicine; experience in workplace health. Passage of an exam is required to become a CIH; the exam is administered by the American Board of Industrial Hygiene.	Industrial hygienists may be involved with the assessment and control of physical, chemical, biological, or environmental hazards in the workplace or community that could cause injury or disease.
Insurance specialists—workers' compensation	Varies—from high school diploma or equivalent to bachelor's degree.	Insurance specialists work for insurance companies that provide workers' compensation insurance. Among their many possible roles, insurance specialists examine and investigate claims for workers' compensation and provide customer service.
Occupational health and safety specialists	Bachelor's degree.	Occupational health and safety specialists analyze many types of work environments and work procedures. Specialists inspect workplaces for adherence to regulations on safety, health, and the environment. They also design programs to prevent disease or injury to workers and damage to the environment.

(Continues)

TABLE 10.3   Careers in Occupational Health and Safety (*Continued*)

Occupation	Required Training and Education	Job Functions
Occupational health and safety technicians	High school diploma or equivalent required.	Occupational health and safety technicians collect data on safety and health conditions in the workplace. They work with occupational health and safety specialists in conducting tests and measuring hazards to help prevent harm to workers, property, the environment, and the general public.
Occupational health nurse	Requires licensure as a registered nurse (college-level education and training; passage of a state board exam, which is necessary for a license to practice) or, alternatively, licensure as a nurse practitioner (a registered nurse who has obtained advanced formal education, usually a master's degree). In addition, occupational health nurses have had experience and additional education in occupational health. Certified occupational health nurses have received certification from the American Board for Occupational Health Nurses after meeting educational and experience standards and passing an occupational health nursing exam.	Occupational and environmental health nursing is a specialty practice that provides for and delivers health and safety programs and services to workers, worker populations, and community groups. This practice focuses on promotion and restoration of health, prevention of illness and injury, and protection from work-related and environmental hazards.
Occupational and environmental medicine (OEM) physician	Doctor of Medicine (MD); Doctor of Osteopathy (DO). Certification in occupational medicine by the American Board of Preventive Medicine (requires additional residency training and passage of an exam).	The major role of the OEM physician is to evaluate the interaction between work and health. As highly trained specialists, OEM physicians and other health professionals enhance the health of workers through preventive medicine, clinical care, disability management, research, and education.

Data from American Association of Occupational Health Nurses. Careers. http://www.aaohn.org/careers /profession-of-occupational-environmental-health-nursing.html. Accessed April 9, 2014; Bureau of Labor Statistics. Occupational health and safety specialists. http://www.bls.gov/ooh/healthcare/occupational-health -and-safety-specialists.htm. Accessed April 9, 2014; American College of Occupational and Environmental Medicine, Physicians new to occupational medicine. http://www.acoem.org/Print.aspx? Accessed April 9, 2014; National Institutes of Health. Office of Research Services. What is industrial hygiene? http://www.ors .od.nih.gov/sr/dohs/aboutDOHS/TAB/Pages/technical_branch_ih.aspx. Accessed April 9, 2014; About.com. Health careers. http://healthcareers.about.com/od/healthcareerprofiles/tp/Occupational-Health-Careers.htm. Accessed April 9, 2014.

Occupational Medicine Physicians

Occupational medicine is "[t]he branch of medicine that deals with the prevention and treatment of diseases and injuries occurring at work or in specific occupations."[43] The rise of occupational medicine can be traced back to the occurrence of medical problems that affected workers employed in large numbers in industry during the Victorian era in England.[44] Today's occupational medicine physicians are increasingly visible regarding prevention of occupational illnesses and promoting workers' health.[45] Their qualifications are described in TABLE 10.4.

Industrial (Occupational) Hygienists

Industrial hygiene (occupational hygiene) is defined as the "science and art devoted to the anticipation, recognition, evaluation, and control of those environmental factors or stresses arising in or from the workplace, which may cause sickness, impaired health and well-being, or significant discomfort among workers or among the citizens of the community."[46(p. 1)] Examples of such environmental stresses are work-related exposures to hazardous agents (biohazards, toxic chemicals, and physical hazards) and other conditions including ergonomic hazards and psychosocial stressors.[47]

During the Industrial Revolution in Western Europe, and especially in England, physicians and other concerned individuals wrote about the deplorable working conditions that existed in many occupations.[48] The field of industrial hygiene can trace its origins in part to mid-1800s writings that documented the appalling hazards in mines and factories of this era. In turn, occupational health now recognizes the importance of industrial

TABLE 10.4 Qualifications Needed by an Occupational and Environmental Health Physician

- Have a general knowledge of worksite operations and be familiar with the toxic properties of materials used by employees and potential hazards and stressors of work processes.
- Be qualified to determine an employee's physical and emotional fitness for work.
- Be capable of diagnosing and treating occupational and environmental diseases and competently handling injuries.
- Possess knowledge of rehabilitation methods; health education techniques; sanitation; workers' compensation laws; local, state, and federal regulatory requirements; and the systems for maintaining medical records.
- Be able to organize and manage the delivery of health services.

Reprinted from American College of Occupational and Environmental Medicine. Physicians new to occupational medicine. Accessed April 9, 2014.

hygiene for preventive medicine. Industrial hygiene specialists must take into account how medical factors may operate in concert with social and economic forces.

Industrial hygiene is a profession that employs rigorous and scientific procedures for control of workplace hazards. Activities may include the identification of potential health hazards and safety issues in an occupational setting, measurement and evaluation of exposures to potentially hazardous agents, and development of recommendations for minimizing such exposures.[47] Among the methods at the disposal of industrial hygienists are environmental monitoring and analytical methods, which aid in the measurement of occupational exposures (**FIGURE 10.8**). An industrial hygienist might, for example, recommend reengineering industrial equipment and modifying work practices to eliminate or minimize potential hazardous exposures.[46]

Occupational Health Nurses

Occupational health nurses are highly trained professionals who perform diverse functions related to health in the workplace. Their responsibilities

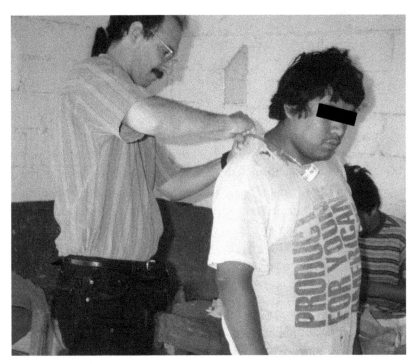

FIGURE 10.8 Occupational hygienist preparing to collect an air sample from a worker in a Mexican manufacturing facility

Courtesy of Centers for Disease Control and Prevention, Public Health Image Library/Aaron L Sussell.

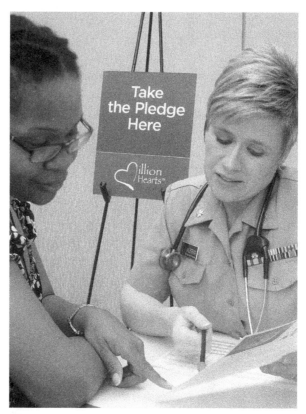

FIGURE 10.9   CDC employee in blood pressure screening exercise conducted by a nurse

Courtesy of Centers for Disease Control and Prevention, Public Health Image Library/Yvonne Green, RN, CNM, MSN.

may involve direct care of employees who have suspected work-related illnesses, development of educational programs, service as an occupational health consultant, and management of corporate-level occupational health activities (**FIGURE 10.9**). Some of these functions complement the work of occupational health physicians through case management, counseling employees and intervening in crises, designing health promotion and risk reduction programs, ensuring legal and regulatory compliance, and detecting of work-related hazards. **TABLE 10.5** lists the roles of occupational and environmental health nurses.

Occupational Safety and Health Technicians

The goal of occupational health and safety technicians is to create safe working conditions by reducing or eliminating deleterious exposures (**FIGURE 10.10**). Technicians are responsible for collecting data on the job environment. In this capacity, they collaborate with other occupational health experts. Entry-level education for technicians is a high-school diploma or equivalent.

TABLE 10.5   Roles of Occupational and Environmental Health Nurses

Case Management

- Occupational health nurses (OHNs) routinely coordinate and manage the care of ill and injured workers.
- Their roles as case managers have grown more sophisticated with the coordination and management of work-related and non-work-related injuries and illnesses, which include aspects related to group health, workers' compensation, and Family Medical Leave Act (FMLA) and short-term/long-term disability benefits.

Counseling and Crisis Intervention

- Besides counseling workers about work-related illnesses and injuries, OHNs often counsel employees on issues such as substance abuse, psychosocial needs, wellness/health promotion concerns, and other health- or work-related concerns.
- OHNs may assume primary responsibility for managing employee assistance programs or handling referrals to employee assistance programs and/or other community resources, and coordinate follow-up.

Health Promotion and Risk Reduction

- OHNs design programs that support positive lifestyle changes and individual efforts to lower risks of disease and injury and the creation of an environment that provides a sense of balance among work, family, personal, health, and psychosocial concerns.
- Immunization, smoking cessation, exercise/fitness, nutrition and weight control, stress management, monitoring of chronic diseases, and effective use of medical services are just a few of the preventive strategies to keep workers healthy and productive.

Legal and Regulatory Compliance

- Whether it is the array of state and federal regulations put forward by OSHA or laws that affect the workplace, such as the FMLA or the Health Insurance Portability and Accountability Act (HIPAA), OHNs work with employers on compliance with regulations and laws affecting workers and the workplace.

Worker and Workplace Hazard Detection

- OHNs recognize and identify hazards.
- OHNs monitor, evaluate, and analyze these hazards by conducting research on the effects of workplace exposures.
- OHNs gather and use health and hazard data to select and implement preventive and control measures as a continual process.
- Examples include an analysis of the effects of toxic chemical exposure, development of plans to prevent work-related accidents, and an analysis of groups, not just individuals, to detect patterns, trends, changes, and commonalities as in pandemic situations.

Reprinted from American Association of Occupational Health Nurses. Careers. http://www.aaohn.org/careers/profession-of-occupational-environmental-health-nursing.html. Accessed April 9, 2014.

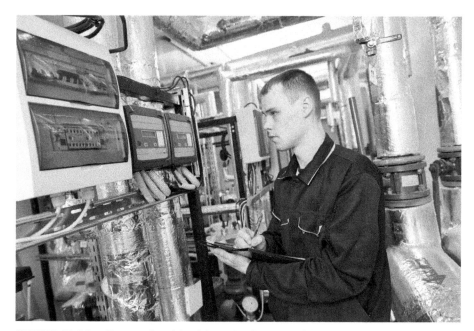

FIGURE 10.10   Occupational health and safety technicians in a representative work setting

Courtesy of Centers for Disease Control and Prevention, Public Health Image Library/Barbara Jenkins, NIOSH.

Ethical Standards for Occupational Health Professionals

Occupational health and safety professionals are obligated to adhere to high ethical standards in the practice of their profession. Examples of these standards are set forth in the International Code of Ethics for Occupational Health Professionals[49] and the American Board of Industrial Hygiene (ABIH) Code of Ethics for industrial hygienists.[50] According to the International Labour Organization (ILO), the International Code of Ethics is premised upon three principles:

> *Occupational health practice* must be performed according to the highest professional standards and ethical principles. Occupational health professionals must serve the health and social well-being of the workers, individually and collectively. They also contribute to environmental and community health.

> *The obligations of occupational health professionals* include protecting the life and the health of the worker, respecting human dignity and promoting the highest ethical principles in occupational health policies and programs. Integrity in professional conduct, impartiality, and the protection of the confidentiality of health data and of the privacy of workers are part of these obligations.

Occupational health professionals are experts who must enjoy full professional independence in the execution of their functions. They must acquire and maintain the competence necessary for their duties and require conditions which allow them to carry out their tasks according to good practice and professional ethics.[49]

The ABIH publishes a set of ethical standards for industrial hygienists and candidates for certification by this organization: "The American Board of Industrial Hygiene ... is a voluntary, non-profit, professional credentialing organization. ABIH certifies qualified industrial hygienists engaged in the practice of industrial hygiene, and who have met the professional knowledge standards established by the Board of Directors."[50] The ABIH's guiding ethical standard is stated as follows:

As professionals in the field of industrial hygiene, ABIH certificants and candidates have the obligation to: maintain high standards of integrity and professional conduct; accept responsibility for their actions; continually seek to enhance their professional capabilities; practice with fairness and honesty; and, encourage others to act in a professional manner consistent with the certification standards and responsibilities set forth [in the detailed code of ethics].[50]

Some Concluding Topics

FIGURE 10.11 shows a historical image of a carpenter who is at work and is not using any personal protective equipment. (He is also smoking while working.) Since this picture was taken, occupational safety standards have advanced greatly in the United States.

This section reviews the public health concept of disease prevention, giving examples of workplace health promotion, responses to societal emergencies, and prevention of substance abuse in the workplace. The connections between public health and occupational health and safety are strong. Consider one of the pillars of the public health model—the triad of primary, secondary, and tertiary prevention—and how it can be applied readily to the promotion of worker safety and health.

Primary prevention in the work setting refers to efforts to reduce the incidence of occupational illnesses. Worksite health promotion programs and emergency preparedness plans can be instrumental in the primary prevention of workers' illnesses. For example, methods for primary prevention include the use of personal protective equipment, substitution of less harmful materials for dangerous chemicals, and redesign of equipment

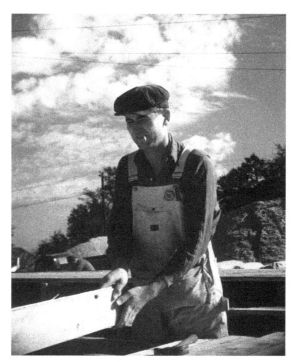

FIGURE 10.11   Male carpenter without protective gear and smoking a cigarette, circa 1943

Courtesy of Centers for Disease Control and Prevention, Public Health Image Library.

to make it safer. The last form of protection, which is called engineering control systems, includes measures such as increasing ventilation to dilute the concentrations of hazardous chemicals and using scrubbing systems to remove airborne pollutants. Engineering control systems are preferred over the use of respirators (one type of PPE), which are a last resort when it is not possible to engineer controls for harmful airborne contaminants.[51]

Secondary prevention involves strategies to reduce the prevalence of occupational diseases. Examples of secondary prevention include careful occupational exposure history taking during medical examinations of employees, screening workers for medical conditions that might have occupational etiologies, and surveillance of occupational illnesses (e.g., sentinel health events).

Tertiary prevention seeks to limit the effects of occupational illnesses through disability limitation and rehabilitation. Programs for tertiary prevention in the workplace include physical therapy for musculoskeletal disorders, treatments for employees who are experiencing workplace-related post-traumatic stress disorder, and interventions for workers who are afflicted by substance abuse issues (e.g., binge drinking). Substance abuse interventions can aid in limiting the sequelae of substance abuse and returning affected workers to productive status.

Workplace Health Promotion

Workplace health promotion is defined "as the combined efforts of employers, employees and society to improve the health and well-being of people at work."[52] Workplace health promotion can be limited to the individual or can encompass the entire work setting. Going beyond the concept of safety, programs for workplace health promotion strive to improve employees' general health status through activities that take place in the work environment. Such health promotion programs could be offered as an employee benefit. In many instances, employees may be receptive to these efforts because they are, in a sense, "a captive audience." Among the many examples of health promotion programs for employees is the Department of Health and Human Services' Million Hearts initiative, which seeks to reduce the impact of cardiovascular risk factors by managing hypertension, cholesterol levels, tobacco use, nutrition, and physical activity.[53] Employers can support this initiative by measures such as creating on-site physical activity facilities and making healthier food choices available in the company cafeteria.

Participation in workplace health promotion activities can be encouraged through incentives such as gift certificates. Some of these programs focus on a single activity, such as smoking cessation, exercise, or modification of heart disease risk factors; others have a broader scope and are devoted to creating a more healthful work environment. EXHIBIT 10.6 presents a case study of a wellness program offered by the Meredith Corporation in Des Moines, Iowa.

Workplace health promotion can help to improve collegial working relationships and raise the esprit de corps of the organization. TABLE 10.6 lists additional benefits for the organization and employee.

The Workplace Health Model

EXHIBIT 10.7 describes the workplace health model for building a workplace health program. The four main steps in program development are assessment, planning, implementation, and evaluation.

Emergency Preparedness

Emergencies caused by natural disasters, severe weather events, and pandemic disease can be extremely hazardous to employees as well as to the community as a whole. Weather-related events may include tornadoes, hurricanes, flooding, and heavy snowfall.[54] In some parts of the United States,

---

EXHIBIT 10.6 Case Study: A Penny Saved—Meredith Corporation Spends to Save

The Meredith Corporation, a media and marketing company based in Des Moines, Iowa, with offices throughout the United States, began its wellness program in 2006 as a way to encourage its employees to be more active and make healthier lifestyle choices. As a part of the program, Meredith offered its employees a fitness club membership. Although the company has offices spread across the country, nearly 40% of the employees went to one franchise club. After crunching the numbers of how often employees who opted for this benefit actually went to the gym, it was determined that few took advantage of the program.

"We realized that we were paying almost $56 per employee visit to offer this benefit," stated Tim O'Neil, Manager of Employee Health and Financial Wellness for Meredith. "It was not in our best interest to offer full-club memberships."

Instead, employees were offered a subsidized membership, the value of which is determined on the basis of the number of visits to the fitness club an employee makes per month. If an employee goes twice per month, he or she gets 25% of the membership subsidized. If the employees goes eight times per month, 100% is subsidized. This change saved the company approximately $200,000 per year, which in turn was reinvested in other wellness areas, and, in fact, resulted in a 10% increase in employees who signed up for the program.

Meredith also offers health risk appraisals for all employees, with a goal of having 85% of the employees take part. After three years, Tim and his colleagues began to look at the impact the programs were having on employee health and the company's bottom line. Of the employees who took part in the company's programs and the health risk appraisal, 97% were in the low to medium health risk category after 18 months. For those employees in the low risk category, there was a 9% decline in insurance claims. For employees in the medium risk category, there was a 39% decline in claims. For the 3% in the high risk category, there was a 30% increase in claims.

The return on investment for Meredith has truly paid off. Reviewing the actual number of dollars, Tim and his colleagues realized that their investment in physical activity and wellness programs over the course of 4 years resulted in a savings of $3.50 for every $1.00 spent.

"Investing in these programs doesn't just make sense," said Tim. "It makes cents. Literally."

Reprinted from Centers for Disease Control and Prevention. Steps to wellness: a guide to implementing the 2008 physical activity guidelines for Americans in the workplace. Atlanta, GA. U.S. Department of Health and Human Services; 2012:13.

---

earthquakes and wildfires can impact the work setting. Adequate preparation for emergencies requires creating a plan for response, worker training, making protective equipment available for the workforce, and, should an emergency occur, having the ability to respond in an organized fashion.[55] A chain of command and modes of communication during an emergency should be established before such an event takes place.

Businesses and other types of employers also need to plan for emergencies caused by pandemic disease, such as pandemic influenza.[56] During a pandemic, many people could die and business operations could be interrupted.

TABLE 10.6   Benefits of Workplace Health Promotion

To the Organization	To the Employee
A well-managed health and safety program	A safe and healthy work environment
A positive and caring image	Enhanced self-esteem
Improved staff morale	Reduced stress
Reduced staff turnover	Improved morale
Reduced absenteeism	Increased job satisfaction
Increased productivity	Increased skills for health protection
Reduced healthcare/insurance costs	Improved health
Reduced risk of fines and litigation	Improved sense of well-being

Reprinted from World Health Organization (WHO). Workplace health promotion. http://www.who.int/occupational_health/topics/workplace/en/index.html. Accessed May 31, 2013.

EXHIBIT 10.7   Workplace Health Model

Building a workplace health program should involve a coordinated, systematic, and comprehensive approach. A *coordinated* approach to workplace health promotion results in a planned, organized, and comprehensive set of programs, policies, benefits, and environmental supports designed to meet the health and safety needs of all employees. A *comprehensive* approach seeks to put interventions in place that address multiple risk factors and health conditions concurrently and recognizes that the interventions and strategies chosen influence multiple levels of the organization, including both the individual employee and the organization as a whole.

Workplace health promotion programs are more likely to be successful if occupational safety and health is considered in their design and execution. In fact, a growing body of evidence indicates that workplace-based interventions that take coordinated, planned, or integrated approaches to reducing health threats to workers both inside and outside the work setting are more effective than traditional isolated programs. Integrating or coordinating occupational safety and health with health promotion may increase program participation and effectiveness and may also benefit the broader context of work organization and environment.

The *systematic* process of building a workplace health promotion program emphasizes four main steps (**FIGURE 10.12**):

1. An assessment to define employee health risks and concerns and describe current health promotion activities, capacity, and needs
2. A planning process to develop the components of a workplace health program, including goal determination, selecting priority interventions, and building an organizational infrastructure
3. Program implementation involving all the steps needed to put health promotion strategies and interventions into place and making them available to employees
4. An evaluation of efforts to systematically investigate the merit (e.g., quality), worth (e.g., effectiveness), and significance (e.g., importance) of an organized health promotion action/activity

Reprinted from Centers for Disease Control and Prevention (CDC). Workplace health model. http://www.cdc.gov/workplacehealthpromotion/model/index.html. Accessed July 29, 2014.

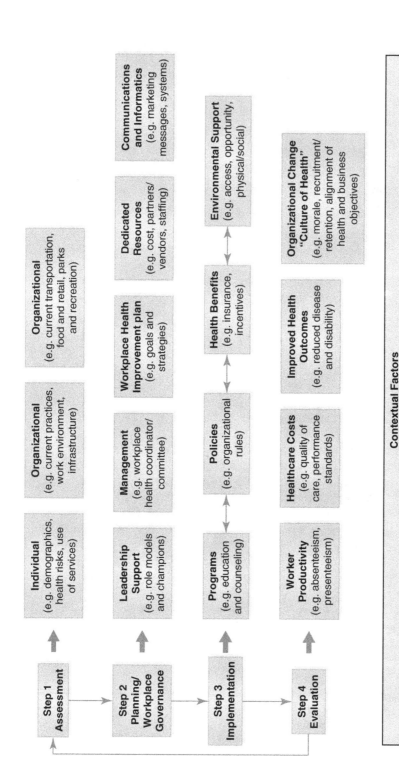

FIGURE 10.12 Workplace Health Model

Employers will need to formulate plans for prevention of transmission of epidemic diseases in the workplace so that vital operations can continue.

Substance Abuse and Work

Use of illicit drugs and heavy use of alcohol have wide-ranging adverse effects among employees and their employers.[57] Most adults who abuse illicit drugs or are binge and heavy alcohol users are employed. The outcomes associated with this type of behavior include lost productivity, absenteeism, increased risk of injuries, lowered health status of workers, and theft and security problems.[58] In the annual National Survey on Drug Use and Health (for the years 2002, 2003, and 2004), 8.2% of workers aged 18 to 64 years reported past-month use of illicit drugs.[59] Almost one-fifth of full-time U.S. workers aged 18 to 25 years reported past-month use of illicit drugs. Consequently, the issue of substance abuse has widespread significance and is greatly concerning to occupational health practitioners. Thus, programs designed for the creation of a drug-free workplace contribute to a healthy job environment.[60]

The U.S. government responded to concerns about substance abuse with the creation of the Drug-Free Workplace Act of 1988. This act

> ... requires *some* Federal contractors and *all* Federal grantees to agree that they will provide drug-free workplaces as a precondition of receiving a contract or grant from a Federal agency. Although all covered contractors and grantees must maintain a drug-free workplace, the specific components necessary to meet the requirements of the Act vary based on whether the contractor or grantee is an individual or an organization. The requirements for organizations are more extensive, because organizations have to take comprehensive, programmatic steps to achieve a workplace free of drugs.[61]

A decade later on June 18, 1998, the U.S. Congress passed the Drug-Free Workplace Act of 1998. The act is addressed particularly to substance abuse in small businesses. Under this act, the Small Business Administration included the following components for the development of a drug-free work setting:

1. "A clear written policy
2. A minimum of 2 hours of training for all employees
3. Additional training for working parents
4. Drug testing by a certified institution
5. Access to an EAP [employment assistant program]
6. A continuing drug and alcohol abuse prevention program"[60(p. 1)]

SUMMARY

Safety in occupational settings is connected inextricably with workers' health. The goal of programs for occupational safety is to create a work environment that is free from exposures and conditions that are injurious to employees; prevention is the core focus of this field. To respond to issues associated with occupationally associated health risks and hazards, occupational health practitioners conduct risk assessments and maintain surveillance of occupational injuries and illnesses. Then they apply risk management procedures for improvement of health in the workplace. Key aspects of such risk management are hazard control and risk communication. Surveillance in occupational health involves collecting information on sentinel health events and occupational health indicators.

The public health model of prevention is helpful for categorizing specific methods of preventing occupational illnesses and improving the health of workers. For example, primary prevention of occupational illnesses and injuries is more cost-effective than programs for secondary prevention, such as screening workers for occupationally associated health conditions.

To create a work environment that is safer and healthier, tomorrow's occupational health experts will need to take on challenging career roles in the field. In addition to careful monitoring of exposures, hazards, and illnesses, their other activities will involve workplace health promotion, development of emergency preparedness plans for employers and employees, and interventions in adverse lifestyle practices that are prevalent in contemporary job settings.

STUDY QUESTIONS AND EXERCISES

1. Define the following terms:
   A. Occupational safety
   B. Workplace health promotion
   C. Risk assessment
   D. Hazard analysis
   E. Surveillance
2. Describe the four procedures for risk assessment as applied to occupational illnesses, injuries, and fatalities.
3. Using your own ideas in addition to those presented in the text, state the strengths and weaknesses of risk characterization.
4. What are the prerequisites of a successful program for occupational health and safety?
5. How do surveillance systems aid in the prevention of occupational injuries? Give examples of surveillance programs that have been designed for use in the occupational setting.
6. Describe the application of occupational health indicators and occupational sentinel health events to the assessment of workers' health.
7. How does workplace hazard communication relate to occupational health risk management?
8. Describe the public health model for prevention and promotion of worker safety as it pertains to the work environment.

9. State the public health levels of prevention represented by personal protective equipment (e.g., dust masks) and engineering controls. Which type—personal protective equipment or engineering controls—is preferred?

10. Describe three occupational roles in the field of occupational health. Meet with a professional occupational health specialist or invite him or her to the classroom to discuss occupational health practice.

REFERENCES

1. Rudolph L, Deitchman S, Dervin K. Integrating occupational health services and occupational prevention services. *Am J Ind Med.* 2001;40:307–318.

2. Dictionary.com. Safety. n.d. http://dictionary.reference.com/browse/safety. Accessed October 21, 2013.

3. U.S. Department of Labor, Occupational Safety and Health Administration (OSHA). *Injury and illness prevention programs.* OSHA FactSheet. Washington, DC: OSHA; 2013.

4. U.S. Environmental Protection Agency. Risk assessment for toxic air pollutants: a citizen's guide. n.d. http://www.epa.gov/airquality/air_risc/3_90_024.html. Accessed April 16, 2014.

5. National Research Council. *Risk assessment in the federal government: managing the process.* Washington, DC: National Academy Press; 1983.

6. U.S. Environmental Protection Agency. Human health risk assessment. n.d. http://www.epa.gov/ncea/risk/health-risk.htm. Accessed October 22, 2013.

7. Porta M, ed. *A dictionary of epidemiology.* 5th ed. New York, NY: Oxford University Press; 2008.

8. Russell M, Gruber M. Risk assessment in environmental policy-making. *Science.* 1987;236:286–290.

9. U.S. Department of Labor, Occupational Safety and Health Administration (OSHA). *Job hazard analysis.* OSHA 3071 2002 (Revised). Washington, DC: OSHA; 2002.

10. Lippmann M, Thurston GD. Exposure assessment: input into risk assessment. *Arch Environ Health.* 1988;43(2):113–123.

11. Ott WR. Human exposure assessment: the birth of a new science. *J Expo Anal Environ Epidemiol.* 1995;5(4):449–472.

12. Lax MB, Grant WD, Manetti FA, Klein R. Recognizing occupational disease: taking an effective occupational history. *Am Fam Physician.* 1998;58(4):935–944.

13. Monson RR. *Occupational epidemiology.* Boca Raton. FL: CRC Press; 1990.

14. U.S. Environmental Protection Agency. Defining biomarkers. n.d. http://www.epa.gov/pesticides/science/biomarker.html. Accessed April 12, 2014.

15. Hyperdictionary. Meaning of sister chromatid exchange. n.d. http://www.hyperdictionary.com/dictionary/sister+chromatid+exchange. Accessed April 12, 2014.

16. Rappaport SM, Symanski E, Yager JW, Kupper LL. The relationship between environmental monitoring and biological markers in exposure assessment. *Environ Health Perspect.* 1995;103(suppl 3):49–54.

17. Landrigan PJ, Carlson JE. Environmental policy and children's health. *Future Child.* 1995;5(2):34–52.

18. Stern PC, Fineberg HV, eds. *Understanding risk: informing decisions in a democratic society.* Washington, DC: National Academy Press; 1996.

19. National Research Council. *Science and judgment in risk assessment.* Washington, DC: National Academy Press; 1994.

20. Yassi A, Kjellström T, de Kok T, Guidotti TL. *Basic environmental health.* New York, NY: Oxford University Press; 2001.

21. Myers ML. Reducing hazards in the work environment. In: Friis RH, ed. *The Praeger handbook of environmental health.* Vol. 4. Santa Barbara, CA: Praeger; 2012:43–67.

22. Covello VT. Risk communication and environmental health: principles, strategies, tools, and techniques. In: Friis RH, ed. *The Praeger handbook of environmental health.* Vol. 1. Santa Barbara, CA: Praeger; 2012:367–389.

23. Lin I, Petersen DD. *Risk communication in action: the tools of message mapping.* EPA/625/R-06/012. Cincinnati, OH: U.S. Environmental Protection Agency; 2007.

24. U.S. Department of Labor, Occupational Safety and Health Administration. Hazard communication. n.d. http://www.osha.gov/dsg/hazcom/index.html. Accessed May 12, 2013.

25. U.S. Department of Labor, Occupational Health and Safety Administration. Personal protective equipment. n.d. https://www.osha.gov/SLTC/personalprotectiveequipment/. Accessed July 17, 2014.

26. U.S. Department of Labor, Occupational Health and Safety Administration. Eye and face protection eTool: selecting PPE for the workplace. n.d. https://www.osha.gov/SLTC/etools/eyeandface/ppe/selection.html. Accessed July 17, 2014.

27. U.S. Department of Labor, Occupational Safety and Health Administration (OSHA). OSHA FactSheet. *Laboratory safety chemical hygiene plan (CHP).* Washington, DC: OSHA; 2011.

28. CPLabSafety. Safety cabinet regulations: choosing a safety cabinet color. n.d. http://www.calpaclab.com/safety-cabinet-regulations-1/. Accessed June 24, 2014.

29. Earnest Orlando Lawrence Berkeley National Laboratory. Chemical hygiene and safety plan: chemical storage. n.d. http://www2.lbl.gov/ehs/chsp/html/storage.shtml. Accessed June 24, 2014.

30. Centers for Disease Control and Prevention (CDC), National Institute for Occupational Safety and Health (NIOSH). *NIOSH pocket guide to chemical hazards.* Cincinnati, OH: CDC, NIOSH; 2007.

31. Morabia A. Annotation: from disease surveillance to the surveillance of risk factors. *Am J Public Health.* 1996;86(5):625–626.

32. Ritz B, Tager I, Balmes J. Can lessons from public health disease surveillance be applied to environmental public health tracking? *Environ Health Perspect.* 2005;113(3)243–249.

33. Thacker SB, Stroup DF, Parrish RG, Anderson HA. Surveillance in environmental public health: issues, systems, and sources. *Am J Public Health.* 1996;86(5):633–638.

34. Thomsen C, McClain J, Rosenman K, Davis L. Indicators for occupational health surveillance. *MMWR.* 2007;56(RR-1);1–7.

35. Levy BS. Editorial: toward a holistic approach to public health surveillance. *Am J Public Health.* 1996;86(5):624–625.

36. Froines J, Wegman D, Eisen E. Hazard surveillance in occupational disease. *Am J Public Health.* 1989;79(suppl):26-31.

37. California Department of Public Health, Occupational Health Branch. Hazard evaluation system and information service. n.d. http://www.cdph.ca.gov/programs/hesis/Pages/default.aspx. Accessed April 14, 2014.

38. Koh D, Aw T-C. Surveillance in occupational health. *Occup Environ Med.* 2003;60:705–710.

39. Rutstein DD, Mullan RJ, Frazier TM, et al. Sentinel health events (occupational): a basis for physician recognition and public health surveillance. *Am J Public Health.* 1983;73:1054–1062.

40. Centers for Disease Control and Prevention, National Institute for Occupational Safety and Health. Occupational sentinel health events SHE(O). n.d. http://www.cdc.gov/niosh/topics/SHEO/. Accessed May 13, 2013.

41. Council of State and Territorial Epidemiologists. Occupational health: indicators. n.d. http://www.cste.org/group/OHIndicators. Accessed May 31, 2013.

42. California Department of Public Health, Occupational Health Branch. Occupational health indicators data tables. n.d. http://www.cdph.ca.gov/programs/ohsep/Pages/IndicatorsList.aspx. Accessed April 14, 2014.

43. The FreeDictionary. Occupational medicine. n.d. http://www.thefreedictionary.com/Occupational+safety+and+health. Accessed August 17, 2013.

44. Lee WR. Emergence of occupational medicine in Victorian times. *Br J Ind Med.* 1973;30:118–124.

45. American College of Occupational and Environmental Medicine. Physicians new to occupational medicine. n.d. http://www.acoem.org/Print.aspx? Accessed April 9, 2014.

46. U.S. Department of Labor (USDOL), Occupational Safety and Health Administration (OSHA). *Industrial hygiene.* OSHA 3143 1998 (Revised). Washington, DC: USDOL, OSHA; 1998.

47. National Institutes of Health, Office of Research Services. What is industrial hygiene? n.d. http://www.ors.od.nih.gov/sr/dohs/aboutDOHS/TAB/Pages/technical_branch_ih.aspx. Accessed April 9, 2014.

48. Abrams HK. A short history of occupational health. *J Public Health Policy.* 2001;22(1):34–80.

49. International Labour Organization (ILO). International code of ethics for occupational health professionals. In: *ILO encyclopaedia of occupational health and safety.* n.d. http://www.ilo.org/oshenc/part-iii/ethical-issues/item/337-international-code-of-ethics-for-occupational-health-professionals. Accessed July 21, 2014.

50. American Board of Industrial Hygiene. American Board of Industrial Hygiene code of ethics. n.d. http://abih.org/sites/default/files/downloads/ABIHCodeofEthics.pdf. Accessed July 21, 2014.

51. Centers for Disease Control and Prevention, National Institute for Occupational Safety and Health. Respirators. n.d. http://www.cdc.gov/niosh/topics/respirators/. Accessed May 13, 2013.

52. World Health Organization. Workplace health promotion. n.d. http://www.who.int/occupational_health/topics/workplace/en/index1.html. Accessed May 31, 2013.

53. Centers for Disease Control and Prevention (CDC). *Cardiovascular health: action steps for employers.* Atlanta, GA: CDC; August 2013.

54. U.S. Department of Labor, Occupational Safety and Health Administration. Emergency preparedness and response. n.d. https://www.osha.gov/SLTC/emergencypreparedness/. Accessed April 14, 2014.

55. U.S. Department of Labor, Occupational Safety and Health Administration. Getting started–general preparedness and response. n.d. https://www.osha.gov/SLTC/emergencypreparedness/gettingstarted.html. Accessed April 14, 2014.

56. U.S. Department of Labor, Occupational Safety and Health Administration. Pandemic influenza. n.d. https://www.osha.gov/dsg/topics/pandemicflu/index.html. Accessed April 14, 2014.

57. National Institutes of Health, National Institute on Drug Abuse. Drug-free work-place resources. n.d. http://www.drugabuse.gov/related-topics/drug-testing/drug-free-workplace-resources. Accessed March 26, 2014.

58. Bush DM, Autry JH 3rd. Substance abuse in the workplace: epidemiology, effects, and industry response. *Occup Med.* 2002;17(1):13–25.

59. Larson SL, Eyerman J, Foster MS, Gfroerer JC. *Worker substance use and workplace policies and programs.* DHHS Publication No. SMA 07-4273, Analytic Series A-29. Rockville, MD: Substance Abuse and Mental Health Services Administration, Office of Applied Studies; 2007.

60. Substance Abuse and Mental Health Services Administration. Components of a drug-free workplace. n.d. http://www.drugabuse.gov/related-topics/drug-testing/drug-free-workplace-resources. Accessed March 26, 2014.

61. U.S. Department of Labor.. Drug-Free Workplace Act of 1988: requirements. n.d. http://www.dol.gov/elaws/asp/drugfree/screenr.htm. Accessed April 14, 2014.

Glossary

additive A combination of two or more chemicals that produces an effect that is equal to their individual effects added together

adjusted rates Summary measures of the rate of morbidity or mortality in populations; statistical procedures have been applied to remove the effect of differences in composition of the various populations

aerosol Small particles, usually in the range of 0.01 to 100 micrometers, dispersed in the air, which include liquid (mist) and small particles (dust)

age standardization A statistical procedure that removes the influence of age from a measure (e.g., death rate)

Agency for Toxic Substances and Disease Registry (ATSDR) Based in Atlanta, Georgia, it is one of 11 federal agencies within the U.S. Department of Health and Human Services. This agency "determines public health implications associated with hazardous waste sites and other environmental releases."

age-specific rate The number of events (e.g., deaths) during a specified time period that occur within an age group of the population divided by the number of persons in that age group times a multiplier

allergic contact dermatitis An inflammation of the skin caused by an immunologic reaction triggered by dermal contact with a skin allergen

alpha particle A subatomic particle made up of the nucleus of a helium atom that is ejected from a radioactive atom

analytic (analytical) epidemiologic study A study that explores the determinants of diseases—that is, the causes of relatively high or low frequencies of diseases in specific populations

antagonistic An instance in which one chemical cancels out the effect of another when the two are administered at the same time

antineoplastic drug   A drug used in cancer chemotherapy

area survey   A measuring of environmental noise levels using a sound level meter to identify work areas where employees' exposures are above or below hazardous levels, and where more thorough exposure monitoring may be needed. The result is often plotted in the form of a "noise map," showing noise level measurements for the different areas of the workplace.

arsenic   A naturally occurring element that is widely distributed in the Earth's crust and which is toxic to humans

arthropod vectors   Insects such as ticks, mites, and mosquitoes that can transmit bacterial, parasitic, or viral agents

asbestos   The name given to a group of six different fibrous minerals (amosite, chrysotile, crocidolite, and the fibrous varieties of tremolite, actinolite, and anthophyllite) that occur naturally in the environment

asbestosis   A type of pulmonary fibrosis that is associated with exposure to asbestos

asphxyiant   A substance that is capable of causing death from suffocation—for example, by decreasing the capacity of the blood to carry oxygen

asthmagen   Asthmagens can be divided into two separate types, namely, inducers and inciters. Inducers are substances that, on single or repeated exposure, cause a previously well individual to develop asthma. In contrast, inciters (or triggers) are substances that can cause symptoms in an individual with pre-existing abnormal airway responsiveness.

audiometry   The testing of a person's ability to hear various sound frequencies

benzene   A colorless liquid with a sweet odor that evaporates into the air very quickly and dissolves slightly in water

beta particle   A particle that is emitted from the nucleus of a radioactive atom

bias   Systematic deviation of results or inferences from truth; processes leading to such deviation; an error in the conception and design of a study—or in the collection, analysis, interpretation, reporting, publication, or review of data—leading to results or conclusions that are systematically (as opposed to randomly) different from truth.

biohazard   Organisms or products of organisms that present a risk to humans

biosafety levels (BSLs)   Level of microbes that relate to their virulence and the degree of hazard that they present

burnout   A syndrome that consists of emotional exhaustion, a sense of depersonalization (e.g., detachment and disengagement), and a feeling that one is less able to be effective in accomplishing goals

byssinosis (brown lung disease)   A lung disorder characterized by reduced lung function and other adverse pulmonary effects associated with breathing cotton dust; it is a form of pneumoconiosis and is both an underlying cause of and a contributing cause to mortality

Caisson disease   A form of decompression sickness that occurs among workers who have been laboring in underground pressurized chambers used in construction projects

carcinogen   A substance or agent that causes cancer in mammals, including humans

carpal tunnel syndrome   When the median nerve, which runs from the forearm into the palm of the hand, becomes pressed or squeezed at the wrist

case-control study   A study in which subjects are defined on the basis of the presence or absence of an outcome of interest

cause-specific rate   A rate that specifies events, such as deaths, according to their cause

chemical hygiene plan (CHP)   A written program stating the policies, procedures, and responsibilities that protect workers from the health hazards associated with the hazardous chemicals used in that particular workplace

chilblains   Swelling and itching of the skin that occurs when it is exposed to cold temperatures

clustering   A closely grouped series of events or cases of a disease or other health-related phenomena with well-defined distribution patterns in relation to time or place or both. The term is normally used to describe aggregation of relatively uncommon events or diseases (e.g., leukemia, multiple sclerosis).

coal workers' pneumoconiosis (CWP; black lung disease)   A serious lung disease caused by breathing coal dust over an extended time period

cohort study   A study wherein subjects are classified according to their exposure to a factor of interest and then observed over time to document the occurrence of new cases (incidence) of disease or other health events

common units   An earlier system of radiation measurement that is often used in the United States

communicable disease   An illness due to a specific infectious agent or its toxic products that arises through transmission of that agent or its products from an infected person, animal, or reservoir to a susceptible host, either directly or indirectly through an intermediate plant or animal host, vector, or the inanimate environment

confined space   A space that has limited or restricted means for entry or exit, and it is not designed for continuous employee occupancy

confounding The distortion of a measure of the effect of an exposure on an outcome due to the association of the exposure with other factors that influence the occurrence of the outcome

contact dermatitis An inflammation of the skin resulting from exposure to a hazardous agent; also called eczema

cross-sectional study A study that examines the relationship between diseases (or other health-related characteristics) and other variables of interest as they exist in a defined population at one particular time. The presence or absence of disease and the presence or absence of the other variables are determined in each member of the study population or in a representative sample at one particular time.

crystalline silica A basic component of soil, sand, granite, and many other minerals; quartz is the most common form

cumulative trauma disorders (CTDs) Chronic disorders involving connective tissue (muscles, tendons) and nerves, often resulting from work-related physical activities

death rate An estimate of the proportion of a population that dies during a specified period

decibels (dBs) The scale for measurement of sound pressure

decision latitude The level of skill and creativity required on the job and the flexibility the worker is permitted in deciding what skills to employ, and also the organizationally mediated possibilities for workers to make decisions about their work

descriptive epidemiologic study A study that characterizes the amount and distribution of disease within a population

dichlorodiphenyltrichloroethane (DDT) An organochloride pesticide. One of the POPs, which has been placed on the list of most dangerous "dirty dozen" chemicals

dioxins A class of structurally and chemically related halogenated aromatic hydrocarbons that includes polychlorinated dibenzodioxins (PCDDs or dioxins), polychlorinated dibenzofurans (PCDFs or furans) and the "dioxin-like" polychlorinated biphenyls (PCBs)

disease surveillance Monitoring distributions and trends of morbidity and mortality data; involves systematic and continuous collection of data

distress Stress that has negative or undesirable consequences

dose The amount of a substance administered at one time

dose–response assessment The process of characterizing the relation between the dose of an agent administered or received and the incidence of an adverse health effect in exposed populations and estimating the incidence of the effect as a function of human exposure to the agent

dose–response curve   A map of associations between exposures and effects

dose–response relationship   A type of correlative association between an exposure (e.g., a toxic chemical) and an effect (e.g., a biologic outcome such as cell death)

dosimetry   The use of body-worn instruments (dosimeters) to monitor an employee's noise exposure over the work-shift

ecologic fallacy   An erroneous inference that may occur because an association observed between variables on an aggregate level does not necessarily represent or reflect the association that exists at an individual level

ecologic study   A study in which the units of analysis are populations or groups of people rather than individuals

employee assistance program (EAP)   A voluntary, work-based program that offers free and confidential assessments, short-term counseling, referrals, and follow-up services to employees who have personal and/or work-related problems. EAPs address a broad and complex body of issues affecting mental and emotional well-being, such as alcohol and other substance abuse, stress, grief, family problems, and psychological disorders.

employee morale   Description of the emotions, attitudes, satisfaction, and overall outlook of employees during their time in a workplace environment

endemic   An infectious disease (or condition) that is habitually present in a geographic area

engineering surveys   Surveys that typically employ more sophisticated acoustical equipment in addition to sound level meters. This equipment furnishes information on the frequency/intensity composition of the noise being emitted by machinery or other sound sources in various modes of operation. These measurements are used to assess options for applying engineering controls.

epidemic   The occurrence in a community or region of cases of an illness, specific health-related behavior, or other health-related events clearly in excess of normal expectancy

epidemiology   The study of the occurrence and distribution of health-related states or events in specified populations, including the study of the determinants influencing such states, and the application of this knowledge to control the health problems

ergonomics   The scientific study of people at work. The goal of ergonomics is to reduce stress and eliminate injuries and disorders associated with the overuse of muscles, bad posture, and repeated tasks.

eustress   Good stress; denotes stress that has positive qualities

executive monkey   A monkey that is exposed to stress via the requirement to press a lever so as to avert an electric shock during an experiment

exposure assessment   A procedure that includes defining populations that have been exposed to a toxicant, measuring the amounts of their exposures, and determining the lengths of their exposures

Fair Labor Standards Act of 1938 (FLSA)   An act of Congress designed "[t]o provide for the establishment of fair labor standards in employments in and affecting interstate commerce, and for other purposes."

fiberglass   A silicate fiber made from very fine strands of glass

formaldehyde   A colorless, flammable gas that has a distinct, pungent smell

frostbite   An injury to the body that is caused by freezing, which most often affects the nose, ears, cheeks, chin, fingers, or toes

fungal diseases   Diseases caused by fungi that are present in the environment

furans   Abbreviated or short name for a family of toxic substances that all share a similar chemical structure; include PCDDs or dioxins and PCDFs or furans

gamma rays   High-energy rays that are part of the electromagnetic spectrum; one of the forms of ionizing radiation

general adaptation syndrome   As specified by Selye, stress is a change in the environment of the organism and the organism's response consists of three stages: alarm reaction, stage of resistance, and stage of exhaustion

General Duty Clause (of the OSH Act)   Requires that "[e]ach employer shall furnish to each of his employees employment and a place of employment which are free from recognized hazards that are causing or are likely to cause death or serious physical harm to his employees"

global outsourcing   The transfer of manufacturing and other operations to countries where they can be performed less expensively

green jobs   Work in agricultural, manufacturing, research and development (R & D), administrative, and service activities that contribute substantially to preserving and restoring environmental quality. Specifically, but not exclusively, this includes jobs that help to protect ecosystems and biodiversity; de-carbonize the economy; and minimize or altogether avoid generation of all forms of waste and pollution

Haddon Matrix   Developed by William Haddon, it is applied widely to the prevention of unintentional injuries and is germane to work-related injuries. This matrix was used originally for categorizing highway safety phenomena, but it is applicable in more general terms to prevention of unintentional injuries.

hand–arm vibration syndrome (HAVS)   The group of symptoms that result from hand-transmitted vibration

hand-transmitted vibration (HTV)   Vibration entering the body through the hands.

hazard   Inherent capability of an agent or a situation to have an adverse effect; a factor or exposure that may adversely affect health

hazard identification   The process of determining whether exposure to an agent can cause an increase in the incidence of a health condition (cancer, birth defect, etc.). It involves characterizing the nature and the strength of the evidence of causation.

health risks   The chances of experiencing an adverse health effect if a person comes into contact with a harmful substance such as a carcinogen or toxic chemical

healthy worker effect   The observation that employed populations tend to have a lower mortality experience than the general population

heavy metal   A metal such as beryllium, cadmium, and chromium that has a high atomic weight with a specific gravity that exceeds the specific gravity of water by five or more times

hertz (Hz)   The number of cycles per second (frequency) associated with the oscillation of a given sound wave, with high and low hertz numbers characterizing high and low tones, respectively

hexavalent chromium   A toxic form of the element chromium

hyperbaric environments   Environments with high ambient air pressures—that is, pressures greater than one atmosphere

hypersensitivity pneumonitis   A disease in which the lungs become inflamed from breathing in foreign substances, such as molds, dusts, and chemicals. These substances also are known as antigens.

hyperthermia   Overheating of the body, possibly due to extreme weather conditions. Unrelieved hyperthermia can lead to collapse and death, particularly in the elderly.

hypobaric environments   Environments characterized by reduced atmospheric pressures, such as those encountered at high altitudes and in outer space

hypothermia   A condition in which the body uses up its stored energy and can no longer produce heat; often occurs after prolonged exposure to cold temperature

incidence   The number of instances of illnesses commencing, or of persons falling ill, during a given period in a specified population

incidence rate   Rate formed by dividing the number of new cases that occur during a time period by the number of individuals in the population at risk

industrial hygiene (occupational hygiene)   The science and art devoted to the anticipation, recognition, evaluation, and control of those environmental factors or stresses arising in or from the workplace and which may cause sickness, impaired health and well-being, or significant discomfort among workers or among the citizens of the community

intentional injuries   Injuries that are caused willfully (on purpose)

International Labour Organization (ILO)   A specialized United Nations agency devoted to the work setting; it was founded in 1919. The main aims of the ILO are to promote rights at work, encourage decent employment opportunities, enhance social protection, and strengthen dialogue on work-related issues.

ionizing radiation   Electromagnetic (X-ray and gamma) or particulate (alpha, beta) radiation capable of producing ions or charged particles

irritant contact dermatitis   A non-immunologic reaction that manifests as an inflammation of the skin caused by direct damage to the skin following exposure to a hazardous agent

isotope   any of two or more species of atoms of a chemical element with the same atomic number and nearly identical chemical behavior but with differing atomic mass or mass number and different physical properties

job demand–control (JD-C) model   A model that postulates an association between job strain and a combination of a high-demand job and low decision latitude

job hazard analysis   A technique that focuses on job tasks as a way to identify hazards before they occur. It focuses on the relationship between the worker, the task, the tools, and the work environment.

job strain   Employees' responses, both physiologic and mental, to exposures to stressors

job stress (occupational stress)   The harmful physical and emotional responses that occur when the requirements of the job do not match the capabilities, resources, or needs of the worker. Job stress can lead to poor health and even injury.

laser   An acronym that stands for "light amplification by stimulated emission of radiation."

latency   The time period between the initial exposure and a measurable response

LD$_{50}$ (lethal dose 50)   The dosage (mg/kg body weight) causing death in 50% of exposed animals

male infertility   A condition caused by low sperm production, misshapen or immobile sperm, or blockages that prevent the delivery of sperm

mercurialism   Poisoning by mercury

musculoskeletal disorders (MSDs)   Injuries or disorders of the muscles, nerves, tendons, joints, cartilage, and disorders of the nerves, tendons, muscles, and supporting structures of the upper and lower limbs, neck, and lower back that are caused, precipitated or exacerbated by sudden exertion or prolonged exposure to physical factors such as repetition, force, vibration, or awkward posture

nanotechnology   The manipulation of matter on a near-atomic scale (1 to 100 nanometers in length) to produce new structures, materials, and devices

National Institute for Occupational Safety and Health (NIOSH)   The federal agency responsible for conducting research and making recommendations for the prevention of work-related illness and injury. Established in 1970 under the Occupational Safety and Health Act of 1970, NIOSH is part of the U.S. Centers for Disease Control and Prevention (CDC) and the U.S. Department of Health and Human Services (DHHS).

National Institute of Environmental Health Sciences (NIEHS)   One of 27 institutes and centers of the National Institutes of Health (NIH). The NIEHS supports a wide variety of research programs directed toward preventing health problems caused by our environment.

noise-induced permanent threshold shift (NIPTS)   A permanent threshold shift that can be attributable to noise exposure

non-ionizing radiation   A series of energy waves composed of oscillating electric and magnetic fields traveling at the speed of light

nuclide   A nucleus with a specific number of protons and neutrons and a specific energy state; it includes radioactive and nonradioactive atoms

obstructive occupational lung diseases   Lung conditions that prevent affected individuals from exhaling air completely, causing air to remain in the lungs

occupational asthma   A disease characterized by variable airflow limitation and/or bronchial hyperresponsiveness due to causes and conditions attributable to a particular working environment and not to stimuli encountered outside the workplace

occupational dermatoses   Those dermatoses for which the cause can be found partly or wholly in the conditions in which the work is carried out

occupational epidemiology   The study of the effects of workplace exposures on the frequency and distribution of diseases and injuries in the population

occupational exposures   Work-related physical conditions (e.g., structural insecurity or deficient lighting), physical stress (e.g., lifting heavy weights or repetitive strain injuries), physical agents (e.g., noise, vibration, or radiation), chemicals (e.g., dusts or solvents), biological agents (e.g., bacteria or viruses) and psychosocial stressors

occupational exposures to blood and body fluids (BBF)   Skin, eye, mucous membrane, or parenteral contact with blood or other potentially infectious materials that may result from the performance of an employee's duties

occupational health   Identification and control of the risks arising from physical, chemical, and other workplace hazards in order to establish and maintain a safe and healthy working environment. These hazards may include chemical agents and solvents, heavy metals such as lead and mercury, physical agents such as loud noise or vibration, and physical hazards such as electricity or dangerous machinery.

occupational health indicators   Measures of health (work-related disease or injury) or factors associated with health (workplace exposures, hazards, or interventions); allow for comparison of its health or risk status across work settings and evaluation of trends over time. These data can help guide priorities for prevention and intervention efforts.

occupational health policy   A plan of action primarily concerned with protecting the health, safety, and welfare of persons at work. These policies typically are designed to protect workers from hazardous work environments by ensuring clean work areas, the use of protective equipment, and ensuring employees are properly trained.

occupational illnesses   Adverse health outcomes—for example, disease and disability—linked with exposures that occur in the work environment

occupational injury epidemiology   A field of research that seeks to describe the distribution and determinants of occupational injuries and to make and test inferences about their prevention

occupational injury or work-related injury   Any damage inflicted to the body by energy transfer during work with a short duration between exposure and the health event (usually < 48 hrs)

occupational lung diseases   A group of illnesses caused by either repeated or extended exposures or a single, severe exposure to irritating or toxic substances that lead to acute or chronic respiratory ailments

occupational medicine   The branch of medicine that deals with the prevention and treatment of diseases and injuries occurring at work or in specific occupations

occupational safety   The creation of a work environment that is free from exposures and conditions that are injurious to employees; prevention is the core focus of this field.

Occupational Safety and Health Act of 1970   Established by Congress "[t]o assure safe and healthful working conditions for working men and women; by authorizing enforcement of the standards developed under the Act; by assisting and encouraging the States in their efforts to assure safe and healthful working conditions; by providing for research, information, education, and training in the field of occupational safety and health; and for other purposes."

Occupational Safety and Health Administration (OSHA)   Established by Congress "to assure safe and healthful conditions for working men and women by setting and enforcing standards and providing training, outreach, education and compliance assistance.... Under the OSHA law, employers are responsible for providing a safe and healthful workplace for their workers."

occupational toxicology   The field that applies the principles and methodology of toxicology to chemical and biological hazards encountered at work

occupationally associated cancers   Cancers hypothesized to be linked to exposures to carcinogens in the work environment

odds ratio (OR)   The measure of association between exposure and outcome used in case-control studies

organic solvent encephalopathy   Long-term neurologic damage from solvent exposure as indicated by headache, memory impairment, and confusion

organic solvent syndrome   A cluster of neurologic symptoms—for example, impaired memory, confusion, restlessness, and insomnia—associated with inhalation of solvents

organization of work (work organization)   The work process (the way jobs are designed and performed) and the organizational practices (management and production methods and accompanying human resource policies) that influence the job design

organochloride pesticide   A pesticide that contains chlorine, carbon, and, sometimes, several other elements

oscillatory vibrations   Noise from sources in the work environment as well as physical vibrations of the human body caused by machinery

OSHA standards Rules that describe the methods employers are legally required to follow to protect their workers from hazards

pandemic An epidemic occurring worldwide or over a very wide area, crossing international boundaries, and usually affecting a large number of people

permanent threshold shift (PTS) Any change in hearing sensitivity that is persistent

permissible exposure limits (PELs) OSHA standards that are subject specific and that provide supporting documentation for promulgation and enforcement of occupational health regulations. They denote an allowable exposure level in the workplace air that is averaged over an eight-hour shift.

persistent organic pollutants (POPs) A group of toxic chemicals that remain for long periods of time in the environment and can accumulate and pass from one species to the next through the food chain

personal protective equipment (PPE) Equipment worn to minimize exposure to workplace hazards that can cause serious injuries and illnesses

pesticide Any substance or mixture of substances intended for preventing, destroying, repelling, or mitigating any pest

pneumoconiosis The accumulation of dust in the lungs and the tissue reactions to its presence

polychlorinated biphenyls (PCBs) Belong to a broad family of man-made organic chemicals known as chlorinated hydrocarbons. Prior to their discontinuation, PCBs were used as an insulating fluid in electrical components such as capacitors and transformers.

polycyclic aromatic hydrocarbons (PAHs) A group of chemicals that are formed during the incomplete burning of coal, oil, gas, wood, garbage, or other organic substances, such as tobacco and charbroiled meat. There are more than 100 different PAHs. PAHs generally occur as complex mixtures (for example, as part of combustion products such as soot), not as single compounds.

popcorn lung A rare, irreversible form of fixed obstructive lung disease that has been identified in workers exposed to flavoring chemicals while working in the microwave-popcorn and flavoring-manufacturing industries

post-traumatic stress disorder (PTSD) A mental health condition that is triggered by a terrifying event. Symptoms may include flashbacks, nightmares, and severe anxiety, as well as uncontrollable thoughts about the event.

prevalence The number of affected persons present in the population at a specific time divided by the number of persons in the population at that time—that is, what proportion of the population is affected by the disease at that time.

primary prevention   Efforts to reduce the incidence of occupational illnesses

psychological stress   A particular relationship between the person and the environment that is appraised by the person as taxing or exceeding his or her resources and endangering his or her well-being

public health   The science and the art of preventing disease, prolonging life, and promoting physical health and efficiency through organized community efforts for the sanitation of the environment, the control of community infections, the education of the individual in principles of personal hygiene, the organization of medical and nursing service for the early diagnosis and preventive treatment of disease, and the development of the social machinery that will ensure to every individual in the community a standard of living adequate for the maintenance of health

pulmonary fibrosis   An occupational lung disease marked by restricted lung volume and increased interstitial pulmonary markings shown in chest X-rays

radiation   Energy traveling through space

radioactivity   The spontaneous emission of radiation from the nucleus of an unstable atom. As a result of this emission, the radioactive atom is converted, or decays, into an atom of a different element that might or might not be radioactive.

radioisotope   A natural or artificially produced isotope that is radioactive

radionuclide   An atom that has an unstable nucleus; when a radionuclide decays, it can emit X- or gamma rays and/or subatomic particles; it is a radionuclide as well as a radioisotope.

recall bias   Refers to the fact that cases may remember an exposure more clearly than controls

relative risk (RR)   The measure of association used in cohort studies; the ratio of the incidence rate of a disease or health outcome in an exposed group to the incidence rate of the disease or condition in a nonexposed group

repetitive motion disorders (RMDs)   A family of muscular conditions that result from repeated motions performed in the course of normal work or daily activities

reproductive hazards   Substances or agents that may affect the reproductive health of women or men or the ability of couples to have healthy children. These hazards may cause problems such as infertility, miscarriage, and birth defects.

risk   The probability of experiencing an adverse effect

risk assessment   The characterization of the potential adverse health effects of human exposures to environmental hazards

risk characterization   Estimates of the number of excess or unwanted health events expected at different time intervals at each level of exposure

risk communication   The two-way exchange of information about risks, including environmental health risks associated with hazardous waste, water contamination, air pollution, and radiation

risk management   The process by which risk-assessment results are integrated with other information to make decisions about the need for, method of, and extent of risk reduction

rotator cuff tendinitis   Irritation of the rotator cuff tendons and inflammation of the bursa (a normally smooth layer) lining these tendons

secondary prevention   Strategies to reduce the prevalence of occupational diseases

selection bias   Distortions that result from procedures used to select subjects and from factors that influence participation in the study

sentinel health event (SHE)   A preventable disease, disability, or untimely death whose occurrence serves as a warning signal that the quality of preventive and/or therapeutic medical care may need to be improved

shiftwork   Working outside the normal daylight hours

SI (System International) units   The International System of Units

silicosis   A lung disease caused by breathing dust containing respirable silica particles

skin sensitizers   Substances that may not cause immediate skin reactions, but repeated exposure can result in allergic reactions; e.g., certain chemicals and proteins from natural materials.

solvent   A substance, usually a liquid, capable of dissolving another substance

sound level meter (SLM)   The basic instrument for investigating noise levels

standardized mortality ratio (SMR)   The ratio of the observed mortality in a population to the expected mortality

stress   A phenomenon that connotes an imbalance between demands originating from the environment and the person's capability to meet these demands

stress management   A set of techniques and programs intended to help people deal more effectively with stress in their lives by analyzing the specific stressors and taking positive actions to minimize their effects. Most stress management programs deal with job stress and workplace issues.

Examples include progressive muscular relaxation, guided imagery, biofeedback, breathing techniques, and active problem solving.

stress-related health outcomes   The more enduring negative health states thought to result from exposure to job stressors

styrene   A colorless liquid that evaporates easily and is used for the manufacture of plastics, rubber, and resins

synergistic   A situation in which the combined effect of several exposures is greater than the sum of the individual effects

synthetic mineral fibers   Fibrous inorganic substances made primarily from rock, clay, slag, or glass

temporary threshold shift (TTS)   A short-term loss in hearing sensitivity that lasts for several hours—for example, 14 hours or longer in certain situations

tertiary prevention   Efforts to limit the effects of occupational illnesses through disability limitation and rehabilitation

tetrachloroethylene   A clear, colorless liquid that has a sharp, sweet odor and evaporates quickly; also called perc or perchloroethylene; widely used in the dry cleaning industry

three core functions of public health   Assessment, policy development, and assurance

threshold   The lowest dose at which a particular response may occur. It is unclear whether exposure (especially long-term exposure) to toxic chemicals at low (subthreshold) levels is sufficient to produce any health-related response

threshold limit value (TLV)   Airborne concentrations of substances that represent conditions under which it is believed that nearly all workers may be unaffected

toluene   A clear, colorless liquid with a distinctive smell that is an excellent solvent and is added to many products including paints, thinners, adhesives, and gasoline

Toxic Substances Control Act (TSCA) of 1976   Allows "EPA to regulate new commercial chemicals before they enter the market, to regulate existing chemicals … when they pose an unreasonable risk to health or to the environment, and to regulate their distribution and use"

toxicants   Toxic substances that are human-made or result from human (anthropogenic) activity (e.g., DDT)

toxicity   The degree to which a substance (a toxin or poison) can harm humans or animals

toxicology The study of the adverse effects of chemicals on living organisms

toxin A toxic substance made by living organisms, including reptiles, insects, plants, and microorganisms

traumatic incidence stress A form of stress that results from experience of a catastrophic event such as a terrorism-linked attack, natural disaster, or act of war

traumatic occupational injuries Injuries caused by traumatic events in the workplace

trench foot A painful and sometimes dangerous condition that occurs when the feet remain wet for long periods

2-butanone (methyl ethyl ketone [MEK]) A colorless liquid with a sharp, sweet odor that has an ability to evaporate rapidly and dissolve many substances; it is used frequently in coatings, paints, cleaners, and glues

unintentional injuries Injuries that occur when there is no deliberate intention for self-harm or harming other people

U.S. Department of Labor (US DOL) The federal government agency charged with administration and enforcement of federal laws that pertain to workplace activities for approximately 10 million employers and 125 million workers.

U.S. Equal Employment Opportunity Commission (EEOC) Enforces regulations that prohibit illegal discrimination against employees

vinyl chloride (vinyl chloride monomer) A colorless gas that burns easily, is unstable at high temperatures, and has a mild, sweet odor; it is used mainly for the manufacture of polyvinyl chloride (PVC)

volatile organic compounds (VOCs) Organic chemical compounds whose composition makes it possible for them to evaporate under normal indoor atmospheric conditions of temperature and pressure

whistleblowing The disclosure by a person, usually an employee in a government agency or private enterprise, to the public or to those in authority, of mismanagement, corruption, illegality, or some other wrongdoing

whole-body vibration (WBV) The form of vibration that occurs when the human body is supported on a surface which is vibrating

work overload The situation in which an employee is assigned more work than he or she is capable of finishing

worker absenteeism Frequent or recurrent absences from a job, often without good cause

workers' compensation programs Provide cash benefits, medical care, and rehabilitation services to workers who experience work-related injuries

workplace bullying   A form of intimidation that often originates from supervisors

workplace chronic diseases   Longstanding illnesses and adverse health effects that arise from occupational exposures

workplace health promotion   The combined efforts of employers, employees, and society to improve the health and well-being of people at work

workplace violence   Any act or threat of physical violence, harassment, intimidation, or other threatening disruptive behavior that occurs at the work site. It ranges from threats and verbal abuse to physical assaults and even homicide. It can affect and involve employees, clients, customers, and visitors.

work-related asthma (WRA)   Asthma that includes work-exacerbated asthma (preexisting or concurrent asthma worsened by factors related to the workplace environment) and occupational asthma (new onset asthma attributed to the workplace environment)

work-related diseases   Adverse health events that arise from the work environment

work-related musculoskeletal disorders (WRMSDs)   MSDs induced or made worse by occupational factors

X-rays   Penetrating electromagnetic radiation whose wavelengths are shorter than those of visible light

zoonosis   An infection or infectious disease transmissible under natural conditions from vertebrate animals to humans. Examples include rabies and plague.

Index

CPSIA information can be obtained
at www.ICGtesting.com
Printed in the USA
JSHW081528171122
33214JS00003B/9